THERAPEUTIC GASTROINTESTINAL ENDOSCOPY

Edited by **Oliviu Pascu** and **Marcel Tantau**

Therapeutic Gastrointestinal Endoscopy
Edited by Oliviu Pascu and Marcel Tantau

Published by InTech
Janeza Trdine 9, 51000 Rijeka, Croatia

Publishing Process Manager Masa Vidovic

Technical Editor Teodora Smiljanic

Cover Designer InTech Design Team

Additional hard copies can be obtained from orders@intechopen.com

Therapeutic Gastrointestinal Endoscopy, Edited by Oliviu Pascu and Marcel Tantau
p. cm.
ISBN 978-953-307-743-7

For EU product safety concerns:
IN TECH d.o.o., Prolaz Marije Krucifikse Kozulić 3, 51000 Rijeka, Croatia,
info@intechopen.com or visit our website at intechopen.com.

Meet the editor

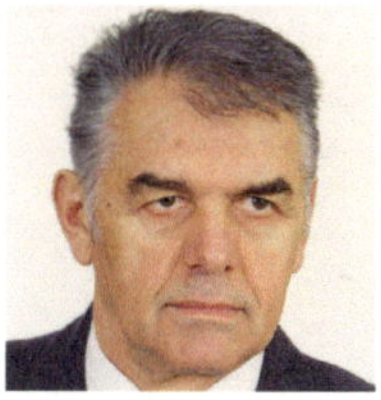

Dr. Oliviu Pascu graduated at the Faculty of General Medicine, Institute of Medicine &Pharmacy in 1963. He became professor of internal medicine and gastroenterology at the IIIrd Medical Clinic, University of Medicine and Pharmacy, Cluj-Napoca, Romania in 1990. From 1990 until 2000 he was dean (Faculty of Medicine) and then rector of the University of Medicine and Pharmacy in Cluj. Until 2009 he acted as president of the Romanian Society of Digestive Endoscopy and is presently honorary president). His first monograph on digestive endoscopy was published in Romania in 1982. while his first textbook on gastroenterology 1996-1997.
He has practiced digestive endoscopy since 1969 and introduced hemostasis and polypectomy in Romania (1975). More than 150 of his articles have been published in Romanian and international medical journals. Dr. Pascu is member of the Academy of Medical Sciences Romania and many Romanian and European scientific societies.

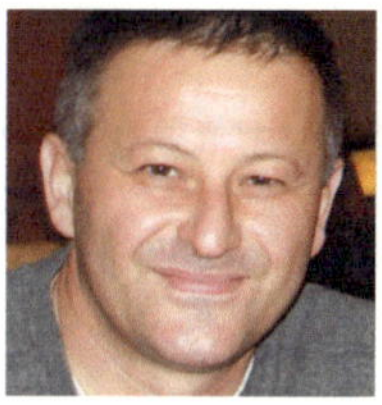

Born at Cluj-Napoca, Dr. Marcel Tantau graduated at the University of Medicine and Pharmacy in his native town in 1990. In autumn of 1992 he passed a formation stage in Royal London Hospital, in Prof. Paul Swain's gastroenterology department. At the end of the same year he was fellow of gastroenterology in CHU Grenoble in 1993 and he got his basic formation of endoscopy. Next year he transferred to CHU Angers, in the service of Prof. Jean Boyer where he perfected advanced endoscopy and ERCP.
Upon returning to Cluj-Napoca in 1995 he began to help the development of therapeutic endoscopy in the gastroenterology department of the 3rd Medical Clinic. In 15 years more than 12.000 ERCPs were performed along with other complex endoscopic interventions such as digestive tube stenting dilatation, complex polyiectomies etc.

Contents

Preface

From the invention of the fiber optic to the modern high-definition CCD chips, endoscopy has been evolving continuously in a strive to improve image. Now it is aiming to see even further into the possibility of immediate histology. With an ever improving and rapid diagnosis, therapy becomes more adapted and aggressive.

This book is an up-to-date overview of new technological achievements in the diagnostic tools of endoscopy. Standard endoscopy needs to be replaced by high definition endoscopy, magnification endoscopy and chromoendscopy for better detection and characterization of lesions. Confocal microscopy is still limited by its cost, but will certainly have a place in the refined assessment of gastrointestinal lesions. The small intestine, the last frontier of endoscopy is now explored more intensively. Its pathology is growing as the examination techniques advances. Capsule endoscopy is very temptive by its acceptance by the patients, still needs certain advances in technology, notably guidance, possibility of biopsy. Because of this, classic endoscopy for small intensive makes progress, and spiral enteroscopy looks promising.

Endoscopy has had a big role in the development of modern gastroenterology. Modern endoscopy will certainly be more therapeutic. It started at the beginning with endoscopic hemostasis and polipectomy, then at the beginning of the 70's with the advent of endoscopic sphincterotomy extended to biliopancreatic pathology and has a huge impact in this difficult pathology.

Plastic stents made the first steps in endoscopic palliation of neoplastic jaundice. Metallic stents, covered or uncovered are better for biliary palliation and can be used also for palliation neoplastic obstruction at different levels of the digestive tube.

Resection of digestive tumors has evolved now to sub-mucosal resection, looking to have one-piece complete resection.

Interventional endoscopy is now very complex and takes a lot of time for the endoscopists to learn these techniques properly.

This book is a very good up-to-date overview of the new techniques of interventional endoscopy for those who want to learn or develop their knowledge in this field.

Different chapters are written by experienced endoscopists in a clear, concise and comprehensive way.

We thank all the authors for their excellent work and we also thank InTech for the idea of this book and the selection of authors.

Lecture of this collection of personal experience of expert endoscopists is very useful for those involved in gastroenterology and digestive endoscopy.

Oliviu Pascu
3rd Medical Department
University of Medicine and Pharmacy 'Iuliu Hatieganu'
Cluj-Napoca
Romania

Marcel Tantau
University of Medicine and Pharmacy"Iuliu Hatieganu" Cluj-Napoca,
Regional Institute of Gastroenterology and Hepatology Cluj-Napoca,
Romania

1

Endoscopic Resection for Undifferentiated-Type Early Gastric Cancer

Yorimasa Yamamoto et al.*
Division of Gastroenterology, Cancer Institute Hospital
Japan

1. Introduction

Currently, endoscopic resection (ER) is the standard treatment for early gastric cancer (EGC), not only in Japan but also in other parts of the world. (Gotoda T et al., 2006)
A new endoscopic resection procedure, called endoscopic submucosal dissection (ESD), allows the direct dissection of the submucosa and has made en bloc resection of large intramucosal or ulcerated lesions feasible. However, at present, the indications for use of ER are limited to EGC without lymph node metastasis.
Gotoda et al. studied surgically resected specimens from EGC patients and decided upon the following four indication criteria for endoscopic resection of EGC without lymph node metastasis. (Gotoda T et al.,2000) (Fig 1)

1. differentiated intramucosal cancer without ulceration, regardless of size
2. differentiated intramucosal cancer with ulceration, 30mm or less in size
3. differentiated minute submucosal penetrative cancer (SM1), 30mm or less in size
4. undifferentiated intramucosal cancer without ulceration, 20mm or less in size

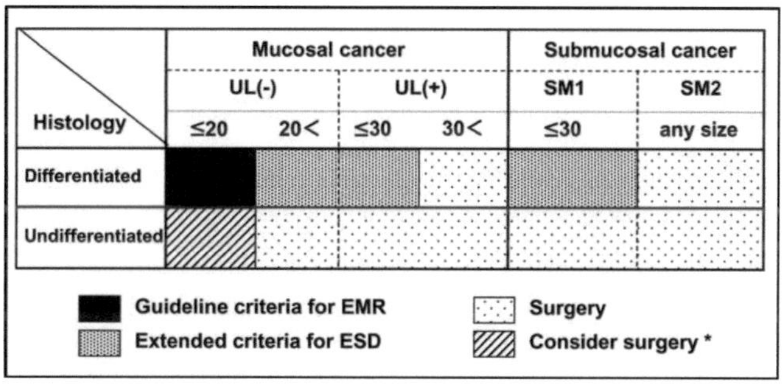

Fig. 1. Extended criteria for endoscopic resection (Tumor size is shown in millimeters).
EMR: Endoscopic mucosal resecton. ESD: Endoscopic submucosal dissection.
UL: ulcerative findings. SM: submucosal

* Junko Fujisaki[1], Toshiaki Hirasawa[1], Takanori Suganuma[1], Masami Omae[1], Kazuhisa Okada[1], Susumu Sawada[2], Akiyoshi Ishiyama[1], Tomohiro Tuchida[1], Etuo Hoshino[1], Hiroshi Takahashi[2] and Masahiro Igarashi[1]
1 Division of Gastroenterology, Cancer Institute Hospital, Japan,
2 Department of Gastroenterology, Showa University Fujigaoka Hospital, Japan.

Expansion of the indications for ER to include undifferentiated-type EGC is not widely accepted at this time because undifferentiated-type EGC has been associated with higher rates of lymph node metastasis than has differentiated-type EGC. (Sano T et al.,1992 ; Yamao T et al.,1996)
Furthermore, it is sometimes difficult to delineate carcinomatous areas in cases where undifferentiated-type EGC is not exposed on the mucosa surface. (Ninomiya Y et al.,2000)
As a result, successful endoscopic resection is reportedly less common in patients with undifferentiated-type EGC compared to those with differentiated EGC. (Miyata M et al.,2000) To avoid invasive surgery, and thereby optimize the patient' s quality of life, it is important to expand the ER indication to include undifferentiated-type EGC in patients at a very low risk of lymph node metastasis.
Recently, several studies for undifferentiated-type EGC treated by endoscopic resection have been reported from different institutions. (Kim JH et al., 2009 ; Kang HY et al.,2010 ; Yamamoto Y et al.,2010) According to these reports, endoscopic resection for undifferentiated-type EGC was technically feasible and might be considered an alternative treatment modality.
In this review, we described the state of diagnostic and therapeutic endoscopy for undifferentiated-type EGC.

2. Undifferentiated-type EGC without lymph node metastasis

Because ER involves only local treatment without lymph node dissection, as a rule, it is performed only if lymph node metastases are not present.
In the study by Gotoda et al., the criteria for undifferentiated-type EGC without lymph node metastasis was intramucosal cancer without ulceration and a diameter of no more than 20mm (expanded-indication lesion). (Gotoda T et al.,2000)
However, this category of tumor was diagnosed in only 141 cases, and the 95% confidence interval for the frequency of positive lymph node metastases was 0-2.6%. This corresponds to a 5-year survival rate worse than the 99% associated with surgically resected intramucosal gastric carcinoma. Therefore, expansion of the indications for ER to include undifferentiated-type EGC was not widely accepted at that time.
Recently, Hirasawa et al. added to Gotoda's findings, by reporting on cases of undifferentiated-type EGC resected at their institutions over the past 9 years; they reported the lymph node metastasis rate and the validity of ER for undifferentiated-type EGC. (Hirasawa T et al,.2009) In the study, the number of expanded-indication lesion reached 310, and no lymph node metastasis was found in any of these cases. (Table 1)

Tumor size	LNM rate(%); UL(-) and LVI(-)
≦10 mm	0.0 (0/105)
11-20 mm	0.0 (0/205)
21-30 mm	1.9 (3/162)
≧31 mm	5.2 (13/249)
Total	2.2 (16/721)

Table 1. Lymph node metastasis by tumor size without UL and LVI in undifferentiated-type intramucosal EGC LNM: lymph node metastasis LVI: lymphatic-vascular capillary involvement UL: ulcerative findings

Thus, the 95% confidence interval decreased to 0-0.96%, with an upper limit of 1% or less. Therefore, it is suggested that the expanded-indication lesion of undifferentiated-type EGC could be considered suitable for curative ER due to the negligible risk of lymph node metastasis.

Several studies have proved that none of the cases of surgically resected expanded-indication lesions was associated with positive lymph nodes. (Ha TK et al.,2008 ; Li C et al.,2008 ; Li H et al.,2008 ; Ye BD et al.,2008 ; Kunisaki C et al.,2009 ; Li H et al.,2010)

However, even if the lesion met the criteria for expanded-indication lesion pathologically, in the previous study, some lesions with lymph node metastasis were reported. In three studies of surgically resected undifferentiated-type EGC that were 20mm or smaller in diameter and had neither ulceration nor lymphovascular invasion, a few were found to have metastasized. Lymph node metastases were found by Abe et al. in two cases with 10-mm or 12-mm lesions, (Abe N et al.,2004) by Nasu et al. in one case with a 13-mm lesion, (Nasu J et al.,2006) and by Park et al. in one case with a 17-mm lesion. (Park YD et al.,2008)

Even though the expanded-indication lesions of undifferentiated-type EGC have a very low risk of lymph node metastasis according to the report of Hirasawa et al, we should remain aware of the fact that a few of the expanded-indication lesion cases may have lymph node metastases.

What kind of mechanism would permit such a lesion to metastasize to the lymph nodes?

In normal gastric mucosa, lymphatic vessels are not found in the upper and middle part of the lamina propria; they exist in the deep lamina propria adjacent to the muscularis mucosa.

These morphologic findings correlate with clinicopathological observations on early gastric cancer. The particularly low incidence of lymph node metastases in the subtype of early gastric cancer that remains confined to the mucosa may be explained by the rarity of lymph capillaries in the mucosa. (Lehnert T et al.,1985 ; Listrom MB et al.,1987)

Sako et al. studied the distribution of lymphatic vessels in the gastric wall by immunostaining for D2-40. (Sako A et al., 2006) The densest distribution of lymphatic vessels was seen in the muscularis mucosa layer. If cancer cells reached the muscularis mucosa layer, they might have the greatest chance of invading the lymphatic vessels.

The morphological detection of intralymphatic tumor cells might be more difficult in undifferentiated-type EGC than differentiated-type EGC. The reason for this was presumed to be that undifferentiated-type EGC are often associated with a loss of glandular formation in the gastric wall, and the cancer cells may be more scattered in the lymphatic vessels.

Therefore, it is possible that if undifferentiated-type EGC reached the deep layer of the mucosa or the muscularis mucosa, the cancer cell could metastasize to the lymph node without invading the general lymphatic system.

However, it is noteworthy that no case with expanded-indication lesions of undifferentiated-type EGC less than 10mm in diameter had lymph node metastases. ER is therefore indicated in such lesions.

We suggest that ER should be used for the treatment of expanded-indication lesions of undifferentiated-type EGC in order to avoid unnecessary invasive surgery and optimize the quality of life.

3. The characteristics of expanded-indication lesion of undifferentiated-type EGC

Most patients with EGC treatable using ER have presented with no cancer related symptom: they have undergone an endoscopy because of symptoms of gastritis or esophagitis, and the cancers have been diagnosed incidentally.

Because an undifferentiated-type EGC indicated for ER has a diameter less than 20mm, it is important for an endoscopist to fully understand the endoscopic finding of such a lesion.

We performed a retrospective analysis of 60 patients who had histologically expanded-indication lesions of undifferentiated-type EGC in whom an ESD was performed at the Cancer Institute Hospital between March 2005 and August 2009. The patient characteristics and the endoscopic findings are shown in Table 2.

mean age±SD (range)	58.3±10.8 (33-78)	Tumor size	
		<10mm	28 (47%)
sex		10mm≦	32 (53%)
M	24 (40%)		
F	36 (60%)	Histology	
		sig	40 (67%)
Tumor location		por	20 (33%)
L	12 (20%)		
M	45 (75%)	Tumor size and histology	
U	3 (5%)	<10mm (n=28)	
		sig	22 (79%)
Gross type		por	6 (21%)
frat	11 (18%)	10mm≦ (n=32)	
depressed	49 (82%)	sig	18 (56%)
		por	14 (44%)
lesion color			
reddish	8 (13%)	H.pylori infection	
discolored	52 (87%)	negative	10 (17%)
		positive	50 (83%)

Table 2. Patient characteristics (n=60)

The mean age of the patients was 58.3±10.8 years (range, 33-81 years), and number of male and female patients was 24 (40%) and 36 (60%) respectively.

The locations of lesions were as follows: lower third of stomach in 12 cases (20%); middle third in 45 cases (75%); upper third in 3 cases (5%).

Regarding the gross type, 11 lesions (18%) were flat, and 49(82%) were depressed, and regarding the tumor color, 52 (87%) were discolored, and 8 (13%) were reddish. Twenty-eight lesions (47%) were less than 10mm in diameter, and 32(53%) were larger than 10mm.

Regarding the histological findings, 40(67%) were signet ring cell carcinoma, and 20(33%) were poorly-differentiated adenocarcinoma.

Regarding the association between tumor size and histological finding, 22 of 28 lesions (79%) less than 10mm in diameter were histologically signet ring cell carcinoma, 18 of 32 lesions (56%) greater than 10mm in diameter were poorly-differentiated adenocarcinoma; lesions greater than 10mm in diameter frequently showed poorly-differentiated adenocarcinoma.

With respect to Helicobacter pylori (HP) infection, 17 of 60 patients (17%) showed no HP infection and no atrophic change in the gastric mucosa, these 17 patients were negative for serum HP antibody and serum pepsinogen; undifferentiated-type EGC was found in the patients who were negative for HP infection.

In summary, undifferentiated-type EGC tended to be found more frequently in females than in males, located in the middle third of the stomach, be 'discolored' in appearance, and was most frequently of the depressed type. (Fig 2)

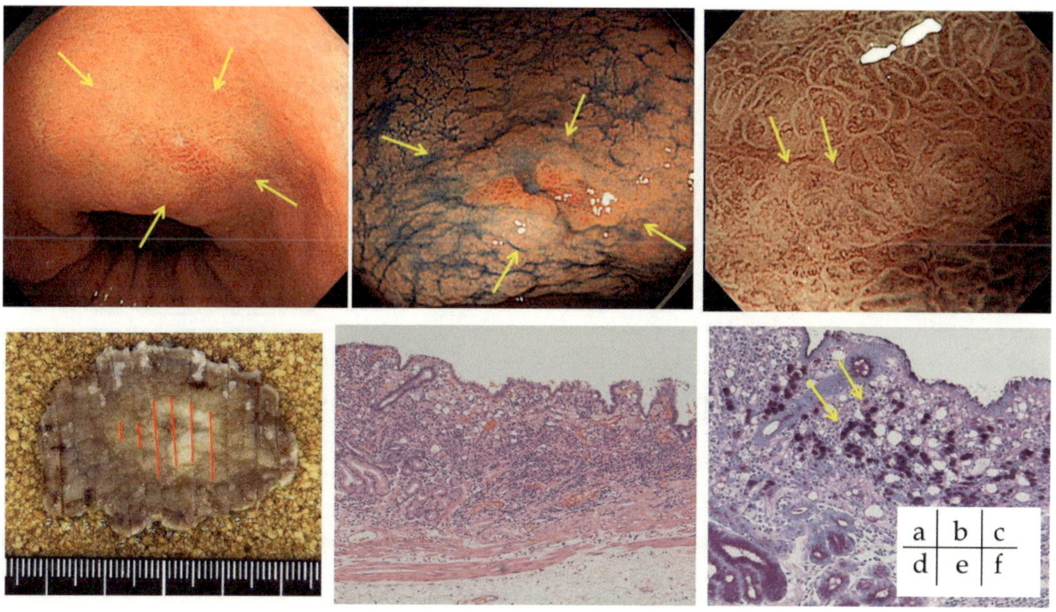

a: Routine observation: A discolored area with biopsy scar in the central was located on the lower-body lesser curvature.. (yellow arrows)

b: Indigo carmine spraying: Dye spraying revealed a discolored lesion with depression. (yellow arrows).

c: Narrow band imaging with magnifying view : NBI showed irregular vascular pattern in the depressed lesion. (yellow arrows)

d: Resected specimen: specimen size 28×23 mm, tumor size 13×9 mm, type 0-IIc, sig, UL(-), pM, ly0, v0, LM(-), VM(-).

e: HE staining: Tubular structure in the lesion was not recognized.

f: PAS staining: Signet-ring cells with PAS staining positive were observed in the middle layer of the mucosa.(yellow arrows)

Fig. 2. Undifferentiated EGC met expand-indication criteria for ESD.

In the development of gastric cancer, it was very interesting that undifferentiated-type EGC was even found in the patients with no evidence of HP infection. (Fig 3)

In a depressed-type EGC, encroachment of the border is one important malignant sign to look for in endoscopic findings. (Oohara et al.,1984 ; Fujii T et al.,1994) However, Takahashi et al. reported that encroachment of the border was found in only 20% patients with undifferentiated-type EGC with diameters less than 10mm. (Takahashi H et al.,2009)

To diagnose undifferentiated-type EGC treatable by ER, an endoscopist should take care when performing an endoscopic examination in order not to overlook a depressed and discolored lesion with no encroachment of the border.

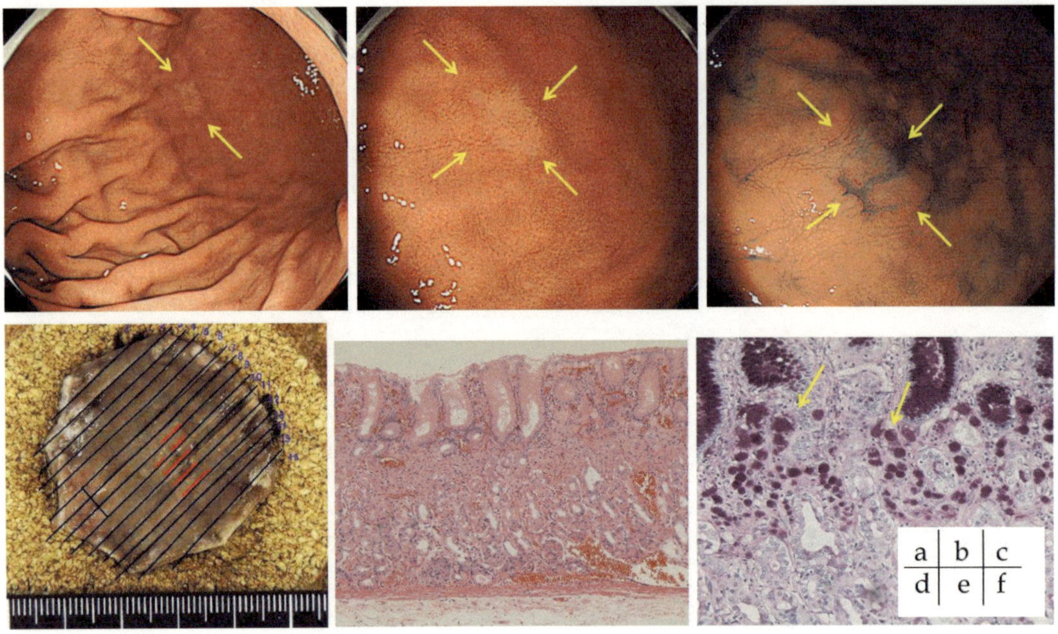

a: Routine observation: A discolored area was located on the lower-body anterior wall. (yellow arrows) This patient had not H.pylori infection

b: Closed view: The border of discolored area was clearly distinguished from the adjacent mucosa.

c: Indigo carmine spraying: Dye spraying revealed a discolored lesion without depression. (yellow arrows). The macroscopic appearance suggested type 0-IIb early gastric cancer.

d: Resected specimen: specimen size 28x23 mm, tumor size 13x9 mm(red line), type 0-IIc, sig, UL(-), pM, ly0, v0, LM(-), VM(-).

e: HE staining: Tubular structure in the middle layer of the lesion was not recognized.

f: PAS staining: Signet-ring cells with PAS staining positive were observed in the middle layer of the mucosa. (yellow arrows)

Fig. 3. A case of undifferentiated EGC without H.pylori infection.

4. Diagnosis of tumor margin and narrow band imaging for undifferentiated-type EGC

Narrow band imaging (NBI) is a new electronic endoscopy system ideally suited to the observation of surface structures, including capillaries. With NBI, short wavelength light radiated through a narrow band filter is strongly absorbed by hemoglobin, thereby allowing surface vascular structures to be distinctly visualized. (Gono K et al.,2004)

The NBI-magnifying endoscopy is capable of predicting the histological characteristics of gastric cancer lesions in not only well-differentiated-type ECG but also in undifferentiated-type.

Nakayoshi et al. reported that microvascular structures can be observed using the NBI magnifying endoscopy, with a fine network pattern visible in well-differentiated-type EGC, and, in contrast, a corkscrew pattern in undifferentiated-type EGC. (Nakayoshi T et al.,2004)

Taken together, these findings suggest that, if a discolored depressed lesion without encroachment found by conventional endoscopy showed a corkscrew pattern by NBI, the lesion is probably undifferentiated-type EGC.

It is well known that it is more difficult to determine the lesion margin in undifferentiated-type EGC than in well-differentiated-type. In some cases of undifferentiated-type EGC, the lesion margin estimated macroscopically with the naked eye differs from that determined by pathology. (Ninomiya et al.,2000)

This difference occurs when the tumor extends along the proliferative zone in the middle layer of the mucosa, leaving normal ducts covering the superficial mucosa. When this extension of cancer cells along the proliferative zone occurs, it is difficult to diagnosis the area of the lesion, even using NBI-magnifying endoscopy. To achieve a more accurate diagnosis, circumferential biopsies of the lesion should be done in all cases of undifferentiated-type EGC.

Recently, we have reported that the width of the proliferative zone in 40 cases of expanded-indication lesion of undifferentiated-type EGC ranged from 0 to 2,390µm (average 605.5µm). (Sawada S et al.,2010) (Fig.4)

In no cases was the width of the proliferative zone over 3mm. (Table 3)

From these results, we recommend that markings around a lesion should be placed 5mm beyond the endoscopically determined lesion margin, and mucosal incisions should be made outside these markings for ER of undifferentiated-type EGC.

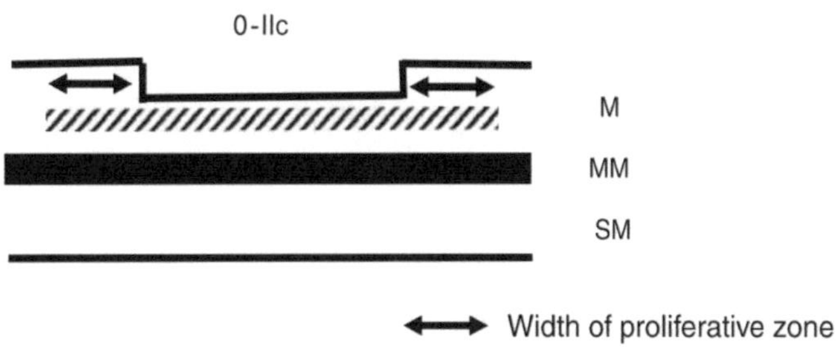

M : mucosa MM : musucularis mucosa SM : submucosa

Fig. 4. Width of proliferative zone

0-1,000 µm	28 (70)
1,001-2,000 µm	11 (27.5)
2,001-3,000 µm	1 (2.5)
Total	40 (%)

n=40, mean=605.5µm

Table 3. Width of proliferative zone (0- II c type undifferentiated-type intramucosal EGC)

5. Therapeutic outcomes of ESD of undifferentiated-type EGC

Endoscopic resections for EGD were divided into two types of procedures, endoscopic mucosal resection (EMR) and endoscopic submucosal dissection (ESD). There are several EMR procedures, including the strip biopsy method (Okazaki Y et al.,1991), double channel method (Takekoshi T et al.,1986), EMR-cap method (Takeshita et al.,1997) These EMR procedures, however, cannot be used for the en bloc resection of lesions larger than 2cm. (Hyun DH et al.,2003)

On the other hand, ESD techniques can make en bloc resection of large lesions or ulcerated lesions feasible. It is important for the success of the ER of undifferentiated-type EGC that the histological findings are evaluated in detail. If the lesion is non-curative pathologically, the patient must undergo additional surgical resection of the stomach. Therefore, ER of undifferentiated-type EGC should be performed with an en bloc resection by ESD procedure.

We reviewed 58 patients with preoperatively diagnosed undifferentiated-type EGC (expanded-indication lesion) who underwent ESD at the Cancer Institute Hospital between September 2003 and August 2008. 9 We carried out ESD using the insulation-tipped diathemic knife method, and glycerol or hyaluronic acid as the local injection material.

The therapeutic outcomes of ESD are shown in Table 4.

The mean diameter of resected specimens was 30mm (range, 15-48mm), the mean diameter of lesions was 11mm (range, 2-28mm), the median operation time was 70 min (range, 23-340 min), the en bloc resection rate was 98 % (57/58 patients), the complete en bloc resection (R0 resection) rate was 90 % (52/58 patients), the curative resection rate was 79 % (46/58 patients).

Bleeding complications occurred in five cases (8.6 %). No cases required blood transfusion or surgery. Perforation occurred in two cases (3.4%), both of which were conservatively and successfully treated by clipping closure. The mean hospital stay was 6.7 days (range, 4-14 days)

Specimen diameter (mm), mean (range)	30 (15-48)
Tumor diameter (mm), mean (range)	11 (2-28)
Operation time (minutes), median (range)	70 (23-340)
One-piece resection rate, n/N (%)	57/58 (98%)
Complete resection rate, n/N (%)	52/58 (90%)
Curative resection rate, n/N (%)	46/58 (79%)
Accurate preoperative diagnosis, n/N (%)	47/58 (81%)
Complications, n (%)	
Bleeding	5 (8.6%)
Perforation	2 (3.4%)
Hospital stay (days), mean (range)	6.7 (4-14)

ESD: Endoscopic submucosal dissection
EGC: Early gastric cancer

Table 4. ESD for undifferentiated-type EGC treatment results (N=58)

Pathological examination revealed that expanded-indication lesions were present in 47 cases and non-indication lesions in 11. The therapeutic outcomes were compared between the two groups, as shown in Table 5.

	Expanded-indication lesions (N=47)	Non-indication lesions (N=11)	*P* value
Specimen diameter (mm), mean (range)	29 (15-48)	33 (15-45)	0.2
Tumor diameter (mm), mean (range)	8.9 (2-18)	18 (8-28)	<0.01
Operation time (minutes), median (range)	65 (23-340)	80 (26-250)	0.55
One-piece resection rate, n/N (%)	47/47 (100%)	10/11 (91%)	0.42
Complete resection rate, n/N (%)	46/47 (98%)	6/11 (55%)	<0.01
Curative resection rate, n/N (%)	46/47 (98%)	0/11 (0%)	
Complications, n (%)			
Bleeding	5 (11%)	0	0.59
Perforation	2 (4.3%)	0	0.82
Hospital stay (days), mean (range)	6.6 (4-14)	7.2 (5-9)	0.3

Table 5. ESD for undifferentiated type EGC treatment results by lesion group (N=58)

With the limited expanded-indication lesions, the mean diameter of the resected specimens was 29mm (range, 15-48mm), the mean diameter of lesions was 8.9mm (range, 2-18mm), the median operation time was 65 min (range, 23-340 min), the en bloc resection rate was 100 % (47/47 patients), the complete en bloc resection rate was 98 % (46/47 patients), and the curative resection rate was 98 % (46/47 patients).

From these results, it can be seen that ESD of expanded-indication lesions for undifferentiated-type EGC was associated with good therapeutic outcomes.

However, non-curative resection was pathologically identified in 12 (21%) of the 58 patients. Eleven of the 12 non-curative resection cases had non-indication lesions. The reasons for incurability were the presence of submucosal invasion in seven cases (12 % of 58 patients), tumor diameter of 21mm or more in five (8.6%), and the presence of ulcer scarring in two (3.4 %); some cases had more than one reason.

The most common factor responsible for non-curative resection was incorrect diagnosis of the depth of invasion. (Table 6)

Factors	n (%)†
Submucosal invasion	7 (12%)
Tumor diameter >20 mm	5 (8.6%)
Ulcer findings	2 (3.4%)
Lymphatic-vascular involvement	2 (3.4%)

*Some patients had more than one causative factor.

† Percentages were calculated based on overall population (N=58).

Table 6. Factors responsible for non-curative resection of non-indication lesions (N=11)*

Six of the seven patients who were found to have submucosal invasion had undergone EUS that resulted in a diagnosis of intramucosal carcinoma.

It has been reported previously that EUS correctly diagnosed the depth of invasion of EGC in 64-78% of cases, and the correct diagnosis rate was lower in cases of undifferentiated-type compared to differentiated-type. (Akahoshi K et al.,1998 ; Hizawa K et al.,2002) Although more accurate diagnosis of the invasive depth is necessary, the currently available assessment methods have limitations in their precision. (Kim JH et al.,2007)

In terms of the technological aspects of ESD, resectable expanded-indication lesions of undifferentiated-type EGC are less than 20mm in diameter and have no ulceration, the ESD procedures are easier than for lesions with diameters greater than 20mm or for ulcerated differentiated-type EGC. Therefore, we consider that the ideal method for diagnosing the invasion depth might be to first carry out ESD followed by pathological examination of resected specimens.

However, if this diagnostic ESD determines that a tumor diameter exceeds 20mm, it is probable that ESD will result in non-curative resection, so more precise preoperative diagnosis of the lesion area using circumferential biopsies is essential.

6. Conclusion

Endoscopic resection of differentiated-type EGC is now standard treatment not only in Japan but also in other parts of the world. Undifferentiated-type EGC has a high rate of lymph node metastasis compared with differentiated-type EGC, and endoscopic resection of undifferentiated-type EGC remains controversial.

However, if the tumor is detected at an early stage and meets the criteria for expanded-indication lesion of undifferentiated-type EGC, then the lymph node metastasis is very rare. We propose that endoscopic resection should be performed on such lesions to avoid unnecessary invasive surgery and optimize the quality of life. In this review, we have described our therapeutic outcomes of endoscopic resection for undifferentiated-type EGC.

An interesting result amongst our cases was the observation that some patients who were H. pylori negative had undifferentiated-type EGC. The rate of H. pylori infection is predicted to decrease in the future. We should take care in the management of cases of undifferentiated-type EGC without H. pylori infection.

It is necessary to study further cases, with a longer follow up period, to prove the validity of the concept of endoscopic resection of undifferentiated-EGC which we have proposed here.

We hope that multicenter, prospective studies will be carried out to asses further this expanded-indication for ER of undifferentiated-type EGC.

7. References

Abe N, Watanabe T, Sugiyama M, et al. (2004), Endoscopic treatment or surgery for undifferentiated early gastric cancer? *Am J Surg*, 188,2,181-4.

Akahoshi K, Chijiwa Y, Hamada S, et al. (1998), Pretreatment staging of endoscopically early gastric cancer with a 15 MHz ultrasound catheter probe. *Gastrointest Endosc*,48, 5, 470-6.

Fujii T, Yoshida S, Abe K, et al. (1994), "Very well differentiated tubular adenocarcinoma" of the stomach: its endoscopic and histopathological characteristics. *Jpn J Clin Oncol*, 24, 3, 128-34.

Gono K, Obi T, Yamaguchi M, et al. (2004), Appearance of enhanced tissue features in narrow-band endoscopic imaging. *J Biomed Opt*, 9, 3, 568-77.

Gotoda T, Yamamoto H, Soetikno RM. (2006). Endoscopic submucosal dissection of early gastric cancer. *J Gastroenterol*,41,10, 929-42.

Gotoda T, Yanagisawa A, Sasako M, et al. (2000). Incidence of lymph node metastasis from early gastric cancer: estimation with a large number of cases at two large centers. *Gastric Cancer*. 2000, 3, 4, 219-25.

Ha TK, An JY, Youn HK et al. (2008), Indication for endoscopic mucosal resection in early signet ring cell gastric cancer. *Ann Surg Oncol*, 15, 2, 508-13.

Hirasawa T, Gotoda T, Miyata S, et al. (2009), Incidence of lymph node metastasis and the feasibility of endoscopic resection for undifferentiated-type early gastric cancer. *Gastric Cancer*, 12, 3, 148-52.

Hizawa K, Iwai K, Esaki M et al. (2002), Is endoscopic ultrasonography indispensable in assessing the appropriateness of endoscopic resection for gastric cancer? *Endoscopy*, 34, 12, 973-8.

Hyun DH, Jeong S, Lee JW, et al. (2003), Usefulness of endoscopic mucosal resection for curative treatment of early gastric cancer. *Korean J Gastroenterol*, 42, 6, 453-60.

Kang HY, Kim SG, Kim JS et al. (2010), Clinical outcomes of endoscopic submucosal dissection for undifferentiated early gastric cancer. *Surg Endosc*, 24, 3, 509-16.

Kim JH, Lee YC, Kim H, et al. (2009), Endoscopic resection for undifferentiated early gastric cancer. *Gastrointest Endosc*, 69, 4, 1-9.

Kim JH, Song KS, Youn YH, et al. (2007), Clinicopathologic factors influence accurate endosonographic assessment for early gastric cancer. *Gastrointest Endosc* , 66, 5, 901-8.

Kunisaki C, Takahashi M, Nagahori Y, et al.(2009), Risk factors for lymph node metastasis in histologically poorly differentiated type early gastric cancer. *Endoscopy*, 41, 6, 498-503.

Lehnert T, Erlandson RA, Decosse JJ. (1985), Lymph and blood capillaries of the human gastric mucosa. A morphologic basis for metastasis in early gastric carcinoma. *Gastroenterology*, 89, 5, 939-50.

Li C, Kim S, Lai JF, et al. (2008), Risk factors for lymph node metastasis in undifferentiated early gastric cancer. *Ann Surg Oncol*, 15, 3, 764-9.

Li H, Lu P, Lu Y, et al. (2008), Predictive factors for lymph node metastasis in poorly differentiated early gastric cancer and their impact on the surgical strategy. *World J Gastroenterol*, 14, 26, 4222-6.

Li H, Lu P, Lu Y, et al. Predictive factors of lymph node metastasis in undifferentiated early gastric cancers and application of endoscopic mucosal resection. *Surg Oncol, 19, 4, 221-6*

Listrom MB, Fenoglio-Preiser CM. (1987), Lymphatic distribution of the stomach in normal, inflammatory, hyperplastic, and neoplastic tissue. *Gastroenterology*, 93, 3, 506-14.

Miyata M, Yokoyama Y, Okoyama N, et al. (2000). What are the appropriate indication for endoscopic mucosal resection for early gastric cancer? Analysis of 256 endoscopically resected lesions. *Endoscopy*, 32, 10, 773-778.

Nakayoshi T, Tajiri H, Matsuda K et al. (2004), Magnifying endoscopy combined with narrow band imaging system for early gastric cancer: correlation of vascular pattern with histopathology (including video). *Endoscopy*, 36, 12, 1080-4.

Nasu J, Nishina T, Hirasaki S, et al. (2006), Predictive factors of lymph node metastasis in patients with undifferentiated early gastric cancers. *J Clin Gastroenterol*, 40, 5, 412-5.

Ninomiya Y, Yanagisawa A, Kato Y, et al. (2000). Unrecognizable intramucosal spread of diffuse-type mucosal gastric carcinomas of less than 20 mm in size. *Endoscopy,* 32, 8, 604-8.

Oohara T, Aono G, Ukawa S, et al. (1984), Clinical diagnosis of minute gastric cancer less than 5 mm in diameter. *Cancer,* 53, 1, 162-5.

Okazaki Y, Tada M. (1991), Endoscopic treatment of early gastric cancer. *Semin Surg Oncol,* 7, 6, 351-5.

Park YD, Chung YJ, Chung HY, et al. (2008), Factors related to lymph node metastasis and the feasibility of endoscopic mucosal resection for treating poorly differentiated adenocarcinoma of the stomach. *Endoscopy,* 40, 1, 7-10.

Sako A, Kitayama J, Ishikawa M et al. (2006), Impact of immunohistochemically identified lymphatic invasion on nodal metastasis in early gastric cancer. *Gastric Cancer,* 9, 4, 295-302.

Sano T, Kobori O, Muto T. (1992). Lymph node metastasis from early gastric cancer: endoscopic resection of tumour. *Br J Surg,* 79, 3, 241-4.

Sawada S, Fujisaki J, Yamamoto N, et al. (2010), Expansion of indications for endoscopic treatment of undifferentiated mucosal gastric cancer: analysis of intramucosal spread in resected specimens. *Dig Dis Sci,* 55, 5, 1376-80.

Takahashi H, et al. (2009), Endoscopic Diagnosis of Early Small and Minute Gastric Cancer. *Gastrointestinal Cancer Atras for Endoscopic Therapy.* Springer, Tokyo, 21-30.

Takekoshi T, Takagi K, Fujii A et al. (1986), Treatment of early gastric cancer by endoscopic double snare polypectomy (EDSP). *Gan No Rinsho.* 32, 10, 1185-90.

Takeshita K, Tani M, Inoue H, et al. (1997), A new method of endoscopic mucosal resection of neoplastic lesions in the stomach: its technical features and results. *Hepatogastroenterology,* 44, 18, 1602-11.

Yamao T, Shirao K, Ono H, et al. (1996). Risk factors for lymph node metastasis from intramucosal gastric carcinoma. *Cancer.* 1996, 77, 4, 602-6.

Yamamoto Y, Fujisaki J, Hirasawa T, et al. (2010), Therapeutic outcomes of endoscopic submucosal dissection of undifferentiated-type intramucosal gastric cancer without ulceration and preoperatively diagnosed as 20 millimetres or less in diameter. *Dig Endosc,* 22, 2, 112-8.

Ye BD, Kim SG, Lee JY, et al. (2008), Predictive factors for lymph node metastasis and endoscopic treatment strategies for undifferentiated early gastric cancer. *J Gastroenterol Hepatol,* 23, 1, 46-50.

Endoscopic Resection of Early Gastric Cancer

Sang Gyun Kim
*Department of Internal Medicine and Liver Research Institute,
Seoul National University College of Medicine, Seoul,
Republic of Korea*

1. Introduction

Endoscopic resection has been accepted as a curative modality for early gastric cancer (EGC) in indication of complete resection without the risk of metastasis. Since conventional endoscopic mucosal resection (EMR) has been introduced from 1984, many improvements of endoscopic accessories and techniques have been achieved. Recently, endoscopic submucosal dissection (ESD) using various electrosurgical knives has been performed for complete resection of EGC, and enables complete resection of EGC which had many technical difficulties in complete resection in the era of conventional EMR.
As the proportion of early gastric cancer has been increasing by early detection with national cancer screening program in Korea (biannual upper endoscopy or barium study for all population over age of 40), endoscopic treatment for early gastric cancer has been expanded with the progress of endoscopic technique and accessories. In this review, endoscopic resection for early gastric cancer would be presented as the history, indication, risk of lymph node metastasis and clinical results.

2. Endoscopic resection for EGC

2.1 History of endoscopic resection for EGC

Since endoscopic resection with electrosurgical snare has been introduced for colorectal polyp in 1973, endoscopic resection has been performed for polypoid-type EGC as curative intent. In 1984, strip biopsy method has been developed for resection of flat-type EGC. In this method, the flat lesion is changed to polypoid lesion by submucosal injection of mixture of normal saline with diluted epinephrine, and resected by grasper forcep and electrosurgical snare through 2-channel endoscope. Although this method had advantages of easy technique, short procedure time and less complication, complete resection rate was around 50 – 70%, which was lower than expected for large-sized or depressed-type EGC (Hirao et al., 1988).
In 1988, EMR-precutting method has been developed, in which after hypertonic saline with diluted epinephrine is injected to submucosal layer around the lesion, circumferential incision around the lesion with needle knife and final resection of the lesion is performed with electrosurgical snare. This method has enabled complete en-bloc resection rather than conventional EMR, but risk of perforation was higher during the circumferential incision, which necessitated higher expertise. Moreover, en-bloc complete resection was still difficult for large-sized or depressed-type EGC.

In 1992, EMR by the cap-fitted method (EMR-C) has been developed, in which en-bloc resection was performed with electrosurgical snare after suction of the lesion by cap-fitted endoscope (Inoue et al., 1993). Although this method was easier and safer than conventional EMR for en-bloc resection of small-sized EGC, en-bloc complete resection was still impossible for larger-sized EGC than diameter of the cap (Akiyama et al., 1997).
To overcome the disadvantages of previous methods, endoscopic submucosal dissection method (ESD) has been developed in late 1990's. In ESD, circumferential incision and direct dissection of submucosal layer of EGC has been possible with various knives, which has enabled en-bloc complete resection even in large-sized or depressed-type EGC. Various knives have been introduced for safe and complete ESD for EGC, and have different advantages/disadvantages according to the lesion. In present, insulation-tipped (IT), triangle-tipped (TT), flex, hook, fork, flush and splash knives are available for ESD.

2.2 Procedure of endoscopic submucosal dissection

Endoscopic submucosal dissection is usually performed under sedation with intravenous midazolam or propofol. With a standard single-channel endoscope, thorough examination is mandatory for the evaluation of whole stomach including the target lesion. After the chromo-endoscopic observation with indigo carmine, marking dots 5 mm outside the tumor margin are made using a conventional needle knife with a forced 20 W coagulation current (VIO 300D; Erbe, Tübingen, Germany) or argon plasma coagulation. Then a mixture of normal saline and indigo carmine with diluted epinephrine (1:100,000) is injected into the submucosal layer along with the marking dots to make the submucosal cushion beneath the lesion. After a small initial incision is made with the needle knife, a circumferential mucosal incision is made around the marking spots, and the submucosal layer is dissected using various knives in 80 W endocut mode. Hemostasis is usually performed for bleeding spots or visible vessels with a coagrasper or argon plasma coagulation. After ESD, the patients is administered proton pump inhibitors intravenously at the day of procedure and then orally for four weeks for the healing of iatrogenic ulcer, pain control and prevention of perforation or post-procedural bleeding

2.3 Selection of knife

Knife is divided into blade- and tip-type according to resection site. Blade-type; needle, insulation-tipped and triangle-tipped knife, Tip-type; flex, hook, fork, flush and splash knife.
Needle knife is usually used in sphincterotomy during endoscopic retrograde cholangiopancreatography, and generates both cutting and coagulation current by electrosurgical unit. It has been used in submucosal dissection for the first time as a simple type.
At first, needle knife is used in marking around the lesion with coagulation current by adjustment of needle length up to 6 mm. Long needle has the risk of bleeding or perforation by attachment of needle to coagulated mucosa. Circumferential incision should be performed with cutting current by step by step for the prevention of perforation. In submucosal dissection, caution should be kept whether dissection is accurately made in submucosal layer.
Needle knife usually necessitates transparent cap at the tip of endoscope for prevention of perforation. Although needle knife has a high speed in resection, longer time can be needed in a beginner for the risk of perforation. Nowadays, needle knife is used for

making the hole at the beginning rather than circumferential incision or submucosal dissection.

IT knife has an insulated tip of 2.2 mm in diameter for the prevention of perforation (Gotoda et al., 1999). Since Hosokawa from Japan has introduced in 1996, IT knife has been used in endoscopic submucosal dissection. It can be used in circumferential incision and submucosal dissection, even in hemostasis of minor bleeding with coagulation current.

After making the incision hole with needle knife, circumferential incision around the lesion is made with IT knife. Insulated tip has an advantage of prevention of perforation even in dead angle. Pull-method with angle of 45 degree from distant part is favorable in incision. In submucosal dissection, full utilization of blade with insulated tip has advantages of shorter procedure time with fast dissection and prevention of perforation even in dead angle. Push-method from nearest part or pull-method from distant part is favorable in submucosal dissection.

The lesion in perpendicular plane such as fundus or greater curvature of upper body is limited in resection with IT knife, and perforation can occur even with insulated tip by whole-blade resection. Although easy procedure and short procedure time can be advantages to experts, unexpected perforation may be a disadvantage to beginners (Ono et al., 2008).

TT knife has a triangle diathermic disc at the tip of 4.5 mm in length, and can be used in marking around the lesion, circumferential incision and submucosal dissection, even in hemostasis of minor bleeding with coagulation current.

After hole-making with TT knife alone, circumferential incision around the lesion is performed with pull-method from distant part. In submucosal dissection, pull-method with diathermic disc is performed from distant part by step by step. Apart from IT knife, dissection with diathermic disc alone needs longer procedure time. The risk of perforation in dead angle can be reduced by fitting transparent cap which enables direct vision of dissection.

Flex knife has a tip of soft semicircular snare, and can be used in marking around the lesion, circumferential incision and submucosal dissection, even in hemostasis of minor bleeding with coagulation current (Kodashima et al., 2006). Soft semicircular snare is contained in soft plastic case, and can be adjusted in length.

After marking, circumferential incision around the lesion is performed with 1 mm in length from distant part. Push-method is used with 1-1.5 mm in length from proximal part in submucosal dissection. The risk of perforation is minimized because of bending of knife with soft nature even in jerky movement. Submucosal dissection by step by step has longer procedure time, and dead angle necessitates fitting transparent cap to prevent perforation. But accurate dissection can be performed by direct vision of dissected submucosa. Also, flex knife with soft nature enables dissection in every direction, even in perpendicular plane. Fixed maintenance of length of knife is indispensible to prevent unexpected perforation in jerky movement.

Hook knife has a hooked tip with 4.5 mm long and 1.3 mm in transverse, and can be used in marking around the lesion, circumferential incision and submucosal dissection, even in hemostasis of minor bleeding with coagulation current. The tip is rotatable in 360 degree to dissect in every direction. Methods of marking, submucosal injection, circumferential incision and submucosal dissection are same as TT knife.

Fork knife developed in Korea has an advantage of marking, incision, dissection, hemostasis, injection and irrigation by one knife without changing accessories (Kim et al.,

2008). Fork knife is composed of needle used in marking and incision and fork used in injection and dissection, which can be handled separately. Methods of marking, submucosal injection, circumferential incision and submucosal dissection are same as flush knife. Major advantage of fork knife is time-saving because of total procedure in one knife without changing accessories. But, needle knife has a risk of perforation during incision, and difficulties in procedure in case of inaccessible location. Submucosal dissection with fork by step by step has longer procedure time, and dead angle necessitates fitting transparent cap to prevent perforation. But accurate dissection can be performed by direct vision of dissected submucosa.

Flush knife has an advantage of marking, incision, dissection, hemostasis, injection and irrigation by one needle-type without changing accessories. Methods of marking, submucosal injection, circumferential incision and submucosal dissection are same as fork knife.

Splash knife has an advantage of marking, incision, dissection, hemostasis, injection and irrigation by one needle-type without changing accessories (Fujishiro et al., 2008). Knife is 2.5 mm long and controllable. Methods of marking, submucosal injection, circumferential incision and submucosal dissection are same as flush knife.

Selection of knife is dependent on the lesion by each characteristic. Although most procedure is performed with one knife, various knives can be utilized for accurate and safe procedure by case by case. Decision factors of knife are location, morphology, size of the lesion and type of procedure. But most of all, familiarity to operator is most important. That is, most important factor of selection of knife is easiness and familiarity to operator.

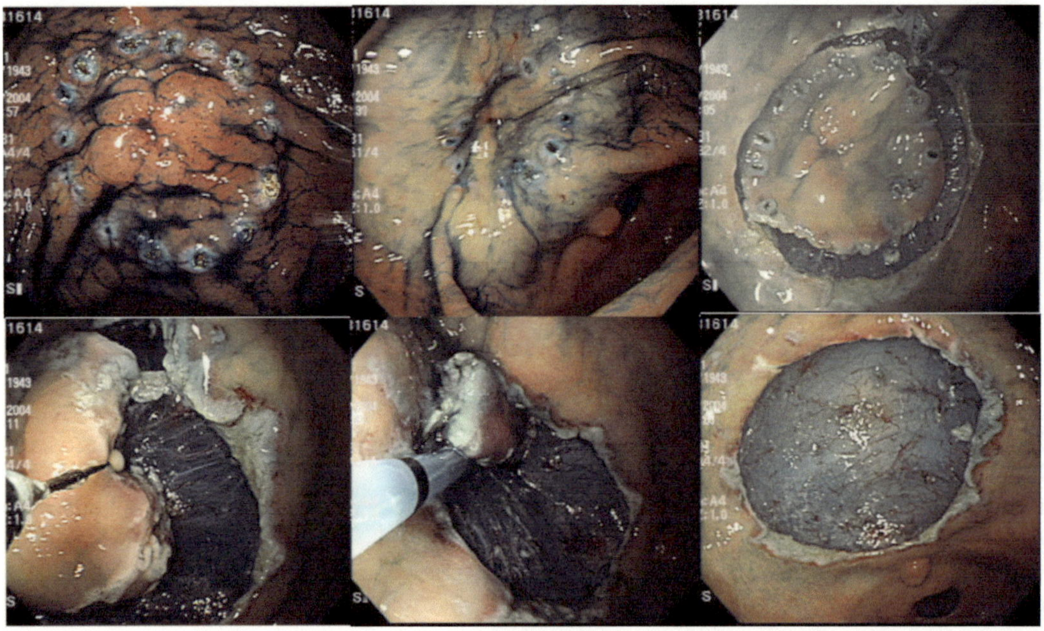

Fig. 1. ESD for EGC from marking, submucosal injection, circumferential incision to submucosal dissection

In cases of stomach, the lesion of greater curvature of high body, fundus and angle is difficult to manage. The lesion of greater curvature of high body and fundus is perpendicular with knife, and is difficult to manage with IT and TT knife. On the other hand, the lesion of angle can be difficult to approach and manage with flex, fork, flush and splash knife which should contact the lesion to dissect because of excessive air inflation during procedure. IT knife has an advantage in management of inaccessible lesion.

Submucosal dissection can be difficult for excessive fibrosis in the lesion with submucosal fibrosis or underlying scar formation. IT knife has an advantage of wide dissection plane and shorter procedure time in experts. To shorten the procedure time for large lesion, IT knife has an advantage of wide dissection plane, and fork, flush or splash knife has an advantage of total procedure with one knife to shorten the procedure time.

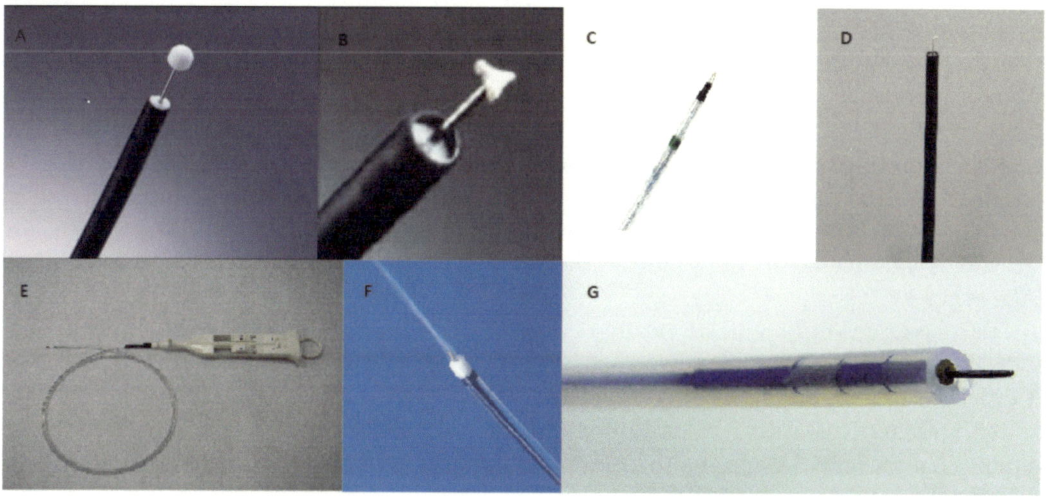

Fig. 2. Various knives used in ESD. A; IT knife, B; TT knife, C; flex knife, D; hook knife, E; fork knife, F; flush knife, G; splash knife

2.4 Conventional indication of endoscopic resection for EGC

As the technical progress has achieved from conventional EMR to ESD, most of limiting factors in complete en-bloc resection have been overcome irrespective of size, shape or location of the tumor, which has resulted in the expansion of the indication of endoscopic resection for EGC. Moreover, ESD has been substituted for surgical resection with increased portion of old age and co-morbidity and importance of postoperative quality of life.

Prior to expansion of indication of endoscopic resection for EGC, the prerequisite is to maintain the quality of life without the sacrifice of survival, which means that the expanded indication should only include EGC without lymph node or distant metastasis, enable complete en-bloc resection without serious complication, and ensure long-term survival not inferior to surgical resection. Therefore, the expansion of indication of endoscopic resection for EGC has a pitfall in the possibility of sacrifice of survival in the setting of insufficient results of long-term survival after endoscopic resection for EGC.

Conventional indication of endoscopic resection for EGC is as follows, 1) differentiated adenocarcinoma confined to mucosa, 2) elevated type ≤ 2 cm, 3) depressed type without ulcer ≤ 1 cm. In this indication, the tumor rarely metastasizes to regional lymph node or distant organ and can be resected endoscopically with negligible risk of recurrence (Ono et al., 2001). Beyond the conventional indication, the tumor in most cases could not be resected completely by conventional EMR with low cure rate in spite of the possibility of candidates of endoscopic resection. Therefore, indication of endoscopic resection was confined to small-sized, superficial tumor which could be resected with en-bloc fashion in the era of conventional EMR.

In the era of ESD, most limiting factors have been overcome in complete resection, and the indication of ESD is decided by the risk factors of lymph node or distant metastasis (Miyata et al., 2000). Although the risk factors of lymph node or distant metastasis are generally accepted as 1) tumor size, 2) differentiation of tumor, 3) invasion depth of tumor, and 4) angiolymphatic invasion of tumor, definite indications of endoscopic resection for EGC are variable according to the studies because of 1) different indication according to studies, 2) retrospective manner, 3) small sample size, and 4) short-term follow-up period.

2.5 Risk factors of lymph node metastasis in EGC

Although the risk of lymph node metastasis in EGC increases with tumor size, depth of tumor invasion and undifferentiated histology, definite indication of endoscopic resection for EGC is variable according to the studies, and the standard indication is not established (Abe et al., 2004).

In a retrospective study with surgically-resected cases with EGC, the expanded indication of endoscopic resection for EGC was proposed with no evidence of lymph node metastasis in; 1) differentiated mucosal cancer without ulcer irrespective of size, 2) differentiated mucosal cancer with ulcer ≤ 3 cm, 3) undifferentiated mucosal cancer ≤ 2 cm, 4) differentiated submucosal cancer ≤ 500 μm depth of invasion (sm1) ≤ 3 cm in size without angiolymphatic invasion (Gotoda et al., 2000).

Histology	Depth					
	m-cancer				sm-cancer	
	Ulcer (-)		Ulcer (+)		≤ sm1	> sm1
	≤ 20 mm	> 20 mm	≤ 30 mm	> 30 mm	≤ 30 mm	Any size
Differentiated	A	B	B	D	B	D
Undifferentiated	C	D	D	D	D	D

Table 1. Expanded indication of endoscopic treatment for early gastric cancer. A, definite indication by guideline; B, expanded indication; C, surgery, but need for more consideration; D, surgery; m, mucosa; sm, submucosa (Soetikno et al., 2005)

On the other hand, lymph node metastasis was found in 4.5% of mucosal cancer and 22.8% of submucosal cancer in another retrospective study with 2173 surgically-resected cases of EGC (Kwak et al., 2000). Of those, lymph node metastasis was found in some of differentiated mucosal cancer without ulcer and 2 cm differentiated mucosal cancer with ulcer, which explains that the risk of lymph node metastasis is not negligible even in the expanded indication of endoscopic resection for EGC.

Although undifferentiated histology is not considered to be the indication of endoscopic resection with higher risk of lymph node metastasis rather than differentiated histology, some portion may be the indication of endoscopic resection with negligible risk of lymph node metastasis. In a retrospective study with 591 surgically-resected cases of undifferentiated EGC, there was no lymph node metastasis in 119 cases with tumor size less than 2.5 cm, confined to mucosa or sm1, and without angiolymphatic invasion, which might be the expanded indication of endoscopic resection (Ye et al., 2008).

In the expanded indication of endoscopic resection for EGC, the pre-evaluation of regional lymph node and distant metastasis is very important with the increment of risk of metastasis (Gotoda et al., 2005). As the risk factors of lymph node metastasis such as accurate tumor size, differentiation, depth of tumor invasion and angiolymphatic invasion cannot be known prior to endoscopic or surgical resection, the risk of lymph node metastasis is restricted to assumption in pretreatment staging. Although endoscopic ultrasonography, computerized tomography, positron emission tomography have been used in cancer staging, diagnostic accuracy for lymph node or distant metastasis varies in 50 - 80%. To expand the indication of endoscopic resection for EGC, new diagnostic modality is mandatory for the evaluation of lymph node metastasis prior to definitive treatment.

Most of all, long-term survival after endoscopic resection should be proven to be not inferior to that after surgical resection to expand the indication of endoscopic resection for EGC. Although conventional EMR for conventional indication have shown long-term survival not inferior to surgical resection in completely-resected cases, long-term survival after ESD has not been established without sufficient data. Long-term prospective study is warranted for long-term survival after ESD for EGC.

2.6 Standardization of risk factors of lymph node metastasis in EGC

Risk factors of lymph node metastasis in EGC are known to be tumor size, depth of tumor invasion, differentiation and angiolymphatic invasion, which have variable criteria according to the studies (Yokoda et al., 2004). In tumor size, discrepancy may exist between surgically-resected and endoscopically-resected specimen. In surgical resection, the tumor size is measured after fixation with formalin, which may be reduced by shrinkage. On the other hand, the specimen is creased and fixed with pin in endoscopic resection, which may be exaggerated in size. Therefore, the study with endoscopically-resected cases may show the result of expanded indication in tumor size rather than the study with surgically-resected cases.

Depth of tumor invasion can be confused in endoscopically-resected cases. On the contrary to surgically-resected specimen, endoscopically-resected specimen does not include all layers of stomach but mucosa and partial submucosa. In the cases of submucosal invasion of tumor, accurate depth of tumor invasion cannot be verified in endoscopically-resected specimen because of lack of muscularis propria which can be the standard of interpretation. Although submucosal layer is divided by 3 with 500 μm, depth of tumor invasion can be much influenced by tissue preparation after endoscopic resection.

Intra- or inter-observer variation among pathologists can exist in the evaluation of differentiation of tumor. High grade dysplasia vs. intraepithelial carcinoma is the main diagnostic problem among the pathologists. In favor of diagnosis of cancer rather than dysplasia, the indication of endoscopic resection may be expanded without the risk of lymph node metastasis. To standardize the risk of lymph node metastasis in EGC, the definition of size, depth of invasion and differentiation of tumor should be also standardized.

2.7 Clinical results of endoscopic resection for EGC

Conventional EMR has shown unsatisfied results in terms of en-bloc complete resection, which lay from 53 – 74% according to size, shape or location of EGC (Kojima et al., 1998). On the other hand, there is no limiting factor in ESD in terms of size, shape or location of EGC. ESD enables en-bloc complete resection of larger-sized, depressed-type with submucosal fibrosis or difficult-located EGC. But ESD has disadvantages of longer procedure time and higher complication rate in terms of bleeding or perforation rather than conventional EMR, and necessitates a longer learning curve and expertise (Choi IJ et al., 2005). Therefore, conventional EMR can be still applied for small-sized, polypoid-type EGC rather than ESD regarding to risk and benefit.

Success rate of conventional EMR was influenced by tumor size, shape and location, and lowered in larger size than 2 cm, depressed type and location of body lesser curvature or posterior wall (Kim et al., 2007). On the contrary to conventional EMR, ESD has much improved the complete en-bloc resection rate. Although complete resection was achieved in 77.6% in a study with conventional EMR, another study with ESD in 1000 cases has revealed en-bloc resection rate of 95.3% and complete resection rate of 87.7% (Chung IK et al., 2009). From 2005 to 2010, a total of 690 cases with EGC were treated by ESD in Seoul National University Hospital. En-bloc resection was achieved in all cases, and complete resection rate was 94.2% in cases with expanded indication.

ESD has a higher risk of complication and longer procedure time than conventional EMR because of larger and deeper dissection. Bleeding and perforation are the most common complication of ESD, which can be reduced by expertise. In a study, major bleeding rate was 0.6% and perforation rate was 1.2% with mean procedure time of 47.8 minutes. Most of bleeding and perforation can be managed by endoscopic hemostasis and clipping without surgical management.

After confirmation of complete resection of EGC at pathological mapping, periodic regular follow-up is performed to detect recurrence. 5-year recurrence free survival is estimated to 99% and overall survival is estimated to 95%, which is comparable to surgical resection. Among 620 cases complete-treated by endoscopic resection in Seoul National University Hospital, 1 case of mortality by cardiovascular event was reported, and disease-free survival was 100% during follow-up. Considering the quality of life after treatment, ESD is a safe and effective treatment for EGC without sacrifice of survival compared to surgical resection.

2.8 Recurrence after endoscopic resection for EGC

Recurrence can be defined as the relapse of previous lesion, which includes local recurrence, synchronous or metachronous lesion, and distant metastasis. However, recurrence of narrow definition is remnant lesions at the site of treatment or metastatic lesions related with previous lesions treated.

Local recurrence is defined as remnant or relapsed cancer at same site after endoscopic resection during follow-up. ESD which enables en-bloc complete resection of larger tumor has reduced the rate of local recurrence of tumor compared with conventional EMR.

Although local recurrence usually develops in a short-term period less than 6 months after initial resection, minute remnant cancer can grow up to gross mass after 1 year.
Local recurrence originates from remnant tumor in incompletely-resected site. In case of positive lateral resection margin at post-resection pathological mapping, remnant tumor around resection margin can grow with healing of iatrogenic ulcer after resection. On the contrary, remnant tumor can infiltrate submucosal or deeper layer in case of positive vertical resection margin in post-resection pathological mapping.
Local recurrence can develop even after complete resection of tumor. Overlooked skipped tumor is not rare around main lesion in EGC, which can lead to local recurrence when the skipped lesion is not included in the resected specimen. To prevent overlooking the skipped lesion, sufficient resection margin should be guaranteed in case of ill-defined tumor margin.
If the post-resection pathological mapping has revealed the positive lateral resection margin, remnant tumor can exist around resection margin. All cases with positive lateral resection margin, however, have not remnant tumor. Mucosal cancers with positive lateral resection margin have been reported to have remnant tumor only in 5.8%. Because cautery effect can ablate the remnant tumor around the circumferential incision during ESD, local recurrence can be prevented even in incomplete resection in terms of lateral margin. Therefore, frequent short-term endoscopic follow-up can be applied for detection of local recurrence in case of minute involvement of tumor in lateral resection margin.
When the local recurrence has developed in case of positive lateral resection margin, definitive treatment should be made for remnant cancer. If the remnant cancer is still confined to mucosa and the result of previous pathologic mapping has shown the negligible risk of lymph node metastasis in criteria of tumor size, differentiation and depth of tumor invasion, additional endoscopic resection can be applied to remnant cancer. However, secondary endoscopic resection could be more difficult in technique because of submucosal fibrosis after healing of iatrogenic ulcer. Sufficient resection margin should be ensured to prevent repetitive recurrence after additional endoscopic resection. Therefore, endoscopic ablation treatment with argon plasma coagulation (APC) can be applied at the site of repeated ESD as additional therapy. If the result of previous pathological mapping has revealed beyond the indication of endoscopic resection such as larger tumor size, positive angiolymphatic tumor invasion or undifferentiated histology, additional gastrectomy with conventional lymph node dissection should be made for the removal of risk of lymph node metastasis as well as remnant cancer.
Endoscopic ablation treatment can be applied to remnant tumor in endoscopically-unresectable and surgically-inoperable cases such as old age or significant co-morbidity. APC is useful for the ablation of superficial tumor and can be repeated with interval until complete resolution of remnant tumor.
When the local recurrence has developed in case of positive vertical resection margin, tumor can infiltrate submucosal or deeper layer because the method of ESD removes most of mucosal and submucosal layer. Therefore, additional gastrectomy and lymph node dissection should be made in case of positive vertical resection margin.
Synchronous lesion is defined as multiple tumors at diagnosis or newly-detected tumor within one year after initial resection. One-year interval is arbitrary because exact time of tumor initiation cannot be resolved. A tumor detected within one year after initial resection might exist at initial diagnosis because conventional endoscopy could not detect minute tumor less than 5 mm in size at initial diagnosis. Especially, tumor more than 5 mm in size

within one year after initial resection could be exist even at initial diagnosis in viewpoint of doubling time of tumor. Metachronous tumor is defined as newly-developed tumor after one year of endoscopic resection. During follow-up after endoscopic resection, metachronous tumor develops at rate of 1 - 3% per year.
The management of synchronous or metachronous tumor depends on status of respective tumor. If the tumor is indicated in endoscopic resection, ESD can be applied for complete resection. On the contrary, surgical resection should be applied in case beyond indication of endoscopic resection.

3. Conclusion

ESD has been a curative treatment modality of EGC in selective indications. The complete resection rate, long-term disease-free results and survival has been comparable to surgical treatment with the progress of endoscopic technique and accessories. After complete resection, regular follow-up examination is mandatory for the detection of metachronous tumor development.

4. References

Abe, N., Sugiyama, M. & Masaki, T. (2004). Predictive factors for lymph node metastasis of differentiated submucosally invasive gastric cancer. *Gastrointestinal Endoscopy*, Vol.60, No.2, (August 2004), pp. 242-245, ISSN 0016-5107

Akiyama, M., Ota, M. & Nakajima, H. (1997). Endoscopic mucosal resection of gastric neoplasms using a ligating device. *Gastrointestinal Endoscopy*, Vol.45, No.2, (February 1997), pp. 182-186, ISSN 0016-5107

Choi, IJ., Kim, CG. & Chang HJ. (2005). The learning curve for EMR with circumferential mucosal incision in treating intramucosal gastric neoplasm. *Gastrointestinal Endoscopy*, Vol.62, No.6, (December 2005), pp. 860-865, ISSN 0016-5107

Chung, IK., Lee, JH. & Lee, SH. (2009). Therapeutic outcomes in 1000 cases of endoscopic submucosal dissection for early gastric neoplasms: Korean ESD Study Group multicenter study. *Gastrointestinal Endoscopy*, Vol.69, No.7, (June 2009), pp. 1228-1235, ISSN 0016-5107

Fujishiro, M., Kodashima, S. & Goto, O. (2008). Successful en bloc resection of superficial esophageal cancer treated by endoscopic submucosal dissection with a splash needle. *Endoscopy*, Vol.40, Suppl.2, (September 2008), E 81-82, ISSN 0013-726X

Gotoda, T., Kondo, H. & Ono, H. (1999). A new endoscopic mucosal resection (EMR) procedure using an insulation-tipped diathermic (IT) knife for rectal flat lesions. *Gastrointestinal Endoscopy*, Vol.50, No.4, (October 1999), pp. 560-563, ISSN 0016-5107

Gotoda, T., Yanagisawa, A. & Sasako, M. (2000). Incidence of lymph node metastasis from early gastric cancer: estimation with a large number of cases at two large centers. *Gastric Cancer*, Vol.3, No.4, (December 2000), pp. 219-225, ISSN 1436-3291

Gotoda, T. (2005) A large endoscopic resection by endoscopic submucosal dissection (ESD) procedure. *Clinical Gastroenterology and Hepatology*, Vol.3, No.7, Suppl.1, (July 2005), S71-73, ISSN 1542-3565

Hirao, M., Masuda, K. & Asanuma, T. (1988). Endoscopic resection of early gastric cancer and other tumors with local injection of hypertonic saline-epinephrine. *Gastrointestinal Endoscopy*, Vol.34, No.3, (May-June 1988), pp. 264-269, ISSN 0016-5107

Inoue, H., Takeshita, K. & Hori, H. (1993). Endoscopic mucosal resection with a cap-fitted panendoscope for esophagus, stomach, and colon mucosal lesions. *Gastrointestinal Endoscopy*, Vol.39, No.1, (January-February 1993), pp. 58-62, ISSN 0016-5107

Kim, HG., Cho, JY. & Bok, GH. (2008). A novel device for endoscopic submucosal dissection, the Fork knife. *World Journal of Gastroenterology*, Vol.14, No.43, (November 2008), pp. 6726-6732, ISSN 1007-9327

Kim, JJ., Lee, JH. & Jung, HY. (2007). EMR for early gastric cancer in Korea: a multicenter retrospective study. *Gastrointestinal Endoscopy*, Vol.66, No.4, (October 2007), pp. 693-700, ISSN 0016-5107

Kodashima, S., Fujishiro, M. & Yahagi, N. (2006). Endoscopic submucosal dissection using flexknife. *Journal of Clinical Gastroenterology*, Vol.40, No.5, (May-June 2006), pp. 378-384, ISSN 0192-0790

Kojima, T., Parra-Blanco, A. & Takahashi, H. (1998). Outcome of endoscopic mucosal resection for early gastric cancer: review of the Japanese literature. *Gastrointestinal Endoscopy*, Vol.30, No.7, (November 1998), pp. 3223-3224, ISSN 0016-5107

Kwak, CS., Lee, HK. & Cho, SJ. (2000). Analysis of clinicopathological factors associated with lymph node metastasis in early gastric cancer review of 2,137 cases. *Journal of Korean Cancer Association*, Vol.32, No.4, (August 2000), pp. 674-681, ISSN 1598-2998

Miyata, M., Yokoyama, Y. & Okoyama, N. (2000). What are the appropriate indications for endoscopic mucosal resection for early gastric cancer? Analysis of 256 endoscopically resected lesions. *Endoscopy*, Vol.32, No.10, (October 2000), pp. 773-778, ISSN 0013-726X

Ono, H., Kondo, H. & Gotoda, T. (2001). Endoscopic mucosal resection for treatment of early gastric cancer. *Gut*, Vol.48, No.2, (February 2001), pp. 225-229, ISSN 0017-5749

Ono, H., Hasuike, N. & Inui, T. (2008). Usefulness of a novel electrosurgical knife, the insulation-tipped diathermic knife-2, for endoscopic submucosal dissection of early gastric cancer. *Gastric Cancer*, Vol.11, No.1, (January 2008), pp. 47-52, ISSN 1436-3291

Soetikno, R., Kaltenbach, T. & Yeh, R. (2005). Endoscopic mucosal resection for early gastric cancers of the upper gastrointestinal tract. *Journal of Clinical Oncology*, Vol.23, No.20, (July 2005), pp. 4490-4498, ISSN 1527-7755

Ye, BD., Kim, SG. & Lee, JY. (2008). Predictive factors for lymph node metastasis and endoscopic treatment strategies for undifferentiated early gastric cancer. *Journal of Gastroenterology and Hepatology*, Vol. 23, No.1, (January 2008), pp. 46-50, ISSN 0815-9319

Yokoda, T., Ishiyama, S. & Saito, T. (2004). Lymph node metastasis as a significant prognostic factor in gastric cancer: a multiple logistic regression analysis. *Scandinavian Journal of Gastroenterology*, Vol.39, No.4, (April 2004), pp. 380-384, ISSN 0036-5521

3

Endoscopic Submucosal Dissection, a New Technique for en Bloc Resection of Large Superficial Tumor in the Esophagus

Makoto Nishimura, Masafumi Sakaguchi, Hideki Kitada, Michio Hifumi and Hiroto Kita
International Medical Center, Saitama Medical University
Japan

1. Introduction

For superficial esophageal cancer, conventional endoscopic mucosal resection with cap (EMRC) has been widely prevailed for reliable and safety treatment[1]. Recent innovations of diagnostic endoscopy including high-resolution endoscopy, narrow band imaging (NBI), and magnified endoscopy allow detect and identify more small lesions of the GI tract, and endoscopist are forced to develop their skills for endocopic treatment. Recently, endoscopic submucosal dissection (ESD) has been developed for en bloc resection of larger superficial tumor in the GI tract than conventional EMR. In this decade, ESD has been widely accepted as a more reliable therapeutic procedure than EMR in Japan, and various devices are developed.
Of the esophageal cancers, squamous cell carcinoma is the most common carcinoma in Japan, and iodine staining endoscopy has been widely used to detect esophageal SCC. Conventional EMRC has been performed for these 10 years, however, since conventional EMRC were carried out with small size cap, 12mm in diameter, there has been the risk to be piecemeal and residual lesions. Recently, newly classification of intrapapillary capillary loop pattern (IPCL) has developed for diagnose the early esophageal neoplasm, and because of these diagnostic innovation, therefore, many endoscopist are forced to remove larger en bloc resection for reliable ESD as well as gastric or colorectal lesions. Therefore, in Japan, ESD for large superficial esophageal neoplasm has been applied; however, esophageal ESD is considered as more difficult and challenging than gastric ESD, and only few studies have elucidated the technical feasibility of ESD in the esophagus.
Needle knife has been used for early gastric and colorectal ESD, and it has been considered causing high complications for esophageal ESD because of its sharpness. For this reason, using other knives, some clinical case series are reported for esophageal ESD, and the safety of esophageal ESD using needle knife is still unclear. In this study, we conducted consecutive esophageal ESD with needle knife and compared EMR to evaluate safety and reliability of needle knife as esophageal ESD device.

2. Patients and methods

Between February 2001 and March 2009, a total of 82 patients with esophageal squamous cell neoplasm were treated by ESD or EMRC at our institution. Data was stored consecutively in the database that include patients information, lesion sizes, histopathologic findings (depth, negative rate of lateral margin, negative rate of vertical margin, lymphovascular invasion), treatment type, complications, and prognosis. Based on initial endoscopic evaluation, patients were selected endoscopic treatment, radiation, chemoradiation, or surgery. Criteria of endoscopic treatment for superficial esophageal tumor at our institution were the follows; (1) previously proven squamous-cell carcinoma (SCC) or dysplasia which cannot rule out concomitant with SCC, up to 75% circumference, (2) supposed to be mucosal or mild submucosal invasion endoscopically, (3) no obvious evidence of lymphovascular invasion echoendoscopically, (4) no prior esophageal surgery, (5) no severe cardiovascular complications. Ulcerated lesion, advanced SCC, adenocarcinoma, 100% circumferential lesion, and patients with severe cardiopulmonary complications were excluded. Written informed consent was obtained from each patient, while conventional surgery or standard chemoradiation with 5-FU/CDDP+RT were offered as options before treatment. After initial treatment, all cases were observed (mean period: 37.2 months, range: 8-103 months), and the local recurrence rate and overall survival period of each group were analyzed.

2.1 Statistical analysis

Data were collected and analyzed. Comparisons between groups were performed χ^2 test for categorical variables. A P value < .05 was considered statistically significant. All analysis were performed on a personal computer by using IBM SPSS version 15 (IBM SPSS 19, IBM, Co, Sorners, NY).

2.2 Cap-EMR technique

With standard panendoscope (GIF-240Z, Olympus Optical, Tokyo, Japan), endoscopic mucosal resection using a cap (EMRC) was carried out under conscious sedation as followed; marking were placed with needle knife, 2) EMR cap was fitted to the tip of standard panendoscope, 3) targeted lesion was elevated by the submucosal injection, 4) the lesion was then sucked into the cap and strangulated by closing the snare, 5) the lesion was resected by the application of electric current.

2.3 ESD technique

For ESD, standard endoscope was used with an attachment (D-201-11804; Olympus, Japan). Briefly, ESD was conducted under conscious sedation as followed; 1) marking were placed with needle knife (KD-10Q-1; Olympus, Tokyo, Japan) around the targeted lesion, 2) 0.5ml normal saline and 1.0% of sodium hyaluronate were injected into submucosal layer, 3) using electrocosurgical generator (VAIO, Erbe Co, Tubingen, Germany), needle knife was used for circumferential cutting and submucosal dissection, and the elevated lesion was performed en-bloc resection. Hemostastic forceps (Coaglaspa, Olympus, Japan) was used for hemostasis. In both groups, all resected specimen were retrieved and histopathologically evaluated.

3. Results

From the database, we corrected 82 patients who underwent esophageal treatment endoscopically. The feature of the patients and lesions are shown in Table 1. Complete resection was achieved in all 82 patients. Sixty-one patients were treated by ESD (57 males, median age 67.5, range 38-87) and 21 patients were treated by EMRC (19 males, median age 66.0, range 46-83). Between both groups, there were no significant differences in patients characteristics; age and sex (p=0.530 vs p=0.653). The tumor size was significantly larger in the ESD group than EMRC group; the mean resected specimen size was 21.4 mm in diameter (range 12-40 mm) for EMRC and 31.3 mm in diameter (range 8-50 mm) for ESD (P<0.001). The en-bloc resection rate was 61.9% and 98.4% in the EMRC and ESD groups, respectively (P<0.01). Histopathologically, there were 52 cases of squamous cell carcinoma (SCC) and 9 dysplasias in the ESD group, while 14 cases of SCC and 7 dysplasias in the EMRC group. The negative horizontal margin rate was 85.7% and 90.1% for the EMRC and ESD groups, respectively (p=0.574). The negative vertical margin rate was 95.2% and 90.8% for the EMRC and ESD groups, respectively (P=0.726). There were 0 cases in the EMRC group and 9 cases of complications in the ESD group (5 cases of stenosis and 4 cases of perforation). Among the patients with perforation in ESD group, 1 case was successfully treated by emergency surgery and others were managed conservatively, however, could not evaluated tumor depth histopathologically because of the patient's status. The local recurrence rate was 5.0 in the EMRC group and 1.6% in the ESD group (P=0.42). 2 patients died from radiative pneumonia and 1 patient died from acute myocardial infarction in the EMRC group, and 1 patient died from pancreatic cancer in the ESD group, and. No patient in either group died from any associated complications or esophageal cancer.

	EMRC	ESD	*P* value
Patients characteristics			
Number of patients	21	61	
Mean age (y)	66	67.5	0.530
Male/ Female	19/2	57/4	0.653
Characteristic of lesions			
Histologic type			0.152
Mild dysplasia	1	0	
Moderate dysplasia	4	4	
Severe dysplasia	2	4	
Squamous cell carcinoma	14	53	

Table 1. Patient characteristics

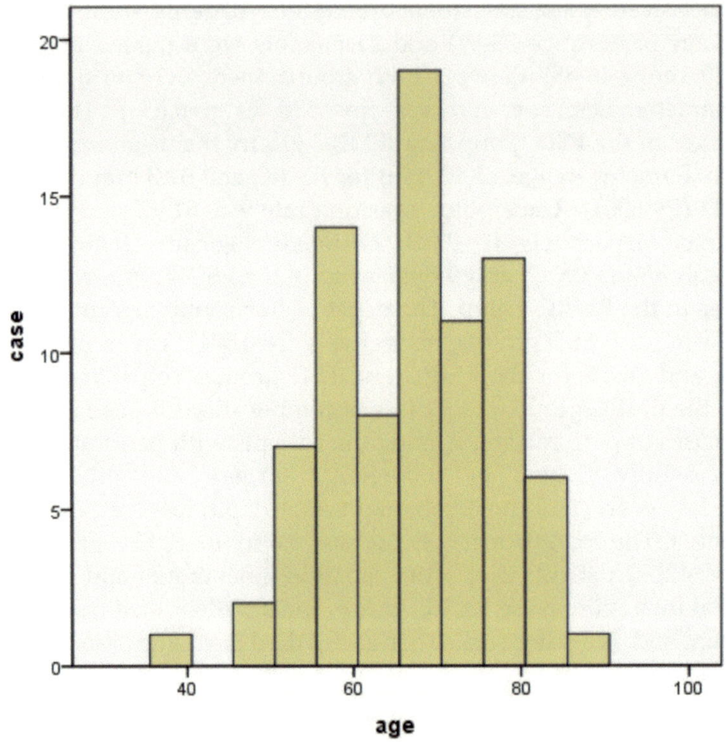
case
age
0
5
10
15
20
40
60
80
100

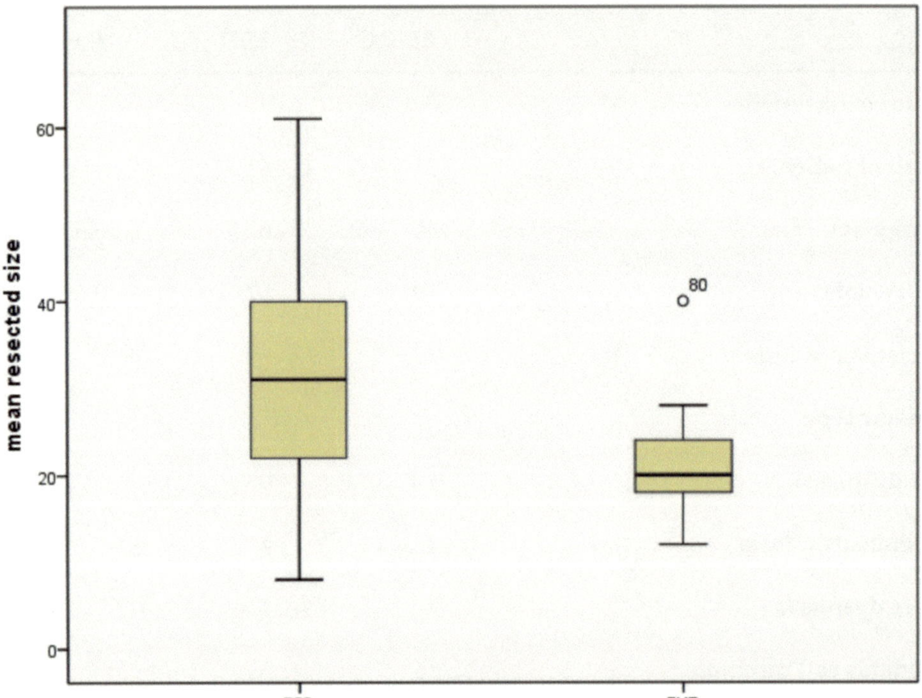
mean resected size
ESD/EMR
ESD
EMR
80
0
20
40
60

	EMRC	ESD	
mean resected size(mean [SD]) (cm)	21.48±2.63	31.34±2.97	p<0.001
en-bloc resection no, rate (%)	13/21 (61.9%)	60/61 (98.4%)	p<0.001
Deapth of the tumos			
Dysplasias	7	9	
m1	2	30	
m2	5	7	
m3	5	9	
sm1	1	2	
sm2	0	3	
sm3	1	0	
unknown		1	
LM negative no, rate (%)	18/21 (85.7%)	55/61 (90.1%)	p=0.574
VM negative no, rate (%)	20/21 (95.2%)	55/61 (90.1%)	p=0.726
local recurrence no, rate (%)	1/20 (5%)	1/61 (1.6%)	p=0.42

Resected size; Manan-Whiteney test p<0.001
En-bloc/piecemeal Peason χ^2 test p<0.001
LM negative rate Peason χ^2 test p=0.574
VM negative rate Peason χ^2 test p=0.726
Prognosis Peason χ^2 test p<0.001
Local recurrence rate Peason χ^2 test p=0.42

Table 2. Results

4. Discussion

In the present study, we have shown that the tumor size and negative horizontal margin rate are superior in ESD than EMRC. ESD is same complication risk as EMRC, however, did not suggest to be able to resect deeper lesions. Our results suggest that ESD is reliable technique for early superficial esophageal tumors.

In the previous study, Ishihara reported ESD using Hook knife has higher curative rate than EMRC or 2-channel EMR[2]. They had carried out ESD later than EMR or c-channel EMR, and they also suggested that continuous improvement of instruments and techniques as our study, however, regarding the limited size of the specimen of EMRC, more reliable resection is possible by ESD than EMRC. In addition, other studies suggests that piecemeal resection with EMR would be risk of local recurrence[3, 4]. Therefore, ESD is considered to be high curative rate for such lesions.

In spite of higher rate of en-bloc, curative resection, low risk of local recurrence and better histopathological evaluation of resected specimen, ESD is time-consuming and technically challenging. In this study, we did not evaluate procedure time. Oka also reported that average operation time was significantly longer in the ESD group than conventional EMR (84.4 minutes versus 12.6 minutes in total average)[5]. Operation time is disadvantage of ESD, therefore, a various technique are improving to overcome this disadvantage. Neuhas indicated that procedure time could be shorten based on the learning curve, especially in ESD rather than EMR[6], and this could be also affect endoscopist's experience, which related to early gastric lesions before esophageal lesions, since esophagus is more limited space and high risk for life-threating complications.

Several different technique using different knives has been reported to overcome the known difficulty of ESD[7-10]. And recently, some comparison study has also reported with various methods[10-12]. Takahashi compared ESD and EMR for early squamous cell carcinoma of the esophagus (SCCE) and reported higher cure rate and safer than conventional EMR, based on the hook-knife ESD method[13]. Oyama also emphasized the advantage of hook-knife ESD for esophageal lesions[9], however, this device is still available only in the limited countries and also require special training because of the uniqueness of its shapes as well as insulated-tip diathermic knife (IT-knife)[14]. On the other hand, needle knife is available all over the world because it is approved as papillotome knife for ERCP already, and has been used without specialized training. Some authors had reported the feasibility and advantage of needle-knife ESD[15, 16], however, many endoscopist still consider that needle knife has higher complication risk for esophageal ESD. Therefore, we conducted the control study using needle-knife, and this is the first large scale, long-term study comparing ESD with conventional EMR of early esophageal neoplasm using needle knife. However, still there is no prospective randomized comparison study between these knives for esophageal ESD, therefore further multicenter study are needed.

The other concern is the risk of complications. Oka also reported that for bleeding and perforation, ESD was higher than conventional EMR (22.6% versus 7.6%, and 6.2 % versus 3.9%, respectively)[5]. Our data also suggests that ESD has high complication risk of perforation; however, all these complications could be managed conservatively in most of the cases because of smaller size of perforation than conventional EMR. More than two of third of the circumferential resection in esophageal ESD is well known to develop delayed stenosis, which could be also safely managed using the balloon type dilator[17].

5. Conclusion

In summery ESD was able to accomplish en-bloc resection and achieved larger resection than conventional EMR for early superficial tumors in the esophagus as well as other GI tract. There are some residual problems of operation time and complication, however, ESD has large advantage to cure the esophageal lesions and indispensable for superficial esophageal neoplasms. Further experiences and multi-center study are needed for compare the various devises.

6. References

[1] Inoue H, Takeshita K, Hori H, Muraoka Y, Yoneshima H, Endo M. Endoscopic mucosal resection with a cap-fitted panendoscope for esophagus, stomach, and colon mucosal lesions. Gastrointest Endosc 1993;39:58-62.

[2] Ishihara R, Iishi H, Uedo N, Takeuchi Y, Yamamoto S, Yamada T, Masuda E, Higashino K, Kato M, Narahara H, Tatsuta M. Comparison of EMR and endoscopic submucosal dissection for en bloc resection of early esophageal cancers in Japan. Gastrointest Endosc 2008;68:1066-72.

[3] Katada C, Muto M, Manabe T, Ohtsu A, Yoshida S. Local recurrence of squamous-cell carcinoma of the esophagus after EMR. Gastrointest Endosc 2005;61:219-25.
[4] Tanabe S, Koizumi W, Mitomi H, Kitamura T, Tahara K, Ichikawa J, Higuchi K, Sasaki T, Nakayama N, Kida M, Saigenji K. Usefulness of EMR with an oblique aspiration mucosectomy device compared with strip biopsy in patients with superficial esophageal cancer. Gastrointest Endosc 2004;59:558-63.
[5] Oka S, Tanaka S, Kaneko I, Mouri R, Hirata M, Kawamura T, Yoshihara M, Chayama K. Advantage of endoscopic submucosal dissection compared with EMR for early gastric cancer. Gastrointest Endosc 2006;64:877-83.
[6] Neuhaus H, Wirths K, Schenk M, Enderle MD, Schumacher B. Randomized controlled study of EMR versus endoscopic submucosal dissection with a water-jet hybrid-knife of esophageal lesions in a porcine model. Gastrointest Endosc 2009;70:112-20.
[7] Ono H, Kondo H, Gotoda T, Shirao K, Yamaguchi H, Saito D, Hosokawa K, Shimoda T, Yoshida S. Endoscopic mucosal resection for treatment of early gastric cancer. Gut 2001;48:225-9.
[8] Yamamoto H, Kawata H, Sunada K, Satoh K, Kaneko Y, Ido K, Sugano K. Success rate of curative endoscopic mucosal resection with circumferential mucosal incision assisted by submucosal injection of sodium hyaluronate. Gastrointest Endosc 2002;56:507-12.
[9] Oyama T, Tomori A, Hotta K, Morita S, Kominato K, Tanaka M, Miyata Y. Endoscopic submucosal dissection of early esophageal cancer. Clin Gastroenterol Hepatol 2005;3:S67-70.
[10] Yahagi N, Neuhaus H, Schumacher B, Neugebauer A, Kaehler GF, Schenk M, Fischer K, Fujishiro M, Enderle MD. Comparison of standard endoscopic submucosal dissection (ESD) versus an optimized ESD technique for the colon: an animal study. Endoscopy 2009;41:340-5.
[11] Nonaka K, Arai S, Ishikawa K, Nakao M, Nakai Y, Togawa O, Nagata K, Shimizu M, Sasaki Y, Kita H. Short term results of endoscopic submucosal dissection in superficial esophageal squamous cell neoplasms. World J Gastrointest Endosc 2010;2:69-74.
[12] Teoh AY, Chiu PW, Yu Ngo DK, Wong SK, Lau JY, Ng EK. Outcomes of endoscopic submucosal dissection versus endoscopic mucosal resection in management of superficial squamous esophageal neoplasms outside Japan. J Clin Gastroenterol 2010;44:e190-4.
[13] Takahashi H, Arimura Y, Masao H, Okahara S, Tanuma T, Kodaira J, Kagaya H, Shimizu Y, Hokari K, Tsukagoshi H, Shinomura Y, Fujita M. Endoscopic submucosal dissection is superior to conventional endoscopic resection as a curative treatment for early squamous cell carcinoma of the esophagus (with video). Gastrointest Endosc 2010;72:255-64, 264 e1-2.
[14] Gotoda T. A large endoscopic resection by endoscopic submucosal dissection procedure for early gastric cancer. Clin Gastroenterol Hepatol 2005;3:S71-3.
[15] Yamamoto H. Endoscopic submucosal dissection of early cancers and large flat adenomas. Clin Gastroenterol Hepatol 2005;3:S74-6.
[16] Kita H, Yamamoto H, Miyata T, Sunada K, Iwamoto M, Yano T, Yoshizawa M, Hanatsuka K, Arashiro M, Omata T, Sugano K. Endoscopic submucosal dissection

using sodium hyaluronate, a new technique for en bloc resection of a large superficial tumor in the colon. Inflammopharmacology 2007;15:129-31.

[17] Mizuta H, Nishimori I, Kuratani Y, Higashidani Y, Kohsaki T, Onishi S. Predictive factors for esophageal stenosis after endoscopic submucosal dissection for superficial esophageal cancer. Dis Esophagus 2009;22:626-31.

4

Endoscopic Treatment of Gastric Adenoma with Argon Plasma Coagulation

Kee Myung Lee and Jin Hong Kim
Ajou University School of Medicine, Korea

1. Introduction

The term gastric adenoma means a benign lesion of the glandular epithelium having variable degrees of cellular atypia and showing papillary or tubular structures. Because long-term follow-up studies of gastric adenomas reveal malignant transformations, it is well known they are premalignant. Since these lesions lie histologically and clinically on the borderline of between whether they are benign or malignant, it is extremely important for clinicians to determine whether they are to be treated or not (Morson, 1980; Kamiya, 1982; Rugge, 1994).

For a long time, there was no specific treatment policy of gastric adenomas and treatment varied from close endoscopic follow-ups to endoscopic resection, considering its heterogeneous clinical consequences (Di Gregorio, 1993; Saraga, 1987). When gastric epithelial dysplasia is classified using the two or three tier system, each group shows a different clinical course. For gastric adenoma with high grade dysplasia (HGD), endoscopic resection has become the standard treatment because of risk of malignant progression and synchronous carcinomas (Lansdown, 1990; Farinati, 1993). Many western publications have recommended close endoscopic follow-up of patients with moderate/low grade gastric epithelial dysplasia (Rugge, 1991, Fertitta, 1993; Rugge, 1991). The frequency of the follow-up has been recommended to be every three to 12 months at least during the first year, but it is still unknown of how long the follow-up should be maintained for when no progression has been detected (Bearzi, 1994; Fertitta, 1993). The disadvantages of endoscopic follow-ups are patient anxiety, risk of disease progression, and low patient compliance for an undefined period (Lansdown, 1990; Rugge, 1991). Though endoscopic resection has become frequently applied for gastric adenoma with low grade dysplasia (LGD), there is ongoing controversy considering its relatively benign natural course and clinical significance. Although endoscopic resection is a less invasive procedure than surgical resection, it still carries the risk of complications and requires hospitalization of several days (Ono 2001, O'Mahony, 2001; Miyata 2000).

Argon plasma coagulation (APC) is a kind of non-contact technique for tissue coagulation, which transfers high-frequency electric current through ionized argon gas to targeted lesions (Grund, 1994; Grunde, 1997). Because APC has an advantage of confining the thermal effect to the superficial layer of the gastrointestinal wall, APC has been used for the treatment of bleeding ulcers, hemorrhagic telangiectasias, and tumors (Chau, 2003;

Cipolletta, 1998; Iacopini, 2007). For the treatment of early gastric cancer, APC has been used on a limited number of patients due to it being impossible to get a pathologic evaluation and to predict the depth of invasion (Sagawa, 2003; Kitamura, 2006). Considering that gastric adenomas are confined to the mucosa and the thermal effect of APC is extended to both the mucosa and submucosa, theoretically the gastric adenoma lesion can be eradicated with APC. APC has the advantage of preventing excessive tissue damage and perforation, due to the coagulation damage of tissue increasing the electrical impedance, in turn decreasing the electrical current and automatically stopping irradiation (Goulet Watson, 2000; Morson, 1980). Based on the above characteristics of APC, it can most probably be the safer and most effective therapeutic option of treating gastric adenomas. However, it has been reported that some endoscopists have experienced an unexpected extension of tissue destruction and even perforation, which could have been due to host and technical factors. Therefore, APC has been proven not to be completely free from the risk of perforation (Hoyer, 1998; Prost, 2004). In this chapter, we will give a brief introduction about the APC procedure after the submucosal saline injection for the treatment of gastric adenomas at the out-patient clinic without any need for hospitalization.

2. Gastric adenoma and its natural course

Most adenomas present a pale surface, and few cases reveal redness on the surface. The frequency of gastric adenomas in different age groups reveals a tendency to increase markedly with aging, especially above the fifth decade. This tendency may have some relation to atrophic changes and especially intestinal metaplasia of the gastric mucosa among the aged (Morson, 1980; Kamiya, 1982; Rugge,1994). In some report, co-existent gastric carcinomas were more frequently found (8%) in the same stomach and meticulous endoscopic evaluation was required. Epidemiological and histopathological studies have shown that intestinal type gastric cancers frequently develop through a sequence of histological events: namely diffuse chronic gastritis, often mucosal atrophy, intestinal metaplasia (complete and/or incomplete), gastric adenoma, and finally invasive carcinoma (Rugge, 1994; Saraga, 1987). Several prospective and retrospective serological studies have now linked *Helicobacter pylori* infection to gastric cancer (Talley, 1991; Parsonnet, 1991; Nomura, 1991). *Helicobacter pylori* infection is clearly associated with the induction of chronic inflammation of the gastric mucosa and the progressive development of metaplastic changes (Asaka, 2006).

Gastric adenoma is known to be a precancerous lesion of intestinal type adenocarcinoma and has diverse outcomes depending on the degree of dysplasia. According to the histological abnormality, gastric dysplasia has been graded using a two or three tier system-high/low or high/moderate/low grade dysplasia. Gastric adenoma with HGD was known to regress in about 5%, to persist in 14%, and to progress in 81–85% of cases (Miyata, 2000; Giovannini 1993). In chronological studies of malignant progression, the time period between diagnosis of HGD and gastric cancer varied and was between less than 1 month to 39 months (Farinati, 1993; Fertitta, 1993). It is suggested the possibility that some of these lesions already contained carcinomatous lesions but the invasive element was not included in the original biopsy sample (Lansdown, 1990; Farinati 1993). Endoscopic resection methods such as endoscopic mucosal resection (EMR) or endoscopic submucosal dissection

(ESD) confirmed this possibility (Miyata, 2000; Giovannini, 1999; Watanabe, 2006). Therefore, gastric adenomas with HGD have to be treated as if it were an early gastric cancer, because of the risk of synchronous carcinoma and high risk of malignant progression (Farinati, 1993; Rugge, 1991).

Gastric adenomas with LGD show a different natural course. Gastric adenomas with LGD have been reported to regress in 38–49%, to be persistent in 19–28%, to progress in 5–21%, and eventually to be diagnosed as gastric adenocarcinoma in 0–5% of cases (Fertitta, 1993; Rugge, 1991). Although many cases of gastric adenomas with LGD do not progress, a number of cases were reported to have done so, progressing to HGD or carcinoma after a median follow-up period ranging from 34.5 to 41.5 months (Fertitta, 1993; Rugge, 1991). This long interval time suggests that gastric adenomas with LGD rarely contain carcinoma at the time of diagnosis (Fertitta, 1993; Rugge, 1991).

Many western publications recommended close endoscopic follow-up of gastric adenomas with LGD, every 3–12 months until no progression is detected (Bearzi, 1994; Fertitta 1993). However, this approach has many problems; patient anxiety, risk of disease progression, and low compliance with frequent and expensive follow-up for an undefined period. Provided that HGD has been confirmed with endoscopic biopsy, many authors suggest surgical or endoscopic resection. Endoscopic resection can offer a non-surgical solution for intramucosal adenocarcinoma with advances in endoscopic localization method (chromoscopy, NBI) and staging techniques (endoscopic ultrasound)(Ono, 2001; O'Mahony, 2001).

3. Endoscopic resection of gastric adenoma

Endoscopic resection methods such as EMR and ESD are already recognized as standard treatments of premalignant lesions and small intramucosal cancerous lesions (Giovannini, 1999; Watanabe, 2006; Takenaka, 2008). Because a lesion is resected by means of electrocautery snaring using the EMR method, EMR is typically used for removal of lesions smaller than 2 cm or piecemeal removal of larger lesions. ESD has been developed for en bloc removal of large lesions (usually more than 2 cm) (Ono, 2001; O'Mahony, 2001). Using the ESD method, a circumferential mucosal incision and submucosal dissection is done with specialized endoscopic electrocautery knives after marking the lesion and then injecting saline into the submucosal layer (Oka, 2006; Takeuchi, 2007, Oka, 2006).

Although EMR and ESD are less invasive procedures than surgical operations, they still carry some risk of complications such as bleeding and perforation, and require hospital admission for a few days (Oka 2006; Takeuchi, 2007). ESD requires the use of expensive specialized knives and a longer procedure time, and runs a higher risk of bleeding or perforation, as compared to EMR (Ono, 2001). Considering the risk of synchronous carcinoma and malignant progression, endoscopic resection is the best therapeutic option of gastric adenomas with HGD (Lansdown, 1990; Farinati, 1993). However, because gastric adenomas with LGD have a relatively benign natural course, endoscopic resection might be an excessive and expensive procedure (Rugge, 1995; Fertitta, 1993). From this point of view, the treatment of gastric adenomas with LGD should be different from the therapeutic option for gastric adenomas with HGD or intramucosal adenocarcinoma. In gastric adenomas with LGD, it can be recommended that therapeutic modalities between the frequent endoscopic follow-up and endoscopic resection be done, because a number of cases were reported to have progressed.

4. Argon plasma coagulation

Argon plasma coagulation (APC) is a non-contact technique for tissue coagulation in which a high-frequency electrical current is transferred to the target tissue by means of ionized argon gas. An APC applicator for endoscopic use was developed in 1994, making it possible to provide tangential irradiation to coagulate a target lesion uniformly (Grund, 1994). APC has been introduced to treat a broad range of gastrointestinal problems, including bleeding ulcers (Chau, 2003; Cipolletta, 1998), Dieulafoy's lesions (Iacopini, 2007), hemorrhagic telangiectasias (Olmos, 2006; Sato, 2005; Rolachon, 2000; Kwan, 2006; Nakamura, 2001), radiation proctitis (Kaassis, 2000; Postgate, 2007) and tumors (Sagawa, 2003; Kitamura, 2006). As the lesion becomes coagulated with APC irradiation, tissue electrical impedance sharply increases and electrical current abruptly decreases and is automatically transferred to surrounding tissue sites with low impedance (Grund 1994; Grund, 1997; Wahab, 1997). Therefore, APC irradiation can safely coagulate large areas of tissue within a short time and the excessive tissue damage can automatically be prevented (Wahab, 1997). This characteristic of APC confines the thermal effect to the superficial portion and is an advantage over conventional endoscopic cauterization. Therefore, APC seems to be the most popular non-contact technique for tissue coagulation in the gastrointestinal field.

5. Argon plasma coagulation and early gastric cancer

As economic development and medical advancement lengthen the life expectancy rate, the number of elderly patients with early gastric cancers who have a serious morbidity of being physically unable to withstand either surgical or endoscopic resection is increasing. Local ethanol injection (Imaoka, 1987), microwave coagulation (Tabuse, 1985), Nd:YAG laser treatment (Yasuda, 1993; Hiki, 1989; Sibille, 1995), and photodynamic therapy(Nakamura, 1990; Ell, 1998; Mimura, 1996) have been applied in such cases. Nd:YAG laser treatment is widely used in treating patients with gastric cancers as a curative or palliative therapy but has the drawback of being impossible of being tangentially irradiated (Tajiri, 1991; Hiki, 1989).

Sagawa et al (Sagawa, 2003) performed ex vivo experiments with swine gastric mucosal tissue in order to set the irradiation conditions of APC for the treatment of early gastric cancers based on histological analysis (Fig. 1). Under all output settings tested from 20 to 100 W, the coagulation front became deeper as the duration of irradiation was prolonged, reaching a plateau after irradiation for 15 seconds with each power setting (Fig. 2). The ex vivo experiment demonstrated that the depth of coagulation could easily be adjusted by changing the irradiation time and current output. They recommended that irradiation at 60 W for 15 seconds (900 J/cm2) is the ideal setting for intramucosal cancer because this setting could cauterize the whole mucosal layer but would not affect the deep submucosal layer. However, there is a concern that the effect of APC observed in the ex vivo experiment would be somehow attenuated in vivo because there is blood flow that may act as a heat sink in living tissue. In addition, there was a concern of chronological changes of coagulation depth within a few days after APC irradiation. They applied the APC technique for the treatment of 27 patients with intramucosal gastric cancers who had no lymph node metastases (T1N0M0). APC showed a very high efficacy (no recurrence in 26/27 patients) after a follow-up period of 18–49 months (median 30 months). High treatment efficacy was obtained in 12 of the 27 patients whose cancers were located at difficult locations for the endoscope to access, the cardia or posterior wall of the gastric body, probably by virtue of tangential irradiation and uniform cauterization over a wide area. With regard to complications, some patients experienced a sense of abdominal fullness and it was easily alleviated by endoscopic suction during the procedure.

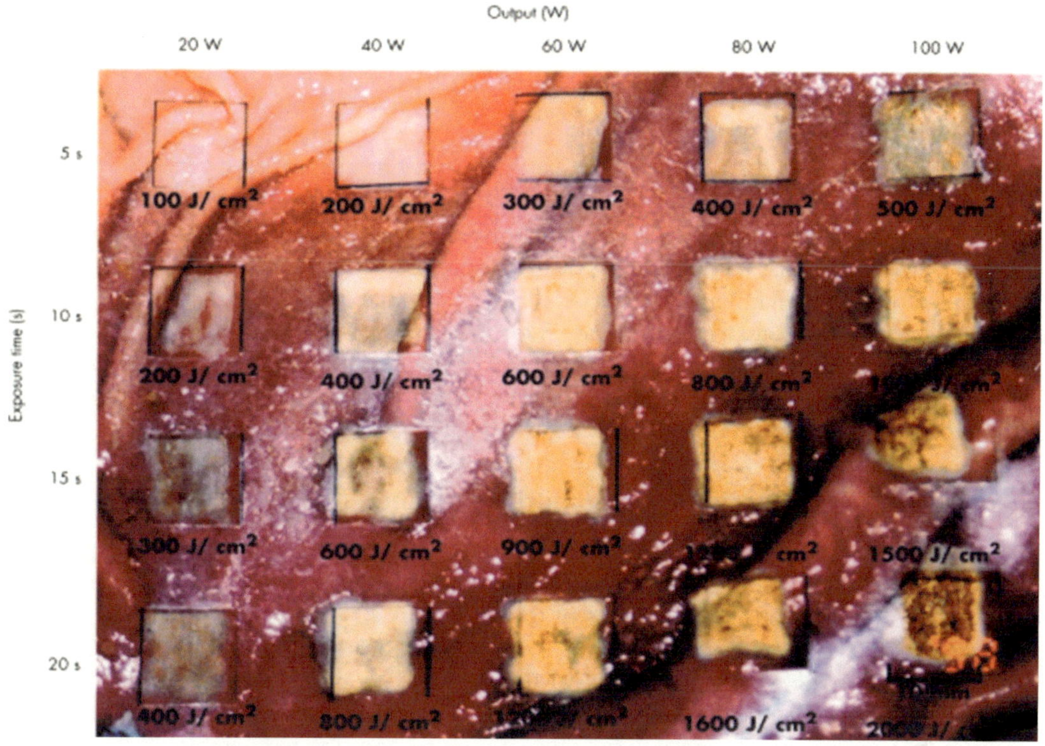

Fig. 1. Macroscopic findings of swine gastric mucosa irradiated by argon plasma coagulation (APC) under various conditions. The effect of APC was macroscopically studied on swine gastric samples at 20, 40, 60, 80, and 100 W, with pulse durations of 5, 10, 15, and 20 seconds. The mucosa exposed to a greater output power of high frequency current and/or for a longer pulse duration underwent a more conspicuous color change from white to brown. (Quotation from Gut 2003;52:334–339 Sagawa T et al)

Kitamura et al (Kitamura , 2006) applied APC for the treatment of early gastric cancers in 40 patients who could not withstand surgical operation and endoscopic resection. There was no residual cancer or recurrence in 35 patients with intramucosal cancer after either a single session or multiple sessions of APC. In contrast, 3 patients (60%), who had large tumors and were treated with a single session of APC, had residual cancers or recurrence among the 5 patients with submucosal cancers after APC treatment. All residual cancers were eradicated after retreatment with additional APC. They also suggested that small early gastric cancers could be successfully treated with only a single session of APC, while large protruding-type tumors or submucosal cancers required two sessions of APC.

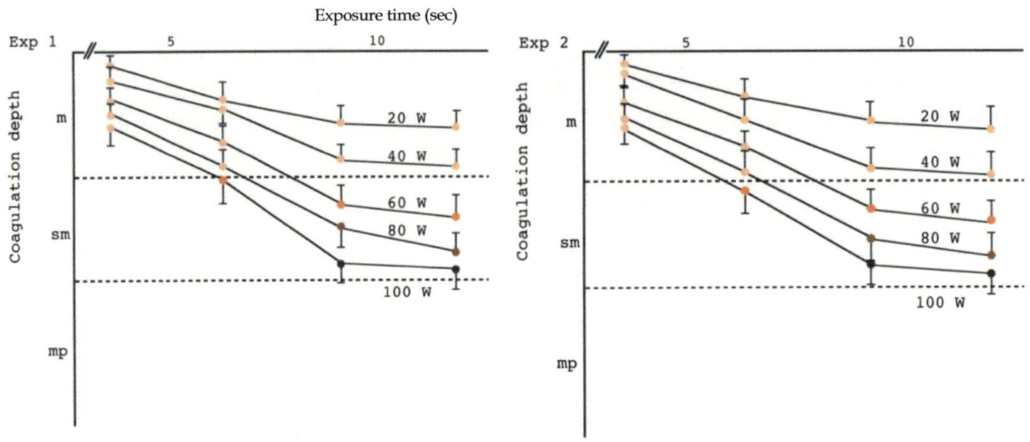

Fig. 2. Coagulation depth under various irradiation conditions based on histological analysis. The experiment was repeated twice using stomach specimens from two separate swine (Exp 1 and Exp 2). The coagulation front became deeper as the duration of irradiation was prolonged, reaching a plateau after irradiation for 15 seconds with each power setting. It was determined that the optimum treatment conditions of APC for clinical studies was a current of 60 W and a maximum irradiation time of 15 s/cm^2, which would not be expected to cause perforation. (Quotation from Gut 2003;52:334–339 Sagawa T et al)

6. Argon plasma coagulation and gastric adenoma

Although APC has been proven to be efficient for the treatment of mucosal and even submucosal cancers, it was only applied to the limited patients who were not suitable for surgical resection or EMR/ESD, because of drawbacks of APC including the inability to be histologically evaluated for the response to treatment immediately after the procedure, because it is impossible for a pathological specimen to be obtained with APC treatment (Sagawa, 2003; Kitamura, 2006). Therefore, either surgical or endoscopic resection is usually preferred to APC treatment for patients whose physical condition is tolerable.

The biologic behavior of adenomas is quite different from that of carcinomas. Because adenomas are limited and confined to the mucosal layer, gastric adenomas with LGD have no capacity to invade or infiltrate into deeper layers of the gastric wall (Di Gregorio, 1993; Saraga, 1987). As APC at optimal setting can totally cauterize the mucosal layer and superficial portion of submucosal layer, theoretically gastric adenomas can be clearly eradicated with APC. Different from gastric adenomas with HGD which should be treated as an early gastric cancer because of the risk of synchronous carcinoma and high risk of malignant progression, gastric adenomas with LGD rarely contain carcinomatous lesions at the time of diagnosis (Farinati, 1993; Fertitta, 1993). Based on these characteristics, APC treatment has many merits over endoscopic resection and frequent endoscopic follow-up; short procedure time, low risk of bleeding and perforation, low procedure cost, and no requirement of hospitalization. Therefore, it could be a reasonable treatment of gastric adenomas with LGD.

APC treatment is characterized by non-contact coagulation, making it possible to provide tangential irradiation to coagulate a target site uniformly (Wahab, 1997; Wahab, 1997, Chau, 2003). This feature is an advantage over other endoscopic cauterization such as local ethanol injection, Nd:YAG laser treatment, photodynamic therapy, and microwave coagulation (Tajiri, 1991; Ell, 1998). APC treatment method of gastric adenomas is similar to that of early gastric cancers. After a circumferential area around the lesion is marked with sufficient distance, irradiation is performed in the manner at 60-90 W for 15 seconds (900-1200 J/cm2), which makes the mucosa surface dry and the tissue to change from white to brown. Different from early gastric cancers in which one or two sessions of cauterization is usually required for eradication, one session of APC irradiation is sufficient for gastric adenomas because the depth of the lesion is limited. Inaccurate identification of boundary and the insufficient distance from the lesion to marking may be a more important factor of residual tumor after APC of gastric adenomas, as opposed to early gastric cancers.

7. Argon plasma coagulation and thermal injury

The thermal injury of APC is known to be confined to the mucosa and superficial submucosa layer and APC can theoretically prevent perforation. However, Kitamura et al (Kitamura, 2006) reported one case of perforation in 40 patients whose early gastric cancers were treated with APC. Fujishiro et al (Fujishiro, 2006; Fujishiro, 2008) investigated thermal tissue damage on the stomach of living minipigs to confirm the safety of APC, including a follow-up case. A minipig was sacrificed without delay after APC application, and a stomach specimen revealed that tissue damage was limited to the shallower submucosal layer regardless of the applied time (Fig. 1 and 2). The other was sacrificed after a one week follow-up, and its stomach specimen showed that granulomatous and fibrotic changes existed in the submucosal layer of the artificial ulcers at the pulse durations of 5 seconds and 10 seconds. However, APC with pulse duration of 20 seconds created the deep ulceration with destruction of the proper muscle layer when examined after one week, which was not detected in the minipig sacrificed soon after APC application (Fig. 3).

The thermal effects of APC have been studied in vitro with resected specimens of the stomach and other organs. Such models are limited to being evaluated to its biologic and healing response to thermal injury and the influence of digestive juices. Exposure of tissue directly to high temperatures causes an inflammatory response, coagulation necrosis, followed by desquamative necrosis. Immediately after exposure to thermal injury, histologic examinations of tissue specimens appeared normal, but necrosis occurred secondarily after formation of a nonvital layer (Fujishiro, 2006; Fujishiro, 2008). The electrical resistance of resected specimens is basically similar to that of the gastric mucosa in vivo. APC was reported to have tissue reaction of shrinkage, desiccation, coagulation, and devitalization from the applied surface to deep portion in order. Histological investigation may not detect the zone of devitalization, which means that tissue damage may be underestimated after APC treatment. APC is not completely safe from the risk of perforation, than we previously thought. This result suggests that we have to be aware of the risk of late perforation, which may occur a few days to a few weeks after APC application.

8. Argon plasma coagulation and submucosal saline injection

Previous experimental studies showed that thermal injury induced by APC was confined to the superficial area and deep tissue destruction caused by perforation was rare (Sagawa, 2003; Watson, 2000). Clinical experiences with endoscopic evaluation also supported the rarity of perforation and safety of APC treatment. However, there is still the possibility of the severe complication of perforation caused by APC as published in some reports (Yoshida, 2005; Fujishiro, 2008). And some studies indicated that APC-induced tissue damage could be extended to the proper muscle layer, which might lead to stricture or deformity of the gastrointestinal tract and also functional disturbance of the sphincter and peristaltic movement.

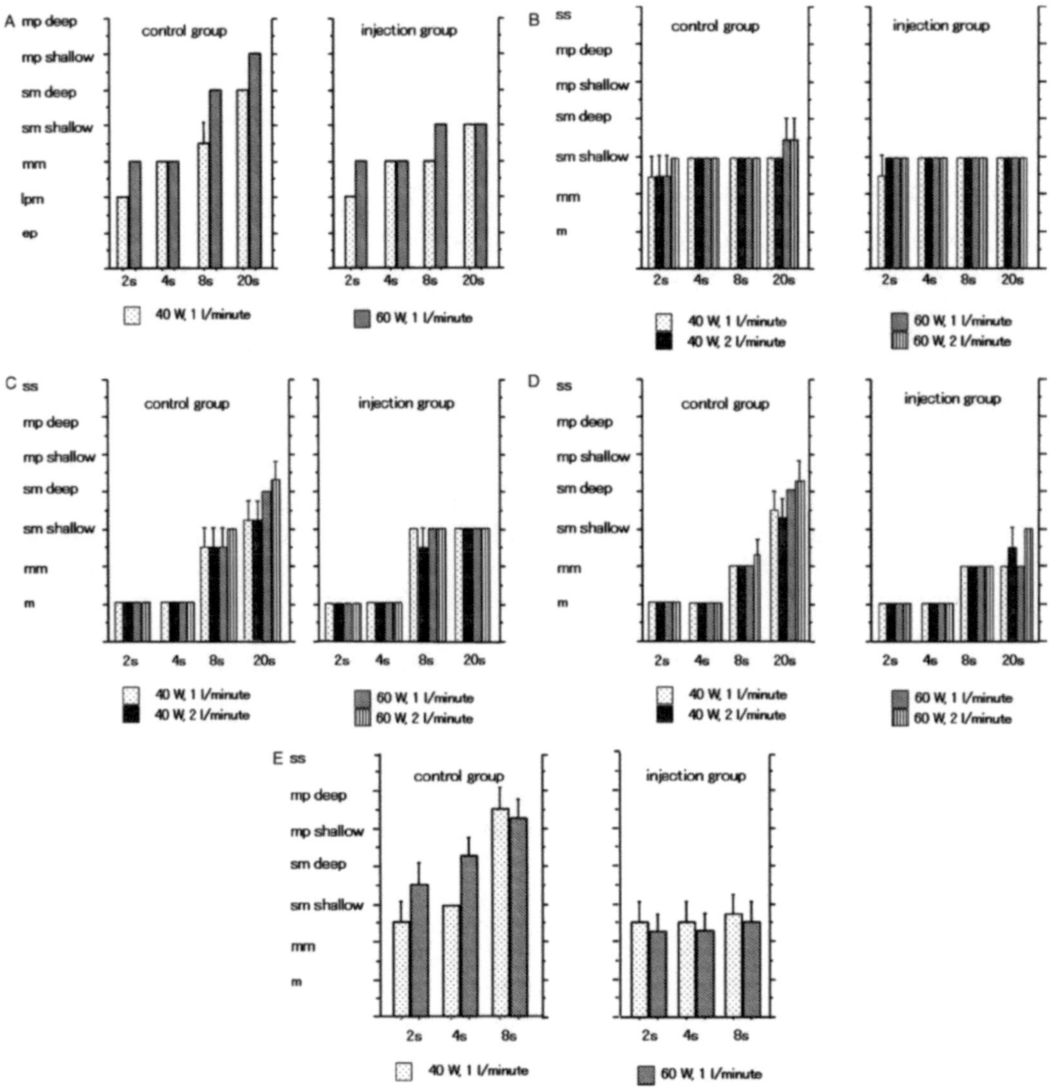

Fig. 3. Correlation between the depth of tissue damage and pulse duration.
The mean depth of the 4 observations is indicated as bars with a standard deviation in each condition. *m, the mucosal layer; ep, the epithelial layer; lpm, the lamina propria mucosae layer; mm, the muscularis mucosae layer; sm, the submucosal layer; mp, proper muscle layer. A, Esophagus. B, Gastric upper third. C, Gastric middle third. D, Gastric lower third. E, Colon.
(Quotation from Surg Laparosc Endosc Percutan Tech. 2006;16:307-11. Fujishiro et al)

Because the risk of deep tissue injury cannot be predicted, meticulous setting of electrical current, flow rate of argon gas, and irradiation duration need to be carefully monitored for a successful APC treatment, taking into consideration anatomical characteristics and patient condition. Differences in the extent of tissue damage due to APC may originate mainly from differences in the wall thickness and in the proportions of the wall components. In an experimental study using porcine tissue, the deepest tissue damage was observed in the colon after APC irradiation at the same setting conditions, probably because the colonic wall is much thinner than that of the other organs. From the parts of the stomach, the deepest tissue damage was observed in the upper third of the stomach at a 2-second pulse duration, which may also be because of the thinness of the mucosal wall (Fujishiro, 2006; Fujishiro, 2008).

Submucosal injection of normal saline is an essential step for polypectomy and EMR for the prevention of bleeding and perforation (Fujishiro, 2004; Yoshida, 2005). The efficacy of submucosal injection of normal saline for the protection from thermal injury during APC was evaluated with animal studies (Norton, 2002; Fujishiro, 2006; Fujishiro, 2008). A minipig was sacrificed immediately after APC application, and its stomach specimen revealed that tissue damage deepened more as the applied time increased, but stayed confined to the mucosa and submucosa whether or not submucosal saline injections were done. The difference of depth of tissue injury was subtle between the two animal models, and the efficacy of submucosal saline injection was inconclusive in the immediate histopathologic evaluation of the specimen (Fujishiro, 2006; Fujishiro, 2008) (Fig. 4). An animal sacrificed one week after APC treatment revealed chronic inflammatory and fibrotic changes in the submucosal layer of the artificial ulcers and no injury of the proper muscle layer regardless of submucosal injection in the case of 5 and 10 seconds of irradiation time. APC irradiation without submucosal saline injections of a longer duration of 20 seconds only deepened the ulceration into the deep proper muscle layer. However, thermal injury after APC treatment of 20 seconds did not extend to the proper muscle layer in the animal with submucosal saline injection (Fig. 5). Therefore, submucosal saline injections are more likely to prevent the occasional deep tissue injury and the significant complication of perforation after long time irradiation of APC (Fujishiro, 2006; Fujishiro, 2008).

The reason of this discrepancy of tissue damage with and without follow-up may be the limitations of histology to evaluate thermal damage, especially the devitalization zone. Histological investigations may not be able to detect the zone of devitalization immediately after tissue damage with APC and it can underestimate the range of damage than the true one. These results have two important clinical meanings. First, there is a risk of deep tissue destruction after APC treatment and follow-up studies are needed to evaluate the damaged lesion. Second, submucosal injection of normal saline before APC may be useful to decrease deep tissue destruction and to prevent perforation in a living body. Other studies using a resected stomach specimen showed the usefulness of submucosal injection before APC. The study of Fujishiro et al (Fujishiro, 2006; Fujishiro, 2008) using a living minipig showed that APC irradiation after submucosal injection can limit thermal injury and prevent perforation not only immediately after procedure but also during the follow-up period.

In practice, some endoscopists' experienced an unexpected extension of tissue destruction and even perforation, which may be affected by various factors; host factors (mucosal and submucosa thickness, blood flow, inflammation, etc), technical factors (the extension of the gastric wall by inflated air, the irradiation angle, the distance between an applicator and tissue, irradiation duration, etc) (Postgate, 2007; Sagawa, 2003). Therefore, submucosal injection of normal saline may be the effective and practical method to prevent extensive damage to the proper muscle layer at any encountered situation.

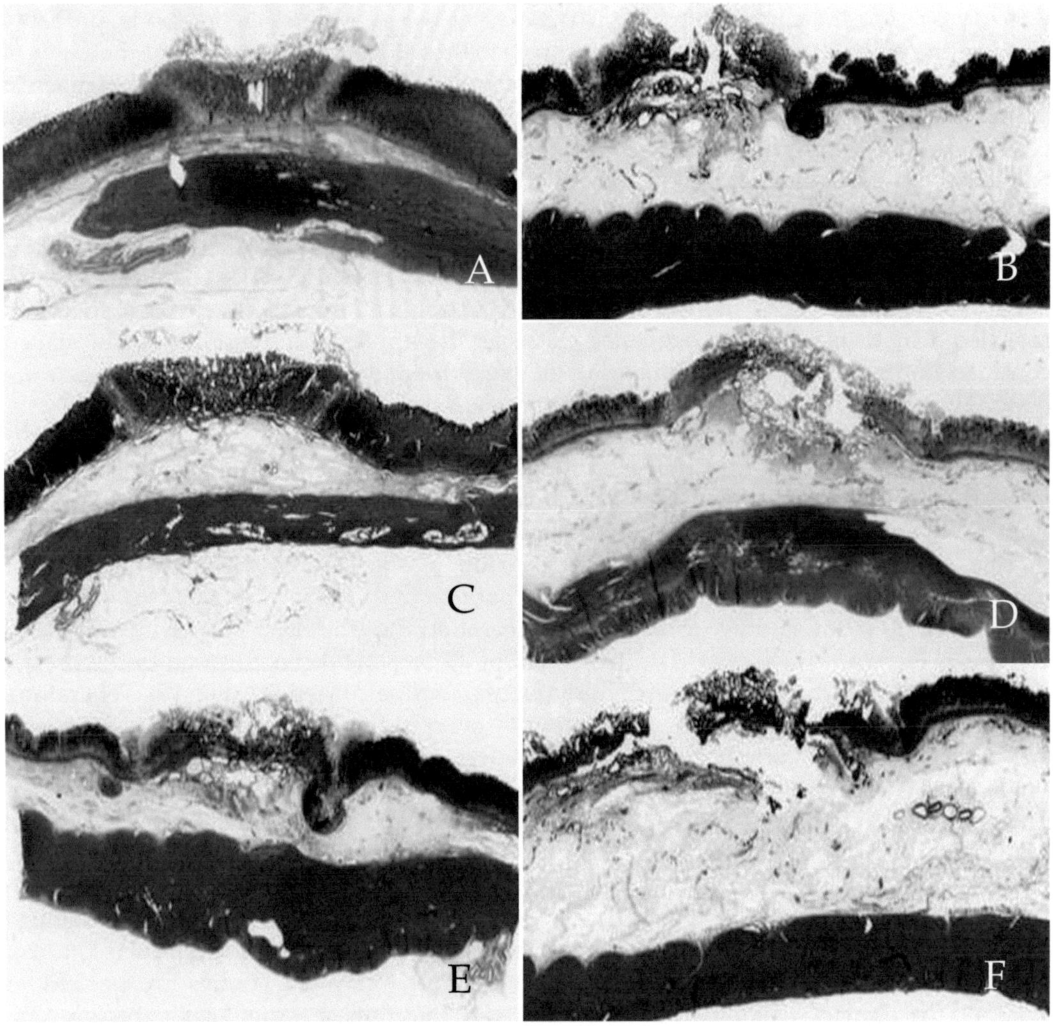

Fig. 4. Tissue injury in a minipig sacrificed immediately after APC. A) APC (5 seconds) without prior submucosal injection. B) APC (5 seconds) after submucosal injection. C) APC (10 seconds) without prior submucosal injection. D) APC (10 seconds) after submucosal injection. E) APC (20 seconds) without prior submucosal injection. F) APC (20 seconds) after submucosal injection. Tissue coagulation was limited to the deeper submucosal layer under all the conditions. The thermal effects tended to deepen with a longer pulse duration and no prior saline injection. With prior saline injection, the increased thickness of the submucosal layer might prevent injury to the deeper submucosal layer. (Quotation from Gut Liver. 2008;2:95-8. Fujishiro M et al)

Since tissue damage up to the submucosal layer is considered sufficient for the treatment of gastric adenoma and intramucosal carcinoma, submucosal injections of saline has a high possibility of becoming the standard preparation prior to APC application in humans.

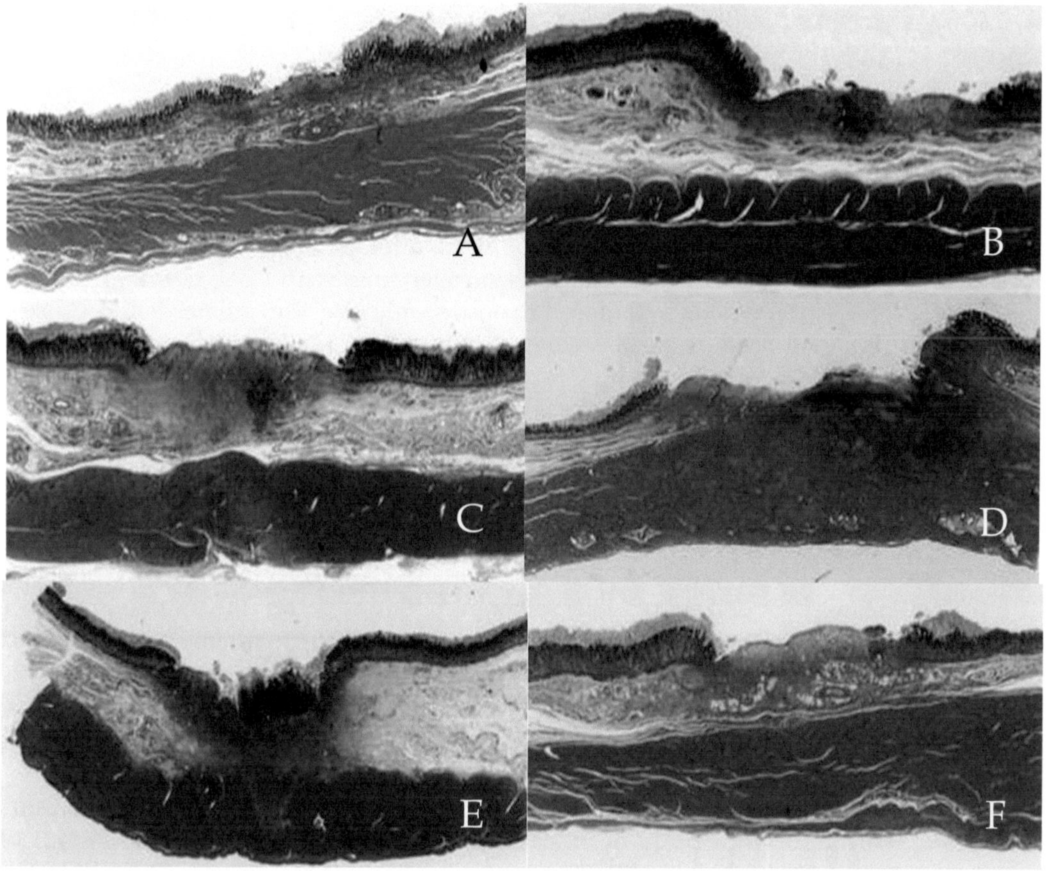

Fig. 5. Tissue damage in a minipig sacrificed 1 week after APC. A) APC (5 seconds) without prior submucosal injection. B) APC (5 seconds) after submucosal injection. C) APC (10 seconds) without prior submucosal injection. D) APC (10 seconds) after submucosal injection. E) APC (20 seconds) without prior submucosal injection. F) APC (20 seconds) after submucosal injection. Under all the conditions except for 20 seconds of APC without prior submucosal injection, granulomatous and fibrotic changes were evident in the submucosal layer of the artificial ulcer, although the actual muscle layer appeared intact. Deep ulceration that destroyed the muscle layer was evident for 20 seconds of APC without submucosal injection.
(Quotation from Gut Liver. 2008;2:95-8. Fujishiro M et al)

9. Gastric adenoma treatment with APC and submucosal saline injection

Gastric adenoma is a precursor lesion of gastric cancer and is usually classified using a two-grade system, divided into LGD and HGD (Lansdown, 1990, Farinati, 1993). Gastric adenoma with HGD has a significant risk of disease progression and containing cancerous lesions, and it should be removed using an endoscopic resection procedure (Lansdown, 1990, Farinati, 1993). Although endoscopic resection is a less invasive procedure than surgical resection, it carries the risk of various complications and requires hospitalization of several days (Watanabe, 2006; Fujishiro, 2004, Yoshida, 2005). Gastric adenoma with LGD is a less progressive disease than HGD; nevertheless, it carries some risk of disease progression (Rugge, 1995; Fertitta, 1993). The risk factors of developing gastric adenoma are chronic atrophic gastritis, intestinal metaplasia, *Helicobacter pylori* infection, old age, cigarette smoking, and alcohol drinking (Talley, 1991; Parsonnet, 1991; Nomura, 1991). These risk factors induce irreversible mucosal changes and can provide an environment for gastric tumors to occur at multiple sites (Talley, 1991; Parsonnet, 1991; Nomura, 1991). Patients at risk also have an increased chance of developing metachronous lesions, and a meticulous endoscopic follow-up should be done after treatment of gastric adenoma. Considering the less progressive nature of gastric adenomas with LGD, new less invasive and feasible treatment methods as opposed to endoscopic resection are needed, because it has a higher risk of procedure-related complications, need for hospitalization and high medical expenses.

Gastric adenomas are confined to the mucosa of the gastric wall but are also located in reach of thermal effect of APC (Morson, 1980; Kamiya, 1982). Although APC is known to be an effective and safe procedure for early gastric cancers, bleeding control, and eradication of vascular lesions, they carry some risk of perforation due to the deep thermal effect. Based on the results of the animal study of Fujishiro et al (Fujishiro, 2006; Fujishiro, 2008), we have opted to use APC with submucosal saline injections (APC–SSI) to treat gastric adenomas with LGD. We have included submucosal saline injections as part of the routine procedure of APC for raising the mucosa and prevention of bleeding and perforation. It can be applied prior to APC to form an insulating fluid cushion in the submucosal layer to limit the thermal effect within the mucosa and superficial submucosal layer. The reduced risk of perforation and bleeding has lead to APC-SSI being available on an outpatient department (OPD) basis without requirement of hospitalization.

We have evaluated the effectiveness of APC–SSI for gastric adenomas with LGD on OPD basis. We conducted a study of 57 patients with a combined total of 64 lesions of gastric adenomas with LGD, including patients who were not suitable for EMR/ESD due to bleeding tendency, serious concomitant disease, poor general condition, and advanced age (Table 1) (Lee, 2009). Gastric adenomas larger than 20 mm, accompanied with surface depression or nodularity, or containing HGD were excluded because of the possibility of co-existing cancerous tissue.

The argon gas flow rate was 2.0 L/min, and the electrical current was set at 60 W. APC treatment was performed under sedation with midazolam and propofol. After spraying indigocarmine solution onto the lesion, the area around the lesion was marked using an APC probe. Normal saline solution was injected into the submucosal layer under the lesion with a standard disposable 25-G injection needle. Sometimes, indigocarmine solution would be mixed with normal saline for better identification of the submucosal layer. Normal saline-mixed solution was injected until sufficient submucosal swelling was achieved. The lesion and neighboring mucosa inside the marked sites were evenly treated with APC until the lesion was completely coagulated and appeared dry under endoscopic examination (Fig. 6).

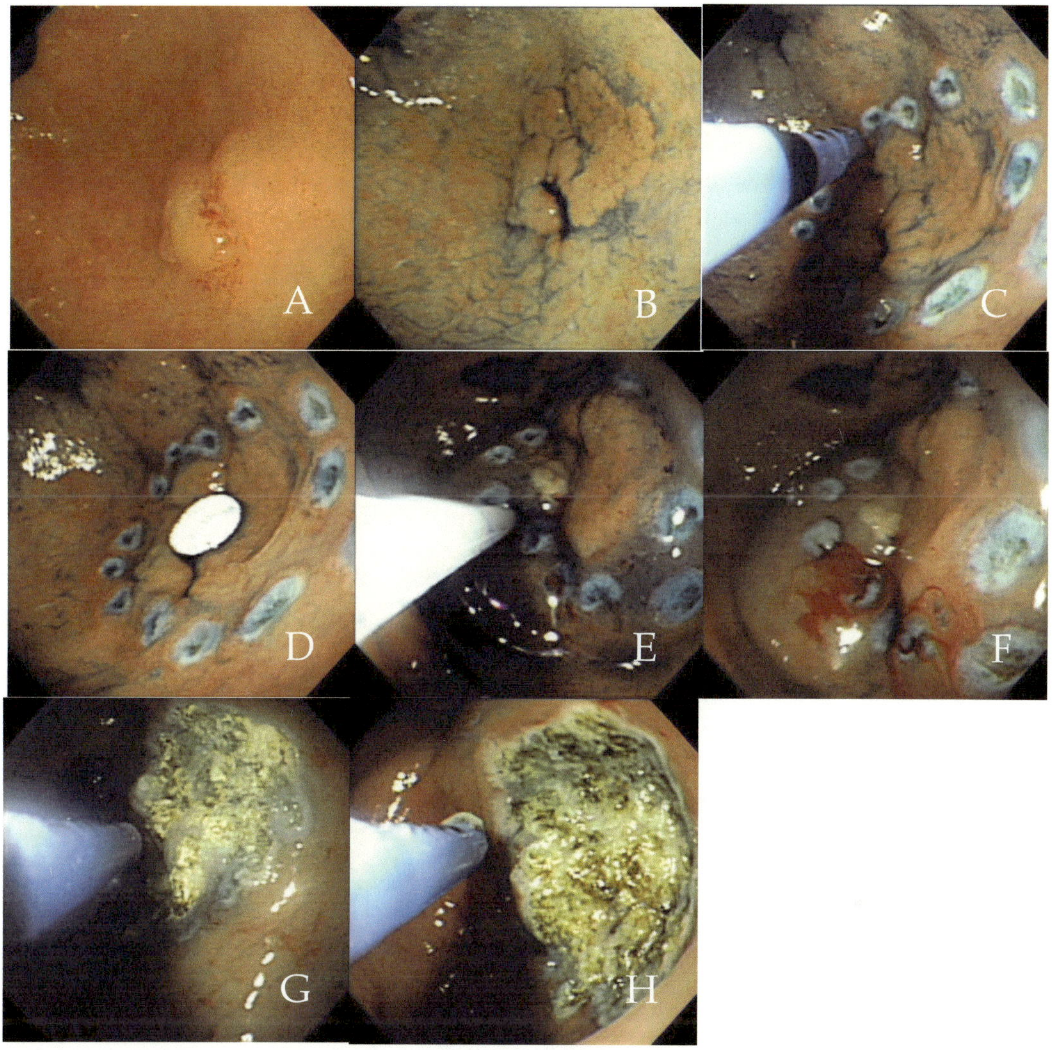

Fig. 6. Endoscopic view of APC-SSI. A) Whitish discolored, flat surfaced, and slightly elevated lesion is noted at the greater curvature side of the distal antrum. B) After indigocarmine solution spraying, the boundary of the lesion is clearly distinct and a granular surface is visible. C) Surrounding markings were done with an APC probe with sufficient distance from the lesion. D) The size of lesion was measured by comparative ratio with 6 mm sized round piece of vinyl. E) Normal saline or sometimes normal saline-indigocarmine mixture solution was injected to the submucosal layer under the lesion with a standard 25-G injection needle. F) Normal saline solution was injected until sufficient submucosal swelling was achieved. G, H) The lesion and neighboring mucosa inside the marked sites were evenly coagulated with APC until the lesion was completely coagulated and appeared dry under endoscopic examination.

After APC–SSI treatment, patients were closely observed. If there was no specific complaint, patients were discharged from hospital with proton pump inhibitor. On the occasion of severe pain or discomfort, patients were admitted to hospital. After discharge, follow- up endoscopic examinations with forceps biopsy was performed at 3, 6, and 12 months and then every 12 months. Lesions found at the same site as the previous lesion were defined as being residual. On the other hand, lesions found at a different site were considered to be metachronous. The treatment outcomes of all patients are shown in Table 1 and 93.7% of gastric adenomas were eradicated with APC–SSI. Four residual lesions (6.3%) were found at previous treated sites and they were gastric adenomas with LGD during mean follow-up time of 5.8 ± 3.2 months (range 3–9 months) (Table 2). Three of these were located at the posterior wall of the upper and mid body. One lesion was located in the prepylorus. The initial lesions were incompletely coagulated probably because their locations were difficult to be accessed with an endoscope. For instance, the prepyloric lesion extending through the pyloric channel into the mucosa of the duodenal side was incompletely treated with APC probably due to the limitation of endoscopic visual field (Fig. 7). All of the residual adenomas were eradicated with additional APC–SSI treatment and did not reappear during follow-up.

Gender (men-women)	45/12
Mean age, yr	59.5 ± 10.9 (34-81)
Macroscopic type	Flat elevated type 58
	Central depressed type 6
Patients with concomitant diseases	32 (56.1%) (COPD, 8; liver cirrhosis, 6; heart failure, 5; renal failure on hemodialysis or peritoneal dialysis, 4; others, 9)
Patients who refused hospitalization for EMR and with a risk of perforation or bleeding	25 (43.8%)

EMR, Endoscopic mucosal resection

Table 1. Characteristics of 57 patients with a combined total of 64 lesions of gastric adenoma treated with APC-SSI

Patient No.	Age, yr	Gender	Location	Pathologic type	Further treatment
1	66	M	P/W of Upper body	Adenoma c LGD	APC-SSI
2	56	M	P/W of Upper body	Adenoma c LGD	APC-SSI
3	70	M	P/W of Mid body	Adenoma c LGD	APC-SSI
4	59	M	G/C of Prepylorus	Adenoma c LGD	APC-SSI

P/W, Posterior wall; G/C, Greater curvature; LGD, Low grade dysplasia; APC-SSI, Argon plasma coagulation with submucosal saline injection

Table 2. Characteristics of 4 patients with residual adenoma

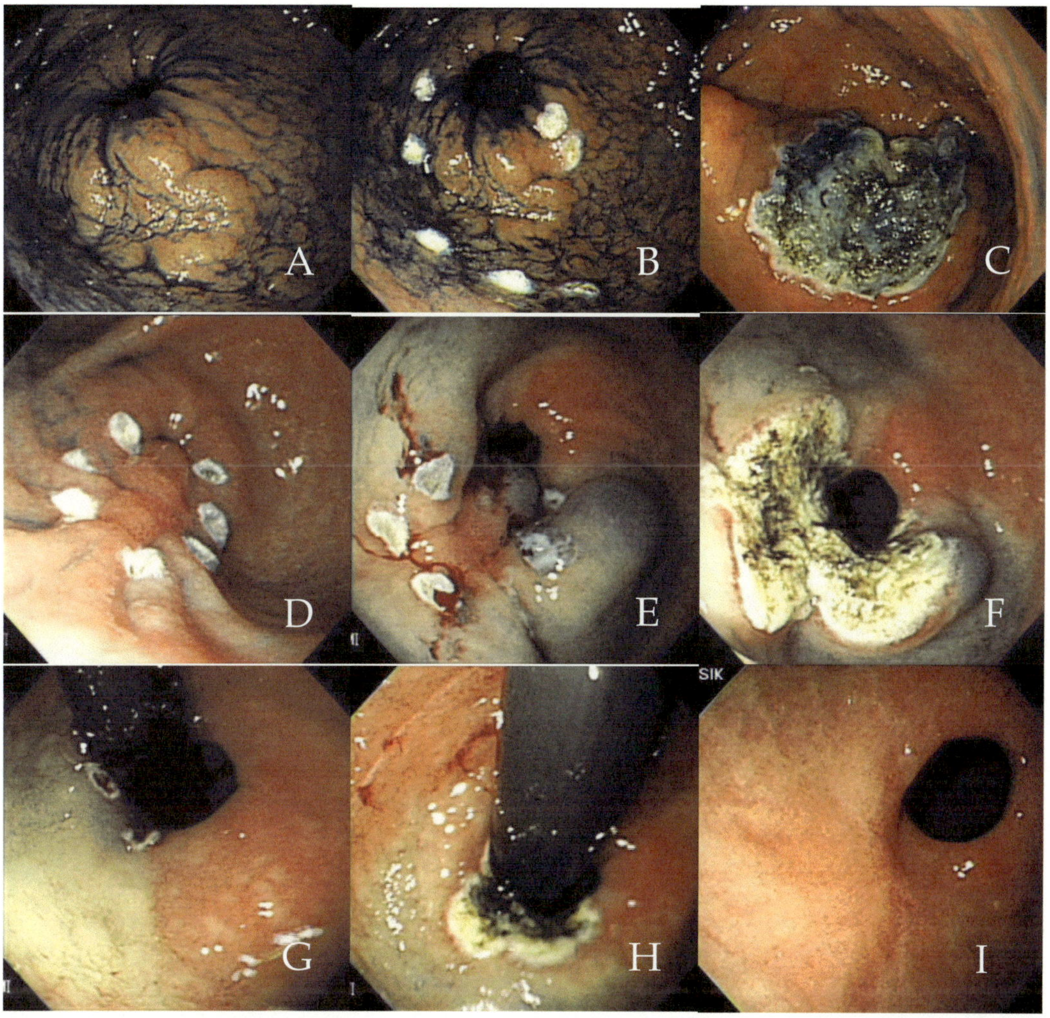

Fig. 7. A case of treatment failure. Residual tumor was found 6 months after APC-SSI for prepyloric lesion. A) Round flat elevated lesion was located at greater curvature side of the distal antrum and prepylorus and has relatively clear margin. B, C) After marking with APC and submucosal saline injection, the lesion and surrounding mucosa was evenly coagulated. D) Follow-up endoscopy at 6 months after APC-SSI, a nodular surfaced elevated mass lesion with fold change was noted. Pathologic examination of biopsy specimen revealed gastric adenoma with LGD. E, F) After marking procedure and submucosal saline injection, the remnant lesion on the antrum was eradicated with APC treatment. G, H) With retroflexion of the endoscope, the lesion had extended into the duodenal bulb. After marking procedure and submucosal saline injection, the remnant lesion on the duodenal side was eradicated with additional APC treatment with retroflexion in the bulb. I) Follow-up endoscopy 1yr after additional treatment revealed healing ulcer scar without tumor recurrence.

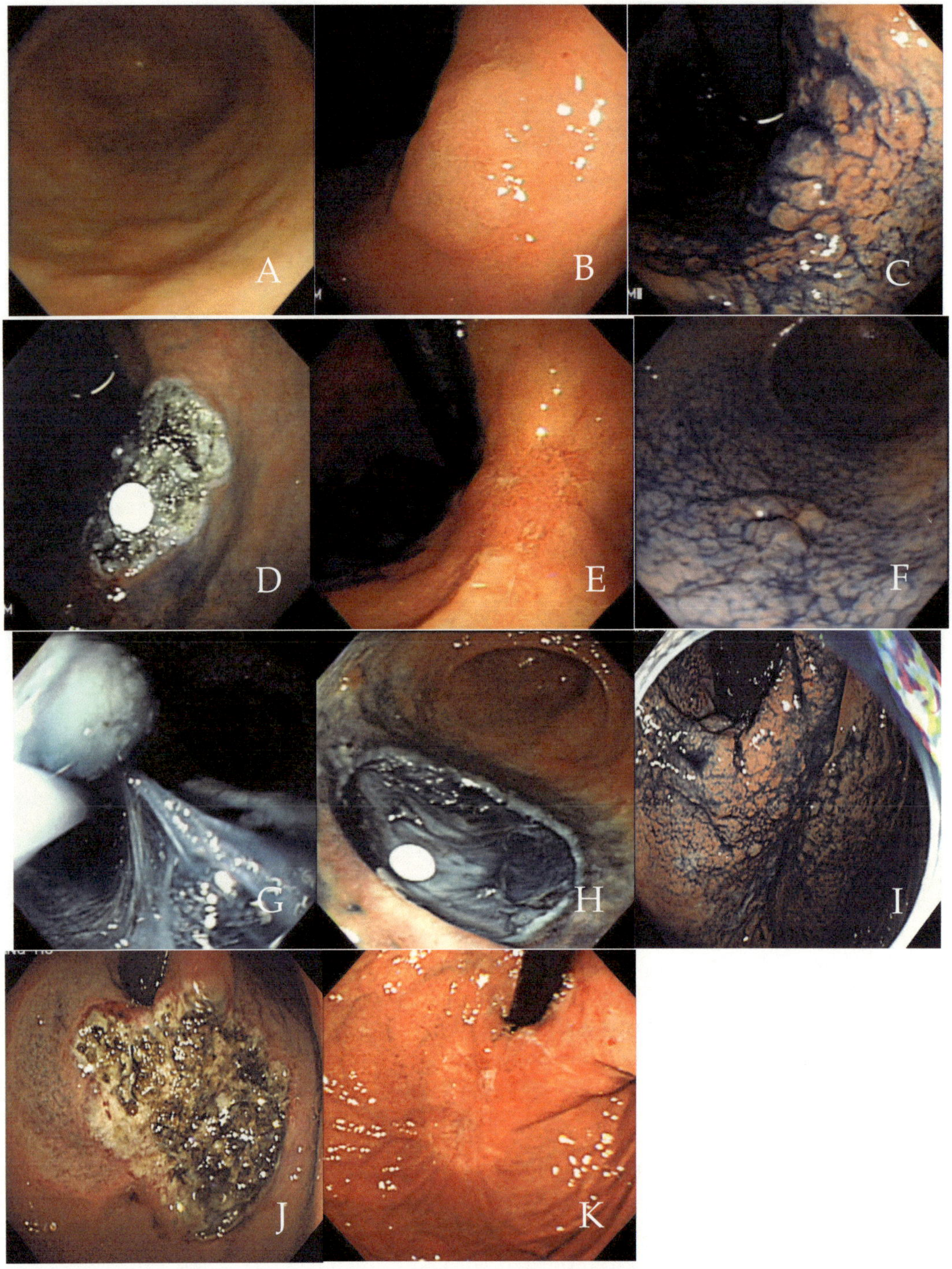

Fig. 8. The case of metachronous intramucosal adenocarcinoma and gastric adenoma after APC-SSI. A) A slightly elevated lesion with smooth surface was noted at the greater

curvature side of the mid antrum. Endoscopic biopsy revealed *Helicobacter* gastritis.
B) Whitish discolored, flat elevated lesion with clear margin was noted at the lesser curvature side of the gastric angle. C) After indigocarmine spraying, its surface revealed a lobular appearance. D) About 25 x 24 mm sized APC-induced round ulceration was noted at the lesser curvature side of the gastric angle. The ulcer base was blue-colored due to the submucosa injection of indigocarmine mixed saline. E) Endoscopic finding at 6 months after APC-SSI showed scarring ulceration with reddish regenerative epithelium.
F) Endoscopic findings at 12 months showed a small elevated lesion with nodular surface at the greater curvature side of the antrum. Forceps biopsy results revealed intramucosal adenocarcinoma.G) For the treatment of the lesion, ESD was done.
H) A large ESD-induced ulcer was seen without bleeding or perforation.
I) A metachronous flat elevated round lesion was found at the lesser curvature side of the cardia during a follow-up endoscopy 2 years later. Forceps biopsy results revealed it was a gastric adenoma with LGD. J) Based on patient age and tumor location, APC-SSI was successfully done to treat the lesion. K) Endoscopic finding at 6 months after the second APC-SSI showed an ulcer scar. There was no evidence of residual tumor with endoscopic biopsy.

Fourteen metachronous lesions were found in eight patients (14.0%) during follow-up (Table 3). Twelve lesions of gastric adenomas with LGD were treated with additional APC–SSI. One lesion of gastric adenoma with HGD was treated with ESD and it was proven to be intramucosal adenocarcinoma (Fig. 8). The other one with intramucosal adenocarcinoma was treated with APC–SSI because of poor general condition and bleeding tendency. Mean interval from treatment to detection of metachronous lesion was 18.1 ± 11.6 months.
Mean procedure time for APC-SSI was 15.0±5.0 (8–30) min. Transient abdominal discomfort occurred in 11 patients. Three complications (4.7%), including Mallory-Weiss tearing, pneumoperitoneum, and delayed bleeding, were noted (Table 4). Mallory–Weiss tearing was successfully controlled using endoscopic hemoclippings. Pneumoperitoneum occurred in a patient with two broad lesions at the lesser curvature side of the mid and upper body after a longer duration of APC-SSI. Endoscopy the next day showed broad ulcerative lesions with a coagulated base without evidence of perforation. The patient was hospitalized and discharged after 2 days of conservative care. Several authors reported one case each of APC-induced pneumoperitoneum after treatment of acute hemorrhagic radiation proctitis (Chung, 2005; Hoyer, 1998; Manes, 2007). Pneumoperitoneum, however, does not necessarily mean perforation. It can be caused by air leakage through a partially coagulated wall by elevated intraluminal pressure. In our study, argon gas flow rate was 2 L/min. The long procedure time of APC inevitably induced marked stomach distention and increased intragastric pressure, probably resulting in air leaking into the peritoneal cavity without a visible perforation site of the gastric wall. Delayed bleeding from the regenerative vessels on the APC-induced ulcer occurred in one patient 2 weeks after the procedure and it was successfully managed with additional APC. APC is an effective noncontact technique for bleeding control (Islam, 2009; Grund, 1994; Grund, 1997) and there was no procedure-related bleeding during and immediately after APC–SSI. This delayed bleeding was not caused by the APC procedure itself but by the healing and regenerative process, indicating that APC may be a safe treatment of gastric adenoma in patients with bleeding risk. This can also bring about stressful retching and Mallory–Weiss tearing. Therefore, frequent suction of

intragastric gas during procedure is helpful for the prevention of marked gastric distention and barotraumas.

Patient No	Age	Gender	Time(mon)	Pathologic type	Further treatment
1	51	M	9	Adenoma c LGD	APC-SSI
2	78	M	6	Adenoma c LGD	APC-SSI
3	49	M	12	Adenoma c LGD	APC-SSI
4	66	M	30	Intramucosal cancer	APC-SSI
5	59	F	5	Adenoma c LGD	APC-SSI
			19	Adenoma c LGD	APC-SSI
6	50	M	6	Adenoma c LGD	APC-SSI
			20	Adenoma c LGD	APC-SSI
7	51	M	12	Intramucosal cancer	ESD
8	49	M	43	Adenoma c LGD	APC-SSI
			12	Adenoma c LGD	APC-SSI
			19	Adenoma c LGD	APC-SSI
			28	Adenoma c LGD	APC-SSI

P/W, Posterior wall; G/C, Greater curvature; LGD. Low grade dysplasia;
APC-SSI, Argon plasma coagulation with submucosal saline injection;
ESD, Endoscopic submucosal dissection

Table 3. Characteristics of 14 metachronous lesions of 8 patients

Mean duration of follow-up (mo)	19.5 ± 15.1 (6-49)
Mean time required for treatment (min)	15.0 ± 5.0
Patients with complications	3 (4.7%)
Mallory Weiss tearing	1
Pneumoperitoneum	1
Delayed bleeding	1
Patients with residual adenoma	4 (7.0%)
Patients with metachronous adenoma	8 (14.0%)

Table 4. Outcomes of endoscopic argon plasma coagulation with submucosal saline injection treatment (n=64)

There are two important viewpoints in this study. One is the importance of the accurate identification of the lateral margin of the lesion. Because gastric adenomas are confined to the mucosal layer and the entire lesion can be ablated with APC, residual lesions may be left near the lateral margin but away from the deep layer (Morson, 1980, Rugge, 1995). Lesion marking should include a sufficient amount of normal tissue around the lesion to ensure a successful APC-SSI, preventing treatment failure, as seen in EMR or ESD. Unlike colorectal or esophageal lesions whose margins are rather easy to delineate with indigocarmine or Lugol spraying, the margins of gastric tumors are sometimes difficult to diagnose, because the background mucosa is affected by acute or chronic inflammation or intestinal metaplasia. Because indigocarmine accumulates in the grooves and emphasizes the surface structural changes of the mucosa, it is difficult to identify the margin of the lesion which surface change is not distinct. Therefore, it could result in incomplete resection with positive lateral margin in EMR or ESD, and also leave residual tissue in those who receive APC treatment for adenomas. Inability to perform histopathologic evaluation of resected specimen is a shortcoming of APC treatment of gastric adenomas and we recommend sufficient margin to be obtained before APC-SSI for the prevention of residual tissue. Therefore, endoscopists should pay more attention to the lesions at difficult sites for endoscopic approach, such as the posterior wall of the upper and mid body, making sure there is sufficient margin from the lesions.

The other viewpoint is the high prevalence of metachronous lesions after APC-SSI for gastric adenomas. We found 14 metachronous lesions in eight patients, and their locations were different from their original lesions during a mean of 19.5 months of follow-up. Those who have risk factors of gastric adenomas, including chronic atrophic gastritis, intestinal metaplasia, *Helicobacter pylori* infection, old age, cigarette smoking, and alcohol drinking, are more likely to develop metachronous lesions even after APC treatment. Chronic atrophic gastritis and intestinal metaplasia are known to be irreversible and may work as a continuous background of gastric cancer to recur at other sites (Talley, 1991; Parsonnet, 1991; Nomura, 1991). Because patients who have risk factors of gastric adenomas have an increased risk of metachronous lesions, meticulous endoscopic follow-up should be done after the treatment of gastric adenomas (Talley, 1991; Parsonnet, 1991; Nomura, 1991).

10. Conclusion

Gastric adenomas are well-known as premalignant lesions of gastric cancer. Gastric adenomas with LGD show a relatively benign natural course and low risk of progression, compared with gastric adenomas with HGD. Though endoscopic resection has become the standard treatment of intramucosal carcinomas and adenomas with HGD, there is controversy about the therapeutic option of gastric adenomas with LGD. APC-SSI is the most reasonable and feasible treatment being safe and effective, which can be done in place of endoscopic resection and repeated endoscopic follow-up.

11. References

Asaka, M. (1997). What role does Helicobacter pylori play in gastric cancer? Gastroenterology, Vol.113, No. 6 Suppl, (September 1996), pp S56-60, ISSN 0016-5085

Bearzi, I. (1994). Gastric dysplasia: a ten-year follow-up study. Pathol Res Pract, Vol.190, No. 1, (August 1993), pp 61-68, ISSN 0344-0338

Chau, C H. (2003). Randomized controlled trial comparing epinephrine injection plus heat probe coagulation versus epinephrine injection plus argon plasma coagulation for bleeding peptic ulcers. Gastrointest Endosc, Vol.57, No. 4, (May 2002), pp 455-461, ISSN 0016-5107

Chung, Y F and W H Koo. (2005). Gastric pneumatosis after endoscopic argon plasma coagulation. Ann Acad Med Singapore, Vol.34, No. 9, (April 2001), pp 569-570, ISSN 0304-4602

Cipolletta, L. (1998). Prospective comparison of argon plasma coagulator and heater probe in the endoscopic treatment of major peptic ulcer bleeding. Gastrointest Endosc, Vol.48, No. 2, (July 1997), pp 191-195, ISSN 0016-5107

Di Gregorio, C. (1993). Gastric dysplasia. A follow-up study. Am J Gastroenterol, Vol.88, No. 10, (January 1993), pp 1714-1719, ISSN 0002-9270

Ell, C. (1998). Photodynamic ablation of early cancers of the stomach by means of mTHPC and laser irradiation: preliminary clinical experience. Gut, Vol.43, No. 3, (October 1997), pp 345-349, ISSN 0017-5749

Farinati, F. (1993). Early and advanced gastric cancer in the follow-up of moderate and severe gastric dysplasia patients. A prospective study. I.G.G.E.D.--Interdisciplinary Group on Gastric Epithelial Dysplasia. Endoscopy, Vol.25, No. 4, (December 1992), pp 261-264, ISSN 0013-726X

Fertitta, A M. (1993). Clinical significance of gastric dysplasia: a multicenter follow-up study. Gastrointestinal Endoscopic Pathology Study Group. Endoscopy, Vol.25, No. 4, (March 1992), pp 265-268, ISSN 0013-726X

Fertitta, A M. (1993). Clinical significance of gastric dysplasia: a multicenter follow-up study. Gastrointestinal Endoscopic Pathology Study Group. Endoscopy, Vol.25, No. 4, (May 1992), pp 265-268, ISSN 0013-726X

Fujishiro, M. (2004). Comparison of various submucosal injection solutions for maintaining mucosal elevation during endoscopic mucosal resection. Endoscopy, Vol.36, No. 7, (June 2003), pp 579-583, ISSN 0013-726X

Fujishiro, M. (2006). Submucosal injection of normal saline may prevent tissue damage from argon plasma coagulation: an experimental study using resected porcine esophagus, stomach, and colon. Surg Laparosc Endosc Percutan Tech, Vol.16, No. 5, (August 2005), pp 307-311, ISSN 1530-4515

Fujishiro, M. (2008). Submucosal Injection of Normal Saline can Prevent Unexpected Deep Thermal Injury of Argon Plasma Coagulation in the in vivo Porcine Stomach. Gut Liver, Vol.2, No. 2, (January 2008), pp 95-98, ISSN 1976-2283

Giovannini, M. (1999). Endoscopic mucosal resection (EMR): results and prognostic factors in 21 patients. Endoscopy, Vol.31, No. 9, (June 1999), pp 698-701, ISSN 0013-726X

Goulet, C J. (2007). In vivo evaluation of argon plasma coagulation in a porcine model. Gastrointest Endosc, Vol.65, No. 3, (May 2006), pp 457-462, ISSN 0016-5107

Grund, K E. (1994). Endoscopic argon plasma coagulation (APC) first clinical experiences in flexible endoscopy. Endosc Surg Allied Technol, Vol.2, No. 1, (April 1993), pp 42-46, ISSN 0942-6027

Grund, K E. (1997). [Argon plasma coagulation through a flexible endoscope. Evaluation of a new therapeutic method after 1606 uses]. Dtsch Med Wochenschr, Vol.122, No. 14, (March 1997), pp 432-438, ISSN 0012-0472 21.

Hiki, Y. (1989). The concepts, procedures, and problems related in endoscopic laser therapy of early gastric cancer. A retrospective study on early gastric cancer. Surg Endosc, Vol.3, No. 1, (September 1988), pp 1-6, ISSN 0930-2794

Hoyer, N. (1998). Massive pneumoperitoneum after endoscopic argon plasma coagulation. Endoscopy, Vol.30, No. 3, (November 1997), pp S44-45, ISSN 0013-726X

Iacopini, F. (2007). Hemostasis of Dieulafoy's lesions by argon plasma coagulation (with video). Gastrointest Endosc, Vol.66, No. 1, (June 2006), pp 20-26, ISSN 0016-5107

Imaoka, W. (1987). Is curative endoscopic treatment of early gastric cancer possible? Endoscopy, Vol.19 Suppl 1, No., (July 1986), pp 7-11, ISSN 0013-726X

Islam, S and K K Tan. (2009). Bleeding inflammatory polyp formation as a complication of argon plasma coagulation therapy on a flat gastric angiodysplasia. Endoscopy, Vol.41 Suppl 2, No., (July 2008), pp E86, ISSN 1438-8812

Kaassis, M. (2000). Argon plasma coagulation for the treatment of hemorrhagic radiation proctitis. Endoscopy, Vol.32, No. 9, (October 1999), pp 673-676, ISSN 0013-726X

Kamiya, T. (1982). Long-term follow-up study on gastric adenoma and its relation to gastric protruded carcinoma. Cancer, Vol.50, No. 11, (January 1982), pp 2496-2503, ISSN 0008-543X

Kitamura, T. (2006). Argon plasma coagulation for early gastric cancer: technique and outcome. Gastrointest Endosc, Vol.63, No. 1, (September 2005), pp 48-54, ISSN 0016-5107

Kwan, V. (2006). Argon plasma coagulation in the management of symptomatic gastrointestinal vascular lesions: experience in 100 consecutive patients with long-term follow-up. Am J Gastroenterol, Vol.101, No. 1, (June 2005), pp 58-63, ISSN 0002-9270

Lansdown, M. (1990). High grade dysplasia of the gastric mucosa: a marker for gastric carcinoma. Gut, Vol.31, No. 9, (April 1989), pp 977-983, ISSN 0017-5749

Lee, K M. (2009). Argon plasma coagulation with submucosal saline injection for gastric adenoma on outpatient basis. Dig Dis Sci, Vol.54, No. 12, (March 2008), pp 2623-2628, ISSN 1573-2568

Manes, G. (2007). Pneumoperitoneum after argon plasma coagulation treatment: perforation or accumulation of air in the cavity? Endoscopy, Vol.39 Suppl 1, No., (April 2006), pp E98, ISSN 1438-8812

Mimura, S. (1996). Cooperative clinical trial of photodynamic therapy with photofrin II and excimer dye laser for early gastric cancer. Lasers Surg Med, Vol.19, No. 2, (May 1995), pp 168-172, ISSN 0196-8092

Miyata, M. (2000). What are the appropriate indications for endoscopic mucosal resection for early gastric cancer? Analysis of 256 endoscopically resected lesions. Endoscopy, Vol.32, No. 10, (June 1999), pp 773-778, ISSN 0013-726X

Morson, B C. (1980). Precancerous conditions and epithelial dysplasia in the stomach. J Clin Pathol, Vol.33, No. 8, (May 1979), pp 711-721, ISSN 0021-9746

Nakamura, S. (2001). Endoscopic induction of mucosal fibrosis by argon plasma coagulation (APC) for esophageal varices: A prospective randomized trial of ligation plus APC vs. ligation alone. Endoscopy, Vol.33, No. 3, (October 2000), pp 210-215, ISSN 0013-726X

Nakamura, T. (1990). Photodynamic therapy for early gastric cancer using a pulsed gold vapor laser. J Clin Laser Med Surg, Vol.8, No. 5, (March 1989), pp 63-67, ISSN 1044-5471

Nomura, A. (1991). Helicobacter pylori infection and gastric carcinoma among Japanese Americans in Hawaii. N Engl J Med, Vol.325, No. 16, (June 1990), pp 1132-1136, ISSN 0028-4793

Norton, I D. (2002). Efficacy of colonic submucosal saline solution injection for the reduction of iatrogenic thermal injury. Gastrointest Endosc, Vol.56, No. 1, (August 2001), pp 95-99, ISSN 0016-5107

Oka, S. (2006). Advantage of endoscopic submucosal dissection compared with EMR for early gastric cancer. Gastrointest Endosc, Vol.64, No. 6, (October 2005), pp 877-883, ISSN 0016-5107

Oka, S. (2006). Endoscopic submucosal dissection for residual/local recurrence of early gastric cancer after endoscopic mucosal resection. Endoscopy, Vol.38, No. 10, (November 2005), pp 996-1000, ISSN 0013-726X

Olmos, J A. (2006). Long-term outcome of argon plasma ablation therapy for bleeding in 100 consecutive patients with colonic angiodysplasia. Dis Colon Rectum, Vol.49, No. 10, (February 2006), pp 1507-1516, ISSN 0012-3706

O'Mahony, S. (2001). Endoscopic mucosal resection for early gastric cancer. Gut, Vol.48, No. 2, (May 2000), pp 151-152, ISSN 0017-5749

Ono, H. (2001). Endoscopic mucosal resection for treatment of early gastric cancer. Gut, Vol.48, No. 2, (June 2000), pp 225-229, ISSN 0017-5749

Parsonnet, J. (1991). Helicobacter pylori infection and the risk of gastric carcinoma. N Engl J Med, Vol.325, No. 16, (September 1990), pp 1127-1131, ISSN 0028-4793

Postgate, A. (2007). Argon plasma coagulation in chronic radiation proctitis. Endoscopy, Vol.39, No. 4, (November 2006), pp 361-365, ISSN 1438-8812

Prost, B. (2004). Unusual complications of argon plasma coagulation. Gastrointest Endosc, Vol.59, No. 7, (August 2003), pp 929-932, ISSN 0016-5107

Rolachon, A. (2000). Is argon plasma coagulation an efficient treatment for digestive system vascular malformation and radiation proctitis? Gastroenterol Clin Biol, Vol.24, No. 12, (July 1999), pp 1205-1210, ISSN 0399-8320

Rugge, M. (1991). Gastric epithelial dysplasia: a prospective multicenter follow-up study from the Interdisciplinary Group on Gastric Epithelial Dysplasia. Hum Pathol, Vol.22, No. 10, (January 1990), pp 1002-1008, ISSN 0046-8177

Rugge, M. (1994). Gastric epithelial dysplasia in the natural history of gastric cancer: a multicenter prospective follow-up study. Interdisciplinary Group on Gastric Epithelial Dysplasia. Gastroenterology, Vol.107, No. 5, (March 1993), pp 1288-1296, ISSN 0016-5085

Rugge, M. (1995). Gastric epithelial dysplasia. How clinicopathologic background relates to management. Cancer, Vol.76, No. 3, (April 1994), pp 376-382, ISSN 0008-543X

Sagawa, T. (2003). Argon plasma coagulation for successful treatment of early gastric cancer with intramucosal invasion. Gut, Vol.52, No. 3, (June 2002), pp 334-339, ISSN 0017-5749

Saraga, E P. (1987). Gastric dysplasia. A histological follow-up study. Am J Surg Pathol, Vol.11, No. 10, (April 1986), pp 788-796, ISSN 0147-5185.

Sato, T. (2005). Efficacy of argon plasma coagulation for gastric antral vascular ectasia associated with chronic liver disease. Hepatol Res, Vol.32, No. 2, (May 2004), pp 121-126, ISSN 1386-6346

Sibille, A. (1995). Endoscopic Nd:YAG treatment of superficial gastric carcinoma: experience in 18 Western inoperable patients. Gastrointest Endosc, Vol.42, No. 4, (June 1994), pp 340-345, ISSN 0016-5107 56.

Tabuse, K. (1985). Microwave tissue coagulation applied clinically in endoscopic surgery. Endoscopy, Vol.17, No. 4, (June 1984), pp 139-144, ISSN 0013-726X

Tajiri, H and Y Oguro. (1991). Laser endoscopic treatment for upper gastrointestinal cancers. J Laparoendosc Surg, Vol.1, No. 2, (August 1990), pp 71-78, ISSN 1052-3901

Takenaka, R. (2008). Risk factors associated with local recurrence of early gastric cancers after endoscopic submucosal dissection. Gastrointest Endosc, Vol.68, No. 5, (March 2007), pp 887-894, ISSN 1097-6779

Takeuchi, Y. (2007). Endoscopic submucosal dissection with insulated-tip knife for large mucosal early gastric cancer: a feasibility study (with videos). Gastrointest Endosc, Vol.66, No. 1, (May 2006), pp 186-193, ISSN 0016-5107

Talley, N J. (1991). Gastric adenocarcinoma and Helicobacter pylori infection. J Natl Cancer Inst, Vol.83, No. 23, (August 1990), pp 1734-1739, ISSN 0027-8874

The EUROGAST study group (1993). An international association between Helicobacter pylori infection and gastric cancer. The EUROGAST Study Group. Lancet, Vol.341, No. 8857, (October 1992), pp 1359-1362, ISSN 0140-6736

Wahab, P J. (1997). Argon plasma coagulation in flexible gastrointestinal endoscopy: pilot experiences. Endoscopy, Vol.29, No. 3, (November 1996), pp 176-181, ISSN 0013-726X

Watanabe, K. (2006). Clinical outcomes of EMR for gastric tumors: historical pilot evaluation between endoscopic submucosal dissection and conventional mucosal resection. Gastrointest Endosc, Vol.63, No. 6, (May 2005), pp 776-782, ISSN 0016-5107

Watson, J P. (2000). The tissue effect of argon plasma coagulation on esophageal and gastric mucosa. Gastrointest Endosc, Vol.52, No. 3, (April 1999), pp 342-345, ISSN 0016-5107

Yasuda, K. (1993). Endoscopic laser treatment for early gastric cancer. Endoscopy, Vol.25, No. 7, (December 1992), pp 451-454, ISSN 0013-726X

Yoshida, T. (2005). The clinical meaning of a nonstructural pattern in early gastric cancer on magnifying endoscopy. Gastrointest Endosc, Vol.62, No. 1, (November 2004), pp 48-54, ISSN 0016-5107

5

Transanal Endoscopic Microsurgery - State of the Art

Pablo Palma[1] and Karoline Horisberger[2]
[1]Division of Colon & Rectal Surgery, University Hospital HUVN Granada,
[2]Department of Surgery, University Hospital Mannheim,
[1]Spain
[2]Germany

1. Introduction

The first description of surgery for rectal cancer was reported by the French surgeon Lisfranc who described a total of nine patients operated trough a perineal-transanal approach (Lisfranc, 1830). Although more recently gaining popularity, transanal techniques have long been used for the treatment of rectal diseases and were promoted by the work of Sir Alan Parks at St. Marks Hospital in London in the 1950s (Parks, 1970). This conventional surgical approach is well suited for the management of selected low rectal lesions; on the contrary, removal of lesions in the middle and upper rectum are less feasible due to the limited accessibility and inadequate exposure afforded by standard instrumentation. For these reasons, those more proximal lesions have historically been tackled by more radical surgical approaches, like abdominal low anterior, abdominoperineal, transsacral, and transsphincteric resections.

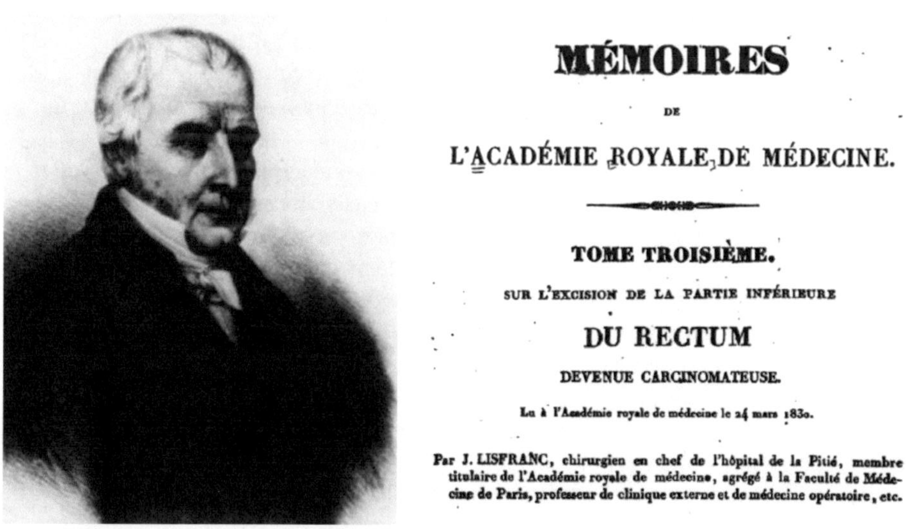
MÉMOIRES
DE
L'ACADÉMIE ROYALE DE MÉDECINE.
TOME TROISIÈME.
SUR L'EXCISION DE LA PARTIE INFÉRIEURE
DU RECTUM
DEVENUE CARCINOMATEUSE.
Lu à l'Académie royale de médecine le 24 mars 1830.
Par J. LISFRANC, chirurgien en chef de l'hôpital de la Pitié, membre titulaire de l'Académie royale de médecine, agrégé à la Faculté de Médecine de Paris, professeur de clinique externe et de médecine opératoire, etc.

Fig. 1. J. Lisfranc's description of surgery for rectal cancer.

Transanal endoscopic microsurgery (TEM) came into practice in Germany, in the early 1980s through the collaboration of the German surgeon Gerhard Buess and the Medical Company Richard Wolf (Buess et al., 1984). Its initial indication was to remove large rectal polyps beyond the reach of standard transanal excision. TEM is a technique for the performance of local excision, by the way of a binocular, magnified operating system. This equipment involves an operating proctoscope, insufflation, and magnified stereoscopic vision. In fact, the three-dimensional amplification, magnified stereoscopic view and lighting within the rectal lumen, allow excellent vision of the operative field, enabling the surgeon to perform an extremely precise excision of rectal lesions, including a full-thickness excision. It has evolved into a valuable, state-of-the-art technology equaling any other technique in terms of reliably positive patient outcome. Its application has expanded beyond the excision of colonoscopically unresectable polyps to the removal of select, early rectal cancers, independent of prior adjuvant chemoradiation therapy. Further fields of use include the treatment of anastomotic strictures, and repair of proximal, complex rectal fistulae. TEM allows greater flexibility and options for the operating surgeon. In addition to extending the surgeon's reach up to the distal sigmoid colon, the four ports of access allow for concomitant use of an illuminated camera, forceps, cautery, suction as well as the freedom to apply common laparoscopic techniques such as suturing and different energy sources.

TEM has been found useful in the treatment of a broad variety of disease processes, both benign and malignant. Though many indications have been described, including excision of carcinoids or even retrorectal tumors, the most common use of TEM remains the resection of colonoscopically unresectable rectal adenomas and carefully selected rectal cancers. It should be stressed that even though TEM extends the reach of conventional transanal resections, it should not lead to any deviation from the established stringent indications for resection, especially in regard to rectal cancer (Palma et al, 2004).

Due to the limited visibility and access inherent to traditional transanal retractors, use of the latter has been restricted to the resection of low rectal polyps and suitably located early cancers. The TEM technique grants access to the entire rectal cavity, facilitating the reach of lesions with their proximal margin located as far as 20 cm from the anal verge. Some of the limitations of TEM are due to the surgeon's personal skills and experience. The conditions treated by TEM, namely, colonoscopically unresectable rectal polyps and early cancers, are far less common in terms of incidence and epidemiology, than those treated by abdominal laparoscopic operations, thus limiting any single surgeon's or institution's volume and operative experience.

Contemporarily several factors have induced a new interest for TEM among practitioners, predominantly due to surging controversy about increased local recurrence rates following standard transanal resection of favorable early stage rectal cancers. TEM bears some advantage over standard transanal excision of neoplasms, including better visualisation of the surgical field and tumor margins. Inflicting fewer traumas, the probability of tumor fragmentation and dissemination diminishes, while additionally enabling resection of the potentially infiltrated mesorectum. As a matter of fact, more and more surgeons are being trained with advanced endoscopic skills. Synergistically these skills make handling the TEM equipment more feasible and surgeons face a less steep learning curve, generally promoting the use of the procedure.

Also, the use of TEM may not be restricted to the anal cavity, but serve as a gateway to the peritoneum for natural orifice transluminal endoscopic surgery (NOTES). Transrectal access to the peritoneum via TEM has the future potential to facilitate the removal of larger organs, maintenance of pneumoperitoneum, endoscopical visualisation of upper abdominal organs and secure suture closure of the proctotomy, by the application of larger, more versatile instruments.

2. TEM Equipment

2.1 Articulated stabilising arm

The proctoscope is aligned using an articulated arm, also known as the Martin arm, which is firmly attached to the operating table (figure 2). There are two ball joints which fully articulate and are locked into place with a single set screw. A bar at the one end of the articulated arm attaches to the rail on the operating table. At the opposite end the articulated arm attaches to the operating proctoscope.

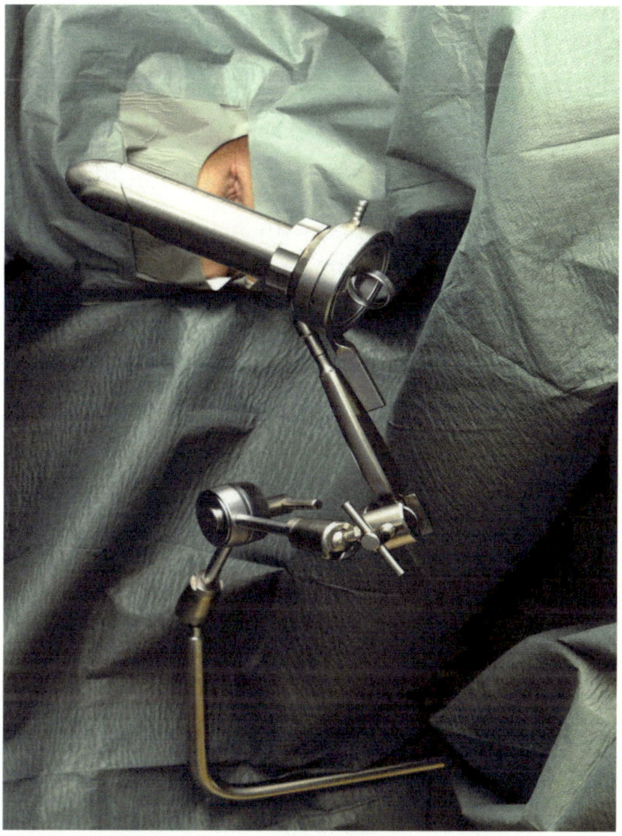

Fig. 2. Martin articulated arm.

2.2 Operative proctoscopes

The diameter of the operating proctoscope is 4 cm, it is available in two different lengths, 10 and 20 cm and allows access throughout the rectum. A rotating collar on the handle locks the scope shaft, creating an airtight seal. The handle comes with a port, allowing the attachment of a hand-bulb insufflator or a tube for monitoring the CO2 pressure (figure 3).

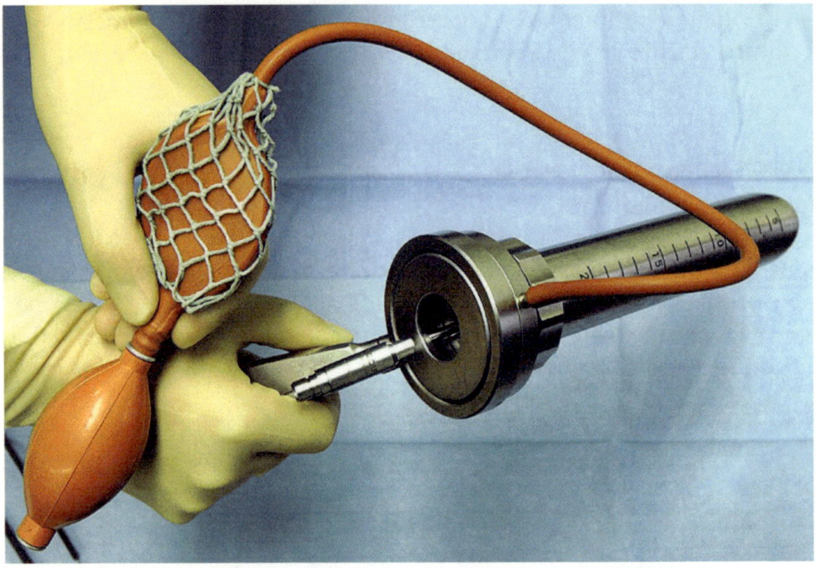

Fig. 3. TEM operating proctoscope (20 cm) with hand-bulb insufflator.

A faceplate is fitted to the handle and locked with an sealed lever. This faceplate has a port for the optics and three rubber caps for the long operating instruments (figure 4). These ports are able to maintain pneumorectum and are fitted with holes of varying size, to accommodate instruments of different diameters. The right-side operating port is slightly larger and thus requires a slightly larger cap. Flap valves in the snap-on multiport piece serve to help prevent gas leaks.

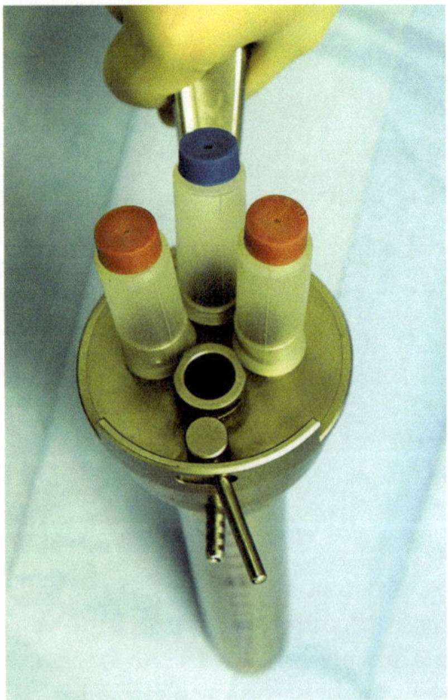

Fig. 4. TEM faceplate with four ports.

2.3 Optics

A 10-mm stereoscope which provides a high-definition, three-dimensional view is used. The stereoscope's long, rigid shaft is inserted into the optic port on the faceplate and extends the entire length of the operating proctoscope.

A 40o, 5-mm scope is inserted into the stereoscope and connected to a camera, allowing a live feed from the rectal cavity to be displayed on a video monitor. The stereoscope also has two ports serving for water irrigation and CO_2 insufflation (figure 5).

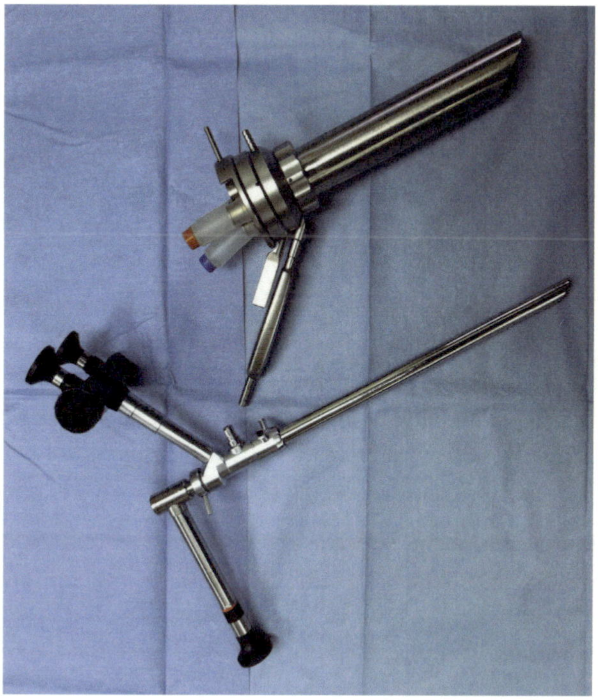

Fig. 5. TEM proctoscope (above) and 10 mm stereoscope (below), attached to a 5 mm scope for video viewing.

2.4 TEM Instruments

Long instruments are needed access the surgical field via the operating TEM proctoscopes (figure 6). The instruments include electrocautery, forceps, scissors, suction probe, clip applier, needle holder, and retractable needle.

There are two variants of forceps, either straight or angled. Both types are provided on instruments with tips facing either left or right. Each instrument may be electrified individually. Also the scissors are provided with the tip facing either left or right, and are mainly used for cutting sutures.

The suction probe is a, double-curved, rigid tube designed to be inserted through the proctoscope and sit on the side of the scope's channel , not to obstruct vision during the procedure.

The needle device has a retractable needle within the tip of the rigid tube and may be extended or retracted with a syringe type handle. The needle holders are available with either a straight or an angled tip. The angled tip provides a slightly wider arc when passing

a needle. In addition the jaws are "self-righting", when the needle is grasped it will rotate into the proper orientation by itself. The needle can be locked into position with a rotating ratchet controlled by the surgeon's thumb. The lock is released by over-squeezing the handle, allowing the surgeon to safely handle the needle.
The clip applier is a unique instrument which crimps a small silver clip onto the suture. Replacing the need for knot tying, clips are placed at the beginning and the end of running suture.

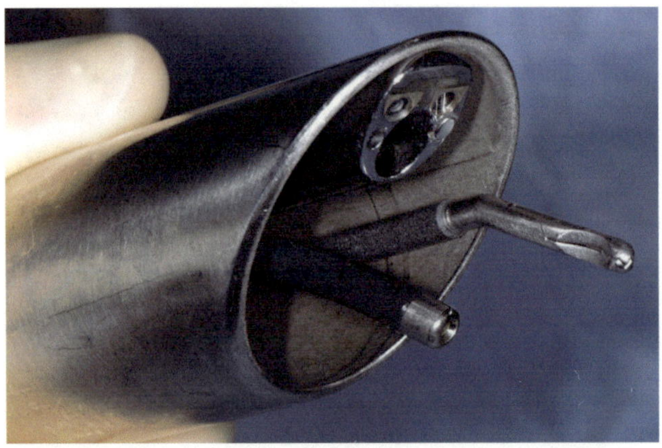

Fig. 6. TEM distal proctoscope opening showing the stereoscope together with forceps and suction probe.

2.5 Specific TEM devices

The specific device providing CO2 insufflation, water injection, and suction is stacked on a suitable portable cart (figure 7) as well as the video monitor, recorder and light source (figure 8). An electrocoagulation unit may be placed in the stack or a separate standard operating room unit may be employed.

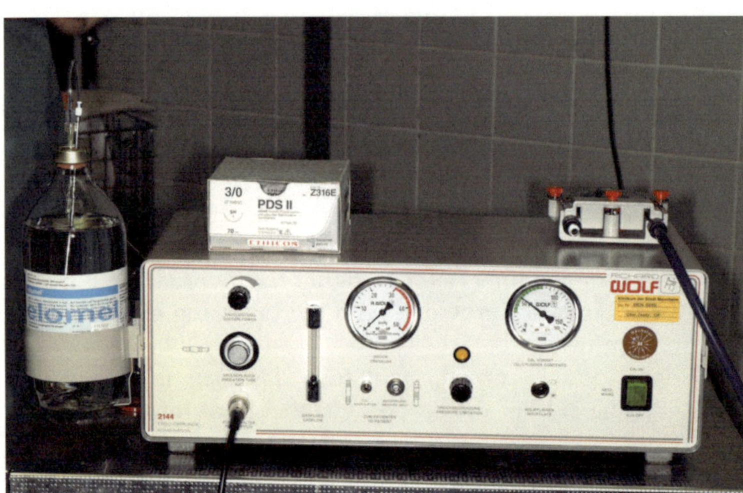

Fig. 7. Specific device for CO2 insufflation, water injection and suction.

The insufflator injects CO_2 via a port on the stereoscope's optic shaft. Lighting is supplied via a fiberoptic cord leading to a connector on the optic probe. Water irrigation may be engaged using a pedal. The water for irrigation flows through the stereoscope's shaft and is diverted across the optic tip, thus keeping the view clear.

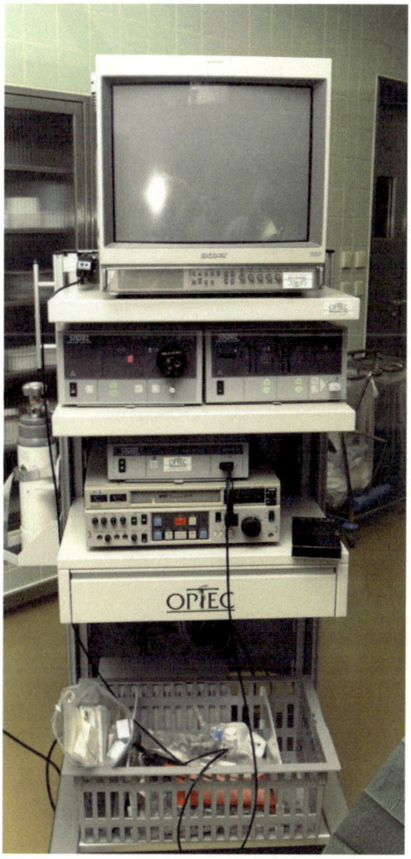

Fig. 8. The video monitor, recorder and light source are stacked on a portable cart.

2.6 Surgical set-up

Assembling the equipment can be time-consuming. The surgeon must position the patient in such way, that the tumor faces down directly towards the operating table; the choice of position is based upon prior examination in the office with a rigid proctoscope locating the tumor at both a specific level and a specific site on the circumference.

The patient may be placed in the lithotomy position, prone, or laterally; for a tumor that is almost circumferential the patient may need to be turned during the procedure. In our experience, the patient must be secured to the table with a bean bag, as the table may need to be rotated to bring the tumor into the center of the field. After positioning the bean bag, the articulated arm is attached to the operating table. The four tubes leaving the insufflation/suction devices must be connected properly.

Figure 9 shows the operation theatre setup with the patient in prone postion in order to reach the neoplasm, located on the anterior rectal wall.

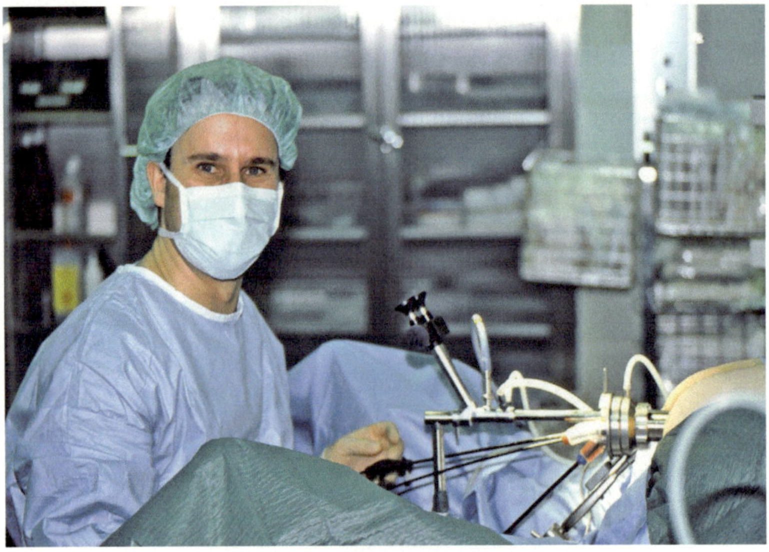

Fig. 9. Surgical setup with the patient in prone position

In conclusion, TEM requires specialized equipment and training. In addition to technical expertise, the dedicated TEM colorectal surgeon should be familiar with the necessary instruments and electronic devices. Expertise in troubleshooting is particularly helpful. There is, however, no substitute for a dedicated operating room team to ensure an efficient and successful TEM procedure.

3. Surgical technique

Preceding the procedure, bowel cleansing and prophylactic antibiosis have to be performed. In the actual procedure, two different operation techniques can be employed. Mucosectomy involves removing the mucosa, including the polyp from the inner circular layer of the muscularis; it represents a suitable technique for sessile adenomas located in the intraperitoneal portion of the rectum.

Full-thickness excision requires removal of all layers of the rectal wall, in the plane located just slightly superficial of the perirectal fatty tissue. This excision is performed for the majority of malignant lesions.

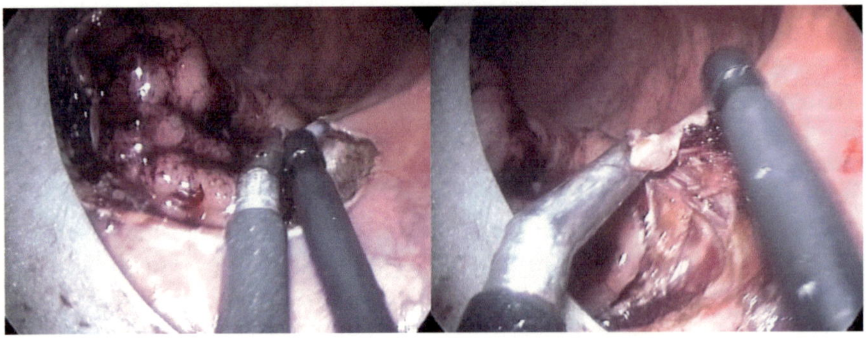

Fig. 10. Surgical dissection of an adenoma with two large TEM instruments.

In cases of malignancy, it is imperative that the procedure includes not only a full-thickness excision but also a 1 cm safety margin of normal mucosa surrounding the lesion.

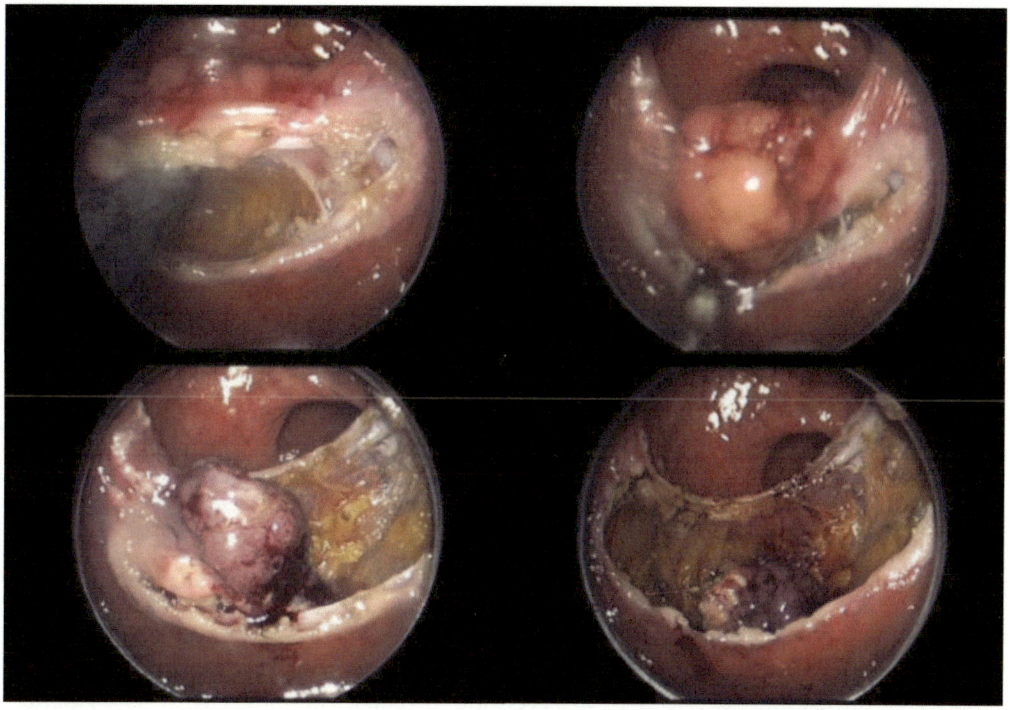

Fig. 11. TEM full-thickness dissection of rectal adenoma, showing the perirectal fatty tissue.

It is of crucial importance to correctly align the specimen on the cork board immediately after resection, to evaluate the safety margins before fixation with formalin. The proximal and distal margins of resection have to be identified to ensure correct histologic examination.

The rectal defect is closed by a running suture with a polydioxanone (3/0) monofilament and has to be performed transversely to prevent stenosis. The application of a silver clip at each end of the suture avoids the need for intraluminal knotting.

Alternatively, recent reports indicate the possibility to leave the defect open for secondary wound repair, especially in cases of partial-thickness excision.

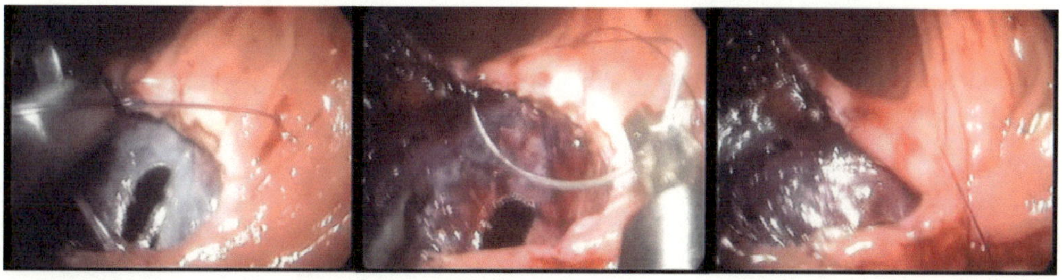

Fig. 12. Rectal wall defect closed by a running suture. Please note the peritoneal opening. Patient in the prone position.

Following the excision of large masses, mobilization of the proximal and distal rectal wall will minimize tension on the suture line (figure 13). Approximating large defects with a single suture at the midpoint, facilitates the closure. Following this, the defect is closed from the peripheral margins to the center in running fashion. In our experience, modern instruments like the endo-stitch™ (Covidien) are well suited to perform the running suture.

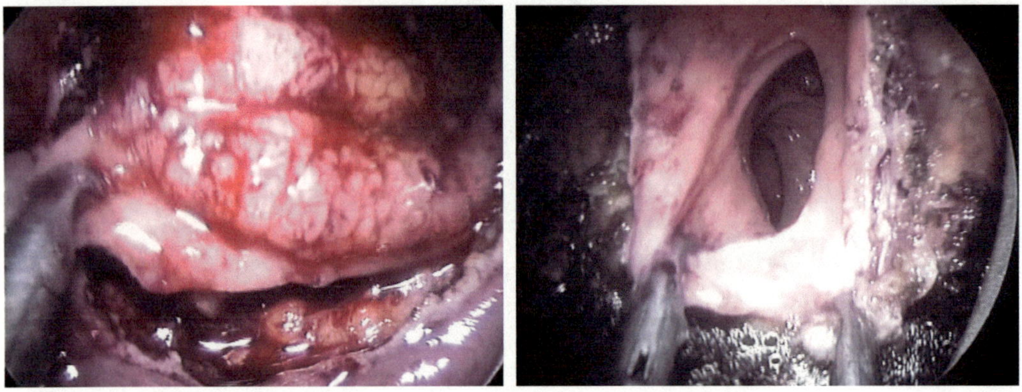

Fig. 13. Large rectal mass excision resulting in a ¾ defect to be closed.

4. Patient selection and staging

Resection of rectal and distal sigmoid adenomas is the most prominent indication for TEM. These benign lesions do not require mesorectal dissection, thus patients can be spared the morbidity of an unnecessary radical intervention. Smaller adenomas without evidence of high-grade dysplasia may be removed by partial-thickness (submucosal) excision. Larger adenomas or those with high-grade dysplasia are at high risk of containing invasive adenocarcinoma loci and should be excised full-thickness with a 10 mm resection margin.

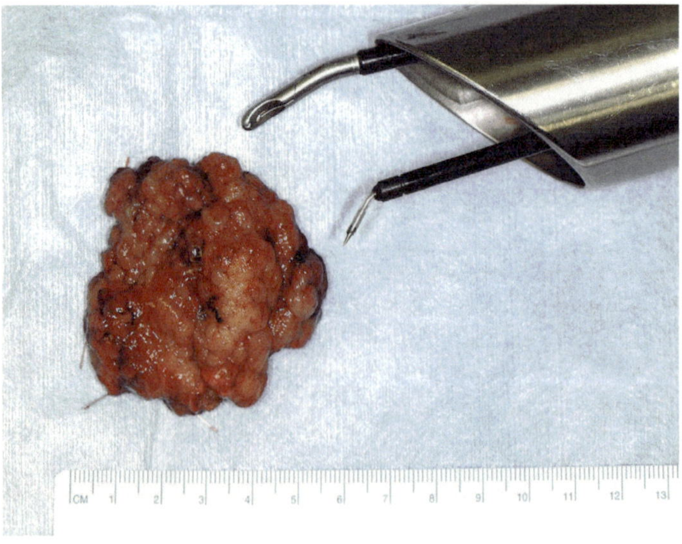

Fig. 14. Adenoma specimen after TEM excision.

Resection of anterior rectal lesions requires special care. Full-thickness excision of the anterior and even lateral rectum carries the risk of unnoticed dissection into the vagina, urethra, or bladder. In this case, failure of adequate closure may lead to a rectourethral or rectovaginal fistula.

Intraperitoneal entry carries a risk of injuring intraabdominal structures, bacterial and potential cytologic contamination, as well as anastomotic leakage. Initially regarded as a complication, intraperitoneal excision with secure closure of the rectal defect has been performed with growing experience, without increased short-term morbidity (figure 12).

In case of a suspicious rectal polyp with unconfirmed malignancy in a patient unfit for or unwilling to undergo major abdominal surgery, TEM can be useful in resecting the entire lesion in one piece for complete histologic assessment. Salvage radical surgery, if indicated, can be performed thereafter without significantly increasing morbidity. TEM may also be useful as a palliative tool in patients with extensive metastatic disease or those medically unfit to withstand radical surgery. Neoadjuvant radiation therapy, when used in conjunction with resection, either aiming for cure or palliation, does not appear to increase complications following TEM.

Accuracy in the preoperative staging is mandatory to correctly select patients eligible for local excision. The routine use of endorectal ultrasound (figure 15), in combination with magnetic resonance imaging (MRI) has revolutionized our ability to perform accurate preoperative staging with respect to rectal wall penetration (T stage) and regional lymph nodes (N stage) (figure 16).

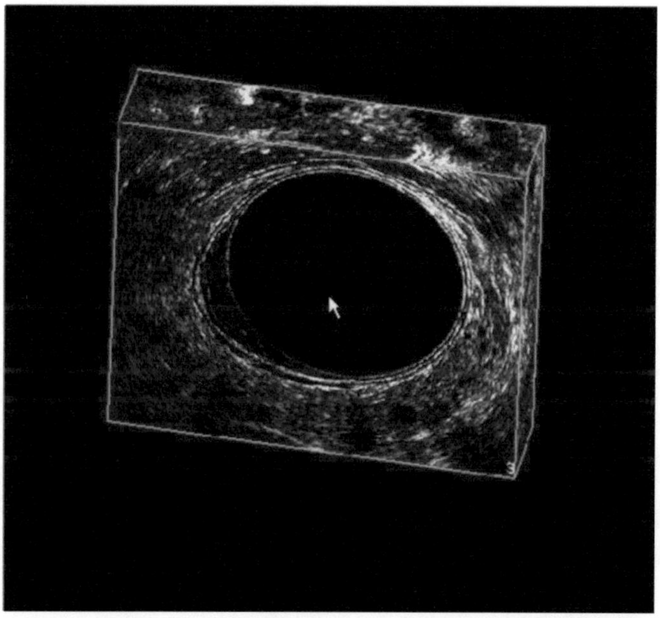

Fig. 15. 3D endorectal ultrsound showing a rectal mass without disruption of any of the rectal wall's layers.

Only patients with negative lymph nodes, a tumor limited to the wall of the rectum, presenting a diameter not exceeding 3 cm (in cases of malignancy), should be considered eligible for local excision.

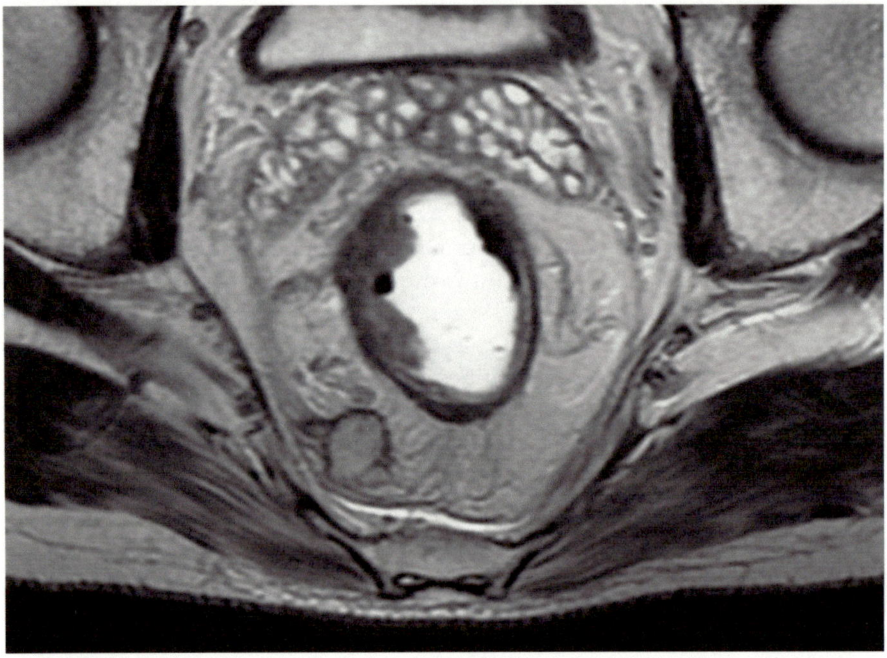

Fig. 16. Pelvic MRI T2 sequence, axial plane showing a rectal mass with a lymph node in the mesorectum.

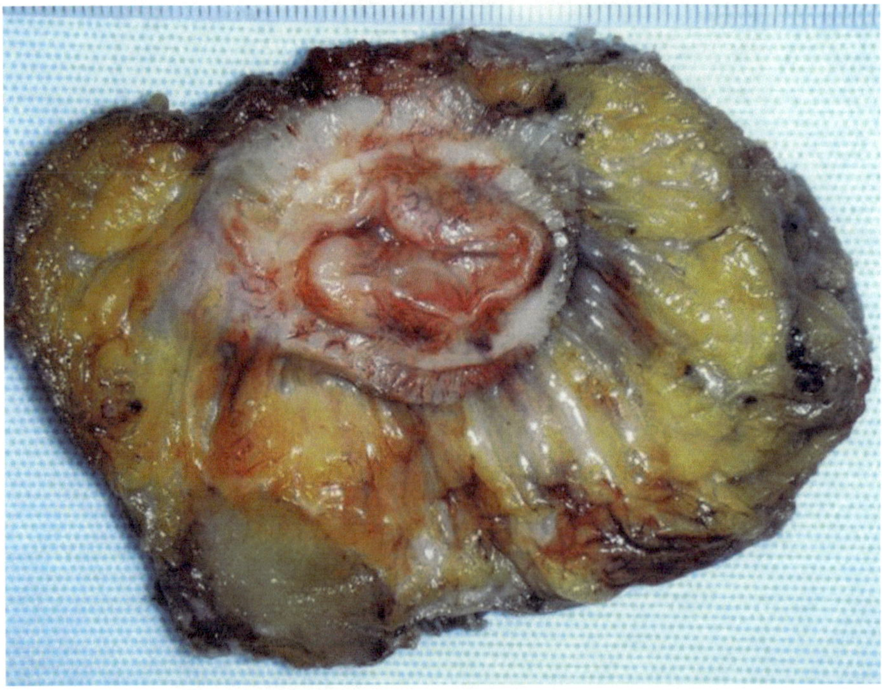

Fig. 17. Histopathological specimen obtained from the patient mentioned above, showing both the rectal mass and the mesorectal lymph node in contact with the mesorectal fascia.

Preoperative staging workup includes:

- Digital rectal examination
- Colonoscopy
- Rectoscopy, to:
  1. Perform biopsies
  2. Measure the distance from the anal verge to the lesion
  3. Evaluate the circumferential position of the tumor
  4. Select an appropriate patient positioning for TEM approach
- Endorectal ultrasound
- Pelvic-MRI
- 18F-FDG PET-CT, specifically in our institution (figure 18).

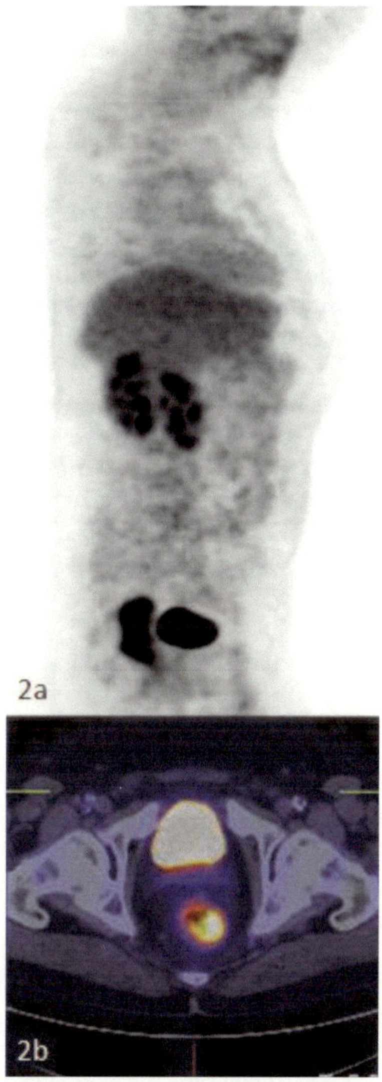

Fig. 18. 18F-FDG PET-CT showing pathologic intense glucose uptake due to rectal cancer.

Each biopsy is examined by a dedicated pathologist to assess the tumor grade, as well as the lymphatic, neural, and blood vessel infiltration.

5. Current indications and results

Results from our experience and others are evaluated in the following chapter

5.1 TEM for benign lesions

Benign rectal tumors that are not suitable for snare diathermy excision are often amenable to removal via the transanal route, employing anal retractors and Parks's method (Parks, 1970). However, this method is limited to the lower third of the rectum. In addition, it may be difficult to visualize the margins of flat adenomas.

Conventional management of higher rectal lesions usually involves transabdominal procedures, posterior trans-sacral (Kraske), or sphincter-splitting (York-Mason) approaches. However, these are major surgical procedures with associated complications and may be unsuitable and unnecessary if the purpose of the intervention is to resect benign lesions or low risk carcinomas.

With the development of TEM by G. Buess (Buess et al., 1984), it is now possible to carry out formal transanal resection by means of a rectoscope, which affords excellent access and vision in the entire rectum.

According to our experience, we recomend a full-thickness resection, to ensure an appropriate margin of safety. In addition, we found that this standard procedure is technically easier to perform than mucosectomy and that it decreases the risk of missing a small rectal cancer which may be located within the villous adenoma. Such 'intraephitelial neoplasia/dysplasia' or 'early invasion' has been reported in up to 31% of cases.

Although it is often difficult to ascertain the precise techniques (full-thickness or submucosal) used, the rates of complete excision at the time of operation and the exact follow up, large published series report a rate of recurrences in up to 27.3% after transanal excision of rectal adenomas (Sakamoto et al., 1991). In contrast the results reported using TEM show a recurrence rate between 3 and 7% with the 5.6% for the adenoma cases of our series pubished in 2004, being well in accordance with previous studies (Palma et al., 2004).

The overall morbidity rate for conventional transanal surgery in reported series varies from 0 to 14.5%, compared with 6% reported in the largest series of a total of 318 adenomas treated by Mentges (Mentges et al., 1996). These results are in accordance with others TEM-series reporting morbidity of up to 4.5% in more than seven hundred patients and with our own experience (7%).

It is of interest that postoperative bleeding is unusual with TEM, whereas it accounts for over half of the complications reported in other series (Sakamoto et al., 1991). Peritoneal entry, on the other hand, as assessed intra-operatively in 8 patient of our published experience (two of them with postoperative pneumoperitoneum), can be a significant source of morbidity with TEM. Presumably the excellent vision afforded by TEM allows more precise haemostasis, whereas the ability to excise high rectal lesions increases the likelihood of peritoneal entry, especially when the tumour is anterior, and thus more likely to be above the peritoneal reflection. In our experience, all perforations were recognized and managed by immediate endorectal suture (fig. 12).

Our results after initial 100 cases with TEM indicate that this technique is reproducible with suitable surgical training.

Interestingly all three protective ileostomies in our series occurred within the first 20 cases indicating a learning curve, despite the fact that all surgeons received a special TEM training.

Regarding the effect of a prolonged anal dilatation with the 40 mm diameter TEM operative rectoscope, manometric studies indicate a decrease in anal sphincter tone ranging from 25% to 37% of pre-operative sphincter pressure, with recovery to clinical continence within 6-16 weeks (Herman et al., 2001). We observed postoperative transitory grade II incontinence in 65 of the 100 patients, with full recovery in 98% of the cases after 12 weeks. There is also evidence indicating a significantly increased risk of diminishing the anal resting pressure by procedures lasting more than two hours. Others found 21% disturbances of rectoanal coordination and rectal perception, depending on the extent and type of resection of the tumor. However, when making continence judgement, it would be necessary to consider the risk of incontinence by using the Parks retractor in conventional surgery, or after a low restorative rectal excision, if those were to be the alternative procedures.

In conclusion, TEM as a minimally invasive technique might be expected not only to benefit a small, specific population of patients in terms of morbidity but also to improve results in terms of completeness of excision and recurrence rates when compared to conventional transanal resection.

5.2 TEM for early rectal cancer

The standard treatment for early rectal cancer has been major surgery by anterior or abdominoperineal resection. After the introduction of total mesorectal excision, results regarding recurrence and survival rates have improved dramatically (figure 19). However, mortality, morbidity, and functional disturbances after major surgery are considerable. Perioperative mortality rates are usually 2 to 3 percent and overall morbidity 20 to 30 percent. Furthermore, anorectal, bladder, and sexual function may be compromised.

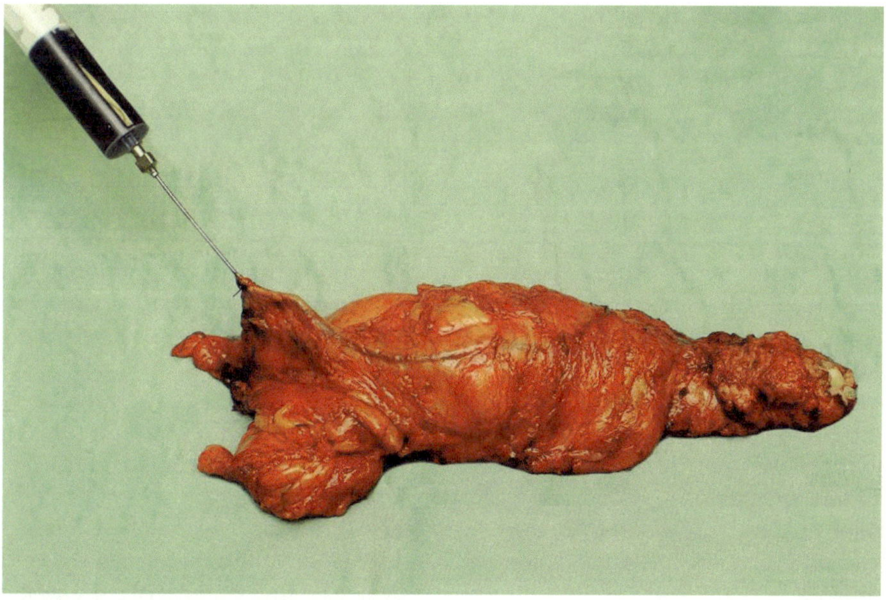

Fig. 19. Total mesorectal excision specimen

Given these side effects, there has been an increasing interest in the locoregional treatment of early rectal cancer. Nowadays local excision for selected rectal neoplasms is an accepted treatment worldwide (Bretagnol et al., 2007). Compared to the gold standard of radical surgery, local procedures of strictly selected early rectal cancers should lead to identical oncological results and even better outcomes regarding morbidity, mortality, and quality of life.

Regardless of this trend, conventional transanal excision of rectal cancer has recently come under close scrutiny because of relatively high rates of local recurrence (Bentrem et al., 2005). In fact, scepticism has been expressed that such treatment may not be in the patient's best interest. Despite all these concerns transanal endoscopic microsurgery has become the current standard procedure for the treatment of large rectal adenomas and early low risk carcinomas with curative intent, mostly in Europe (Demartines et al., 2001, Palma et al., 2004).

As already assessed and in contrast to conventional transanal excisions using anal retractors, TEM offers an exceptionally good overview of the whole rectal cavity, allowing the precise removal of lesions not only in the lower and middle rectum but also in the upper region or even the retrorectal space, and obviates the need for major surgery.

Despite the limitations and the lack of power of clinical studies to detect differences in outcome such as survival and complication rates, TEM does appear to result in less local recurrence than other usual methods of local excision.

Furthermore, after local excision of early rectal cancer by TEM, recurrence and survival rates are comparable to those seen after major surgery, and complication rates and functional results are even superior when put into contrast with those seen after major surgery (Middleton et al., 2005).

Since the introduction of TEM in our Division of Colon & Rectal Surgery a majority of patients with adenomas and T1 low-risk rectal cancer have been treated with local excision by this technique (Palma et al., 2004).

In 2009 we ran a single center report to evaluate the safety and oncological outcomes of TEM excision compared to radical surgery (RS) in the treatment of T1 low-risk rectal cancer. We found no statistical differences between RS and TEM in terms of local recurrence and disease free survival rates (Palma et al., 2009).

Today, various surgical techniques are still under discussion for the treatment of early rectal carcinomas. The historical gold standard procedures, such as anterior and abdominoperineal resection, show excellent results regarding local recurrence and survival rates, but are dearly paid for by a high incidence of complications and impaired quality of life (anorectal, sexual, and urinary dysfunction). Additionally, some of the patients require temporary diverting enterostomies. On the other hand, there are conventional, sphincter-preserving techniques, such as conventional transanal resection with Park's retractor (Parks, 1970), which are associated with an almost unacceptably high local recurrence rate of up to 29% (Madbouly et al., 2005).

The primary factor limiting the effectiveness of local treatment for early rectal cancer is lymph node invasion. Depths of invasion into the rectal wall, grade or degree of differentiation, vascular, lymphatic and neural invasion are independent predictors of the risk of nodal metastasis.

Since initial studies by Morson (Morson, 1985) and Hermanek (Hermanek & Marzoli, 1994) large series of resected rectal cancers have shown that well-differentiated tumors confined to the submucosa (T1) without vascular, lymphatic or neural invasion carry a 4% risk of nodal metastasis.

Although the reported rate of recurrence for early rectal cancers (pT1) resected by TEM is between 4- and 14%, follow-up and differentiation between low- and high-risk features are variable among series reported. In fact, the only published prospective study comparing TEM with radical resection for T1 low risk rectal cancer showed no statistical difference between local excision and radical resection regarding local recurrence and metastasis rate (Winde et al., 1996). These results are in accordance with our observations. We assessed two recurrences in the TEM group compared to none in the RS group. Local control is therefore undoubtedly better assessed after RS, but on the other hand it is interesting to underline that there was no statistically significant difference in overall survival and disease-free survival depending on the operation performed.

In an outstanding systematic review published recently, both comparative and case-series studies were examined to assess evidence related to the safety and efficacy of TEM compared with radical resections and conventional local excisions ((Middleton et al., 2005). Despite limited evidence the authors pointed out the unequivocal tendency of TEM to achieve better results in well-selected cases than conventional local excision, without being less effective than radical resection. The question arising is, whether TEM represents the only adequate alternative to radical resection for early rectal cancer.

The reason for the superiority of TEM over other transanal conventional techniques is the use of an optical system with 3D-view, 6-fold magnification, and human eye resolution; the creation of a stable pneumorectum, and specially designed instruments that allow full-thickness excision under excellent view conditions not only in the lower but also in the middle and upper parts of the rectum. Furthermore, full-thickness excision allows proper histological examination.

Recently we showed the ability and advantages of this technique to approach tumors located in the retrorectal space (Zoller et al., 2007).

The advantage of TEM has already been observed in the lower rate of recurrences for adenoma excision (up to 7%) when compared to recurrence rate after transanal conventional excision (up to 27.3%). Even for adenomas, completeness of excision is an important predictor for early recurrence. Furthermore, the literature reported a lower morbidity rate when using TEM for adenoma excision (7% complication rate compared to 14.5% for conventional transanal surgery) (Ganai et al., 2006).

Surprisingly many publications still advocate for caution in the local excision of rectal cancer. However, these studies are questionable regarding selection criteria, use of endorectal ultrasounds preoperatively, proper *"in toto"* excision, and histological examination (R-Status, differentiation, and lymphovascular invasion).

In addition, some data is compromised by mainly retrospective analyses over extended time periods, and by a lack of standardized pathology reports.

The main argument explaining the high rate of local recurrences after conventional local excision could be a technically inadequate operation in which margins are insuficcient, inadequate depth of resection, or shedding and implantation of tumor cells into the surgical field (Cataldo, 2006).

Moore (Moore et al., 2008) compared 82 patients after TEM with another 89 after conventional transanal excision for rectal neoplasms. He found clear margins in 71 percent of specimens in the conventional group compared with 90% in the TEM group. Furthermore, non fragmented specimens were more likely to be found after TEM than after conventional surgery (94 *vs.* 65 percent). In our hands the rate of Rx and R1 after local excision was 5.88 and 2.94%, respectively.

We believe that strict patient selection criteria, together with full-thickness and margin-free excision is crucial for patient outcome. The strong correlation between incomplete tumor resection and poor outcome is widely accepted. In our experience, positive excision margins should not be regarded as a risk factor for recurrence but should be viewed as insufficient therapy requiring further treatment.

Therefore, accurate pathological examination after corkboard fixation of the specimen, and intensive, close cooperation between surgeon and pathologist cannot be overemphasized.

Although local recurrence was only observed after local excision, patients treated with TEM in our hands showed no significant differences in terms of overall survival and disease-free survival, as compared to patients who underwent RS. As local excision represents a minimally invasive technique in terms of morbidity, mortality and functional outcome, TEM should be offered as a valid option for well-selected patients with early rectal cancer.

Despite the difficulty to perform further studies in the future, comparing different methods of local excision with more radical procedures and the possible combination of neoadjuvant chemoradiation for better local and distant control even for high risk tumors (Borschitz et al., 2008), we can conclude following our published experience, that TEM should be considered as best practice to perform a local excision of well selected cases of early rectal carcinoma.

5.3 TEM in rectal cancer after chemoradiation

Although adjuvant or neoadjuvant chemoradiotherapy seems to improve the prognosis after local excision, the indications for any kind of therapy following local resection of rectal cancer by TEM remain controversial. In fact, local treatment of rectal cancer is limited by the impossibility of removing the potentially positive lymph nodes, supporting the concept of adjuvant radiotherapy, chemotherapy, or both to achieve local control of the lymph nodes.

Borschitz (Borschitz et al., 2008) published a review of the findings of neoadjuvant chemoradiation (nCRT) and local excision (LE) for T2–3 rectal carcinoma. He found a total of 237 patients in seven different studies available for analysis, which did in fact permit an assessment of the recurrence rates in relation to histopathological tumor response.

Patients with systemic metastases were excluded, and lymph node status was provided by only a few authors.

In most studies analysed, clinical staging before nCRT identified a T2/3 rectal carcinoma (T1 2%; T1–2 14%; T2 34%; T3 50%).

The studies reported different therapeutic concepts, tumor locations, and intervals from completion of nCRT to surgery. Nevertheless, the analysis by Borschitz identified a number of similarities among them. These were predominance of cT2–3 carcinomas and the occurrences of local recurrence (LR). Patients with response at the submucosa level (ypT1) consistently showed low LR rates of 2% (0%–6%).

Less clearly defined were the results of ypT2 findings, which ranged from 6% to 20% LR rates. Clearly unfavorable were the findings in patients, whose disease did not respond to therapy (ypT3), for whom a mean LR rate of 21% was calculated. The widely divergent LR rates of ypT2 findings may be increased as a result of to nonuniform time intervals from nCRT to surgery.

The study by Borschitz confirms prior findings observed after nCRT and conventional resection. Almost no LR were reported for CR after nCRT of advanced (T3/4) tumors. Critical prognostic parameters are tumor response and tumor- free lymph nodes. LR and systemic recurrence rates ranging 0% to 23% and 8% to 22% were determined for this constellation. For lesions that did not respond to therapy and for persistent nodal disease, far higher LR rates ranging from 16% to 58%, and metastases ranging from 35% to 58% were reported.

Neoadjuvant CRT followed by LE may represent a viable alternative to rectum extirpation in patients with low T2–3 rectal carcinoma. Despite an optimized surgical technique made available by total mesorectal excision, less favorable results were reported for tumors in the lower rectum.

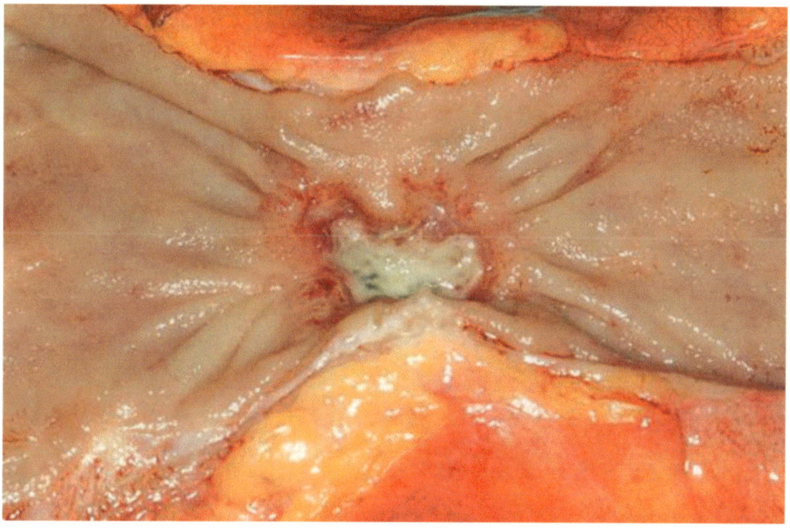

Fig. 20. Rectal cancer after neoadjuvant chemoradiation showing areas of fibrosis indicating good response

The distal mesorectum, described by Morson (Morson et al., 1963) as a "bare area," attenuates distally and is characterized by a circumferential decrease in healthy tissue surrounding the tumor, leading to a loss of tissue layers and a restricted field of view. For this region, incomplete mesorectal excision has been suggested as the cause of higher LR rates.

Local full-thickness excision may be performed as an adequate therapeutic measure for complete response (CR) after nCRT.

The described concept has been taken one step further by Habr-Gama (Habr-Gama et al., 2004) who did not find a need for subsequent surgery in patients with clinically complete responses. In her retrospective, long-term, follow-up study which so far has remained unique, she reports a LR rate of only 3% in 100 patients.

The question whether radical surgery, LE, or close-meshed follow-up alone may be appropriate in these patients, still remains largely unanswered. Furtherly it needs to be clarified, whether after nCRT with clinical confirmation of complete response, possibly remaining but vital tumor cells require surgical removal. These cells may have been damaged by irradiation and thus rendered unable to proliferate. Alternatively, some tumor cells surviving nCRT may represent resistant hypoxic clones that build the basis for development of recurrence later on.

In summary, the findings of the revision made by Borschitz support the proposition, that the indication for LE after nCRT may be extended to distal cT2–3 rectal carcinoma. The strongest prognostic parameter for favorable oncological outcomes is an effective tumor response without residual tumor (ypT0) or with response to at least the submucosa level (ypT1) in the excised specimen. For ypT2 tumors, the interpretation of the heterogeneous results should be performed with caution. But an extrapolation may be possible from LE alone, without nCRT. LE is not adequate in patients whose tumors exhibit no response or weak response to nCRT. These patients should be treated conventionally, that is, using radical surgery.

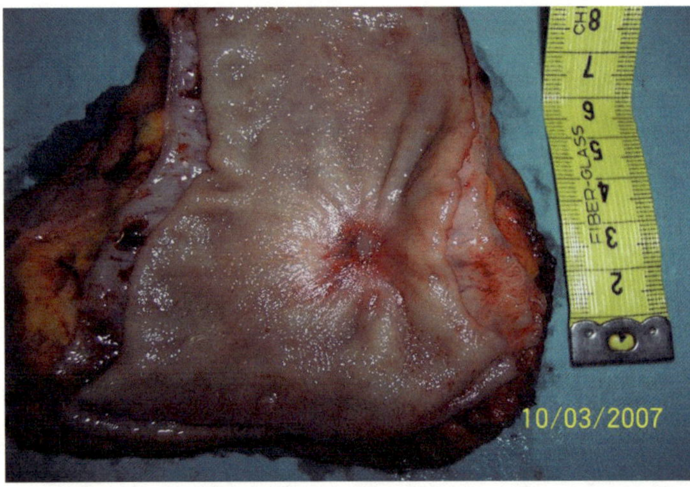

Fig. 21. Rectal cancer after neoadjuvant chemoradiation showing complete response (ypT0)

6. Conclusion

Transanal Endoscopic Microsurgery is a fairly new variant of transanally performed surgery of the rectal cavity, developed in Germany during the 1980's. In comparison to preceding techniques, it has largely expanded the spatial range and resolution of transanal procedures by employing state-of-the-art optics and endoscopic instruments, enabling the surgeon to reach parts of the rectum that were previously unaccessible by transanal approach.

Repassing the findings throughout the manuscript, it is evidence based to conclude that TEM currently is and prospectively will be playing an important role in the management of lower rectal neoformations.

When used in select cases of adenoma or low-grade adenocarcinoma and in accordance with the stringent indications governing more radical interventions, already in place, patients are due to benefit from less morbidity and mortality, including shorter recovery times.

Within its constraints, TEM has also shown a more favorable incidence of local recurrences compared to standard transanal surgery, while being able to parallel local recurrence rates of more extended invasive interventions, like anterior resection and abdominoperineal approaches, outlining its qualities in curative treatment of rectal cancer.

It has to be stressed, that the suitability of TEM must be determined in a meticulous preoperative staging and grading process, including MRI imaging and endorectal ultrasound, to tackle the thin red line separating availible approaches case by case.

Apart from that, TEM may also serve as a last line measure for patients unfit or unwilling to undergo laparotomy, adding to its value in managing palliative instances.

Aditionally, in multimodal therapy schemes, including neoadjuvant chemoradiotherapy, the indication of TEM could expand, in the near future, to those patients showing a complete response.

7. References

Bentrem DJ, Okabe S, Wong WD, Guillem JG, Weiser MR, Temple LK. (2005) T1 adenocarcinoma of the rectum: transanal excision or radical surgery? *Ann Surg*; 242: 472-7.

Borschitz Th, Wachtlin D, Moehler M. (2008). Neoadjuvant Chemoradiation and Local Excision for T2-3 Rectal Cancer. *Annals of Surgical Oncology*, 15:712–720.

Bretagnol F, Merrie A, George B, Warren BF, Mortensen NJ. (2007) Local excision of rectal tumours by transanal endoscopic microsurgery. *Br J Surg*; 94: 627-33.

Buess G, Hutterer F, Theiss J, Boebel M, Isselhard W, Pichlmaier H. (1984) Das System fuer die transanale endoskopische Rectumoperation. *Chirurg*; 55: 677–80.

Cataldo PA. (2006) Transanal endoscopic microsurgery. *Surg Clin N Am*; 86: 915–25.

Demartines, N, von Flue MO, Harder FH. (2001) Transanal endoscopic microsurgical excision of rectal tumors: indications and results. *World J Surg*; 25: 870-5.

Ganai S, Kanumuri P, Rao RS, Alexander AI. (2006) Local recurrence after transanal endoscopic microsurgery for rectal polyps and early cancers. *Ann Surg Oncol*; 13: 547-56.

Habr-Gama A, Perez RO, Nadalin W, et al. (2004). Operative versus nonoperative treatment for stage 0 distal rectal cancer following chemoradiation therapy: long-term results. *Ann Surg*; 240:711–7.

Herman RM, Richter P, Walega P, Popiela T. (2001) Anorectal sphincter function and rectal barostat study in patients following transanal endoscopic microsurgery. *Int J Colorectal Dis*; 16: 370–6.

Hermanek P, Marzoli GP. (1994) Lokale Therapie des Rektumkarzinoms. Verfahren in kurativer Intention. Berlin Heidelberg New York: Springer.

Lisfranc J. (1833) Memoire sur l'excision de la partie inferieure du rectum devenue carcinomateuse. *Paris, Mem Ac R Méd.*

Madbouly KM, Remzi FH, Erkek BA, Senagore AJ, Baeslach CM, Khandwala F. (2005) Recurrence after transanal excision of T1 rectal cancer: should we be concerned? *Dis Colon Rectum*; 48: 711-9.

Mentges B, Buess G, Schaefer D, Manncke K, Becker HD. (1996) Indications and results of local treatment of rectal cancer. *Dis Colon Rectum*; 39: 886–92.

Middleton PF, Sutherland LM, Maddern GJ. (2005) Transanal endoscopic microsurgery: a systematic review. *Dis Colon Rectum*; 48: 270-84.

Moore JS, Cataldo PA, Osler T, Hyman NH. (2008) Transanal endoscopic microcurgery is more effective than traditional transanal excision for resection of rectal masses. *Dis Colon Rectum*; 0: 1-5.

Morson BC, Vaughan EG, Bussey HJR. (1963) Pelvic recurrence after excision of rectum for carcinoma. *Br Med J*: 13–8.

Morson BC. (1985) Histological criteria for local excision. *Br J Surg*: 53-4.

Palma P, Freudenberg S, Samel S, Post S. (2004) Transanal endoscopic microsurgery: indications and results after 100 cases. *Colorectal Dis*; 6: 350–5.

Palma P, Horisberger K, Joos A, Rothenhoefer S, Willeke F, Post S. (2009) Local excision of early rectal cancer: is transanal endoscopic microsurgery an alternative to radical surgery? *Rev Esp Enferm Dig*; 101: 172-178.

Parks AG. (1970) A technique for the removal of large villous tumours in the rectum. *Proc R Soc Med* ; 63: 89-91.

Sakamoto GD, MacKeigan JM, Senagore AJ. (1991) Transanal excision of large rectal villous adenomas. *Dis Colon Rectum*; 34: 880–5.

Winde G, Nottberg H, Keller R, Schmid KW, Buente H. (1996) Surgical cure for early rectal carcinomas (T1). Transanal endoscopic microsurgery vs. anterior resection. *Dis Colon Rectum*; 39: 969-79.

Zoller S, Joos A, Dinter D, Back W, Horisberger K, Post S, Palma P. (2007) Retrorectal tumors: excision by transanal endoscopic microsurgery. *Rev Esp Enferm Dig*; 99: 547-550.

6

Diagnostic and Therapeutic Endoscopy in the Biliary Tract and Pancreas

Ian C Roberts-Thomson and Nam Q Nguyen
Departments of Gastroenterology and Hepatology
The Queen Elizabeth Hospital and Royal Adelaide Hospital, Adelaide
Australia

1. Introduction

The development of fiberoptic endoscopes between 1960 and 1970 was an important event in the evolution of the specialty of gastroenterology. Several of these endoscopes had side-viewing or oblique-viewing lenses that provided reasonable views of the ampulla of Vater. Cannulation of the ampulla and retrograde pancreatography was first reported in 1968 (McCune et al., 1968). Subsequent developments largely occurred in Japan and led to a more detailed description of endoscopic retrograde cholangiopancreatography (ERCP) in 1970 (Takagi et al., 1970). This was soon followed by a description of endoscopic sphincterotomy by independent groups in Germany and Japan in 1974 (Classen & Demling, 1974; Kawai et al., 1974).

By the mid-1970's, ERCP had been adopted by several major centers but was not widely accepted because it was perceived as either "too difficult" or "too prone to complications". The major complication was that of pancreatitis. This occurred in up to 10% of patients and was associated with significant morbidity and at least some mortality. Even today, risks for pancreatitis remain significant despite a large number of studies that have attempted to reduce the risk using procedural modifications or various drugs.

The next milestone in therapeutic ERCP was a description of endoscopic stents for malignant biliary obstruction (Soehendra and Reynders-Frederix, 1979). This was followed by a description of therapeutic procedures in the pancreas including stents for strictures in the main pancreatic duct, endoscopic extraction of pancreatic stones, endoscopic drainage of pancreatic pseudocysts and endoscopic stents for pancreatic fistulae and pancreatic ascites. By the mid-1980's, ERCP had been widely adopted and was recognized as the therapeutic procedure of choice for bile duct stones, particularly after cholecystectomy.

Developments since 1990 include the use of self-expanding metal (metallic) stents for malignant biliary obstruction and the development of ultrathin endoscopes for direct cholangioscopy and pancreatoscopy. Although endoscopic ultrasound (EUS) was first described in 1976 (Lutz and Rosch, 1976), it has only recently been widely applied to pancreatic and biliary disorders, largely because of technical developments including the opportunity for tissue sampling using fine-needle aspiration.

The purpose of this report is to provide an outline of diagnostic and therapeutic procedures in the biliary tract and pancreas. We will also include endoscopic procedures currently under evaluation that might have a role in future therapy.

2. Diagnostic procedures

2.1 Historical and technical aspects

Prior to 1970, options for cholangiography included intravenous cholangiography and percutaneous transhepatic cholangiography. The former was unhelpful in the presence of jaundice and, in the absence of jaundice, had a relatively high frequency of false positive and false negative results. Percutaneous cholangiography was largely restricted to patients with jaundice and was usually performed as a pre-operative procedure because of the risk of a bile leak. Although ultrasound (US) and computed tomography (CT) scans were introduced in the late 1970's and early 1980's, respectively, these investigations did not have a major impact on the frequency of diagnostic procedures until the late 1980's. Magnetic resonance imaging (MRI) scans were introduced in the late 1990's but have only become widely available in the past decade.

Surprisingly, the endoscopes and ancillary equipment necessary for ERCP were largely developed in the 1970's. The principle was placement of a catheter in the orifice of the ampulla followed by the injection of contrast into the desired duct. The procedure was performed using intermittent fluoroscopy and radiographs were taken of appropriate images. In most patients, the desired duct is the bile duct but, unfortunately, it is often easier to outline the main pancreatic duct. Because of this, various techniques have been used to promote biliary cannulation including the use of a partly-opened papillotome, use of appropriately placed guide-wires and, under some circumstances, use of small endoscopic incisions (pre-cuts) to facilitate bile duct cannulation. The latter technique should probably be restricted to experts because of higher risks for pancreatitis (Hochberger et al., 2003). Endoscopic and radiologic images of selected biliary and pancreatic disorders are shown in figures 1 and 2.

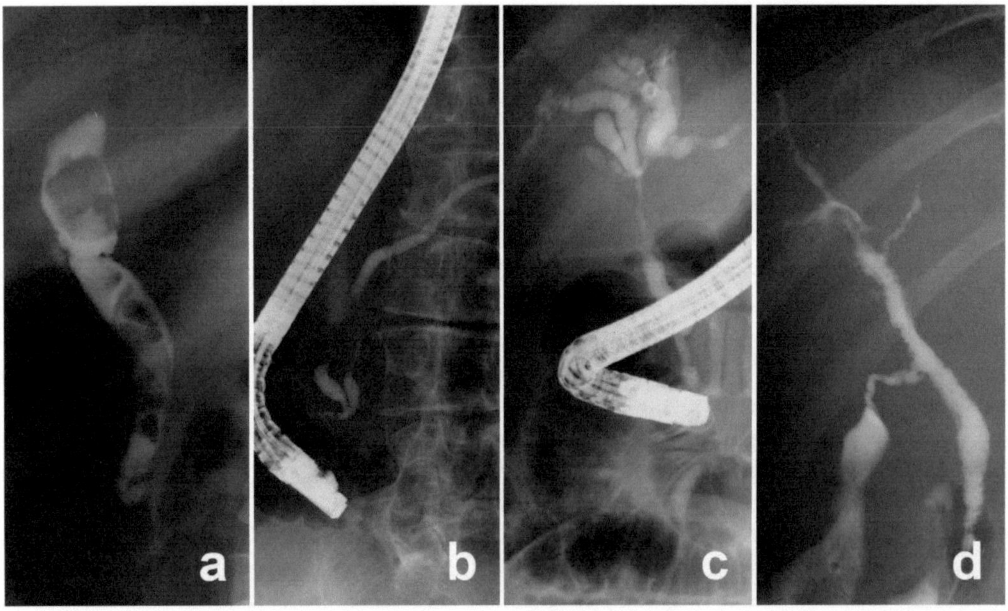

Fig. 1. Miscellaneous cholangiograms. (a) Multiple bile duct stones. (b) Carcinoma of the head of pancreas with strictures in the lower bile duct and main pancreatic duct. (c) Bile duct cancer involving the common hepatic duct. (d) Typical features of sclerosing cholangitis.

2.2 Bile duct stones

The preferred diagnosis for both patient and endoscopist is that of choledocholithiasis. In this setting, cannulation of the ampulla is often relatively easy and stones are outlined as mobile filling-defects within the bile duct. The cystic duct and gallbladder can also be outlined. For most of these patients, the sequence of investigations is an upper abdominal ultrasound study followed by ERCP. For patients with a probability of bile duct stones of 80% or less, additional useful information may be obtained by magnetic resonance cholangiopancreatography (MRCP) or EUS.

2.3 Ampullary, biliary and pancreatic neoplasms

Duodenal endoscopy is helpful for at least some neoplasms. In particular, most ampullary neoplasms can be diagnosed at duodenal endoscopy and confirmed by biopsy. Furthermore, approximately 5% of biliary and pancreatic cancers infiltrate or ulcerate into the second part of the duodenum and can also be confirmed by biopsy. Typical pancreatic cancer with obstructive jaundice (but without duodenal infiltration) results in strictures in both the main pancreatic duct and bile duct. This is usually associated with proximal dilatation of both ducts. In the absence of jaundice, the typical appearance is a stricture in the main pancreatic duct with proximal dilatation or complete obstruction of the duct. Similarly, in bile duct cancer, the typical appearance is an irregular biliary stricture that is normally associated with proximal dilatation including dilatation of intrahepatic ducts.

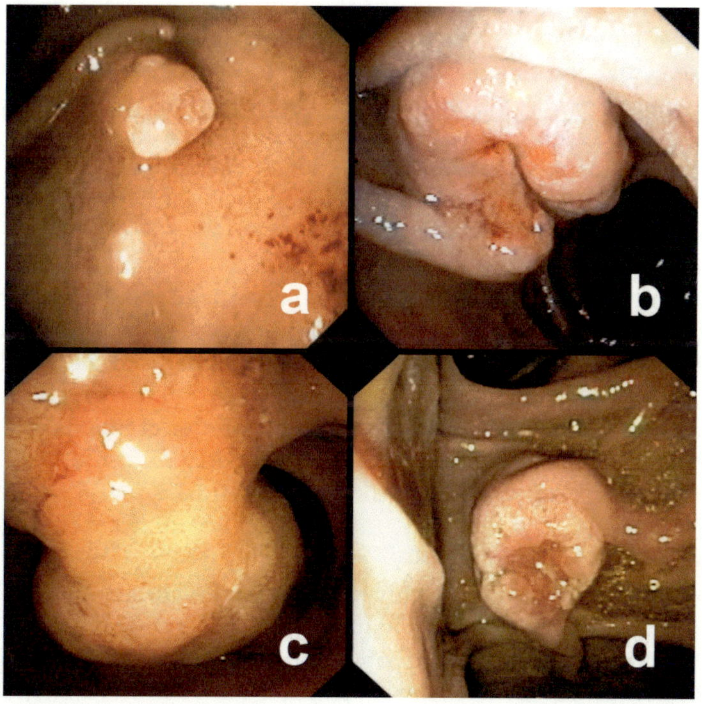

Fig. 2. Neoplasms of the ampulla of Vater. (a) Tiny adenomas of the ampulla associated with familial adenomatous polyposis. (b) Neuroendocrine neoplasm (carcinoid tumor) of the ampulla. (c) Large polypoid carcinoma of the ampulla. (d) Small ulcerated carcinoma of the ampulla.

At a clinical level, it may be difficult to differentiate pancreatic cancer from autoimmune pancreatitis and some cases of chronic pancreatitis. Although malignant biliary strictures without pancreatic duct strictures are usually caused by bile duct cancer (60%-70%), alternative possibilities include gallbladder cancer that spreads to the bile duct and metastatic cancer or lymphoma in subhepatic lymph nodes. Rarely, the differential diagnosis can also include benign biliary strictures such as post-operative strictures and sclerosing cholangitis.

2.4 Pancreatitis and its complications

Prior to the mid-1980's, ERCP was widely used for the diagnosis of non-calcific chronic pancreatitis and for the diagnosis of complications of pancreatitis such as pseudocysts and biliary obstruction. The diagnosis of chronic pancreatitis largely rested on radiological changes in the main pancreatic duct and side-branches. In relation to pseudocysts, at least 70% could be outlined at pancreatography although there was a small risk of conversion of a pseudocyst into a pancreatic abscess. Today, modern imaging techniques have largely replaced pancreatography for the diagnosis of most pancreatic disorders. However, pancreatography may still have a role in uncommon disorders such as idiopathic relapsing pancreatitis and pancreatic ascites (Petersen, 2002).

2.5 Role of endoscopic ultrasound

EUS is being increasingly used to enhance the diagnostic accuracy of traditional ERCP. Arguably, the most important development is the contribution of fine-needle aspiration to the histological or cytological diagnosis of various neoplasms. However, it is also being used to confirm the diagnosis of bile duct stones, to diagnose non-calcific chronic pancreatitis and to delineate the size and spread of various neoplasms (Figure 3a-e). In relation to bile duct stones, endoscopic ultrasound may be more sensitive than ERCP and MRCP for the detection of small stones, <5 mm in diameter (Kondo et al., 2005). It may also have a role in acute biliary pancreatitis where bile duct stones can pass spontaneously into the duodenum after induction of pancreatitis.

Endoscopic ultrasound is also being used for the diagnosis of mild chronic pancreatitis that is not associated with ductal dilatation, calcification or cysts. Various EUS criteria have been developed to reflect changes in pancreatic parenchyma that may be more sensitive than ductal changes at ERCP (Gleeson and Topazian, 2007). For pancreatic neoplasms, EUS provides high-resolution images of the pancreas that can detect lesions as small as 2-3 mm in diameter. Similar results have been obtained for bile duct cancer although the quality of images for distal tumors is superior to that for proximal tumors.

2.6 Tissue sampling

Although radiologic appearances are highly associated with various cancers, some surgeons and most oncologists are reluctant to embark on major therapies without histologic confirmation. As noted above, a minority of tumors can be identified at duodenal endoscopy and confirmed by duodenal biopsy. For the majority, options include percutaneous fine-needle aspiration with cytology and the histologic or cytologic evaluation of tissue taken at endoscopy. One endoscopic option is the cytologic evaluation of fluid aspirated from the main pancreatic duct or bile duct (Tanaka and Kida, 2009). In general, results from these studies have been disappointing. A variation is that of brushing cytology of these strictures. This has been helpful in some studies but results in bile duct cancer have been disappointing, perhaps because many cancers are sclerotic with only a minority of malignant cells (Tanaka and Kida, 2009). Another endoscopic approach is to take biopsies of the stricture using routine or modified biopsy forceps. This can be technically demanding but, when biopsies are obtained, confirmation of cancer has been reported in approximately 50% of cases (Howell et al., 1996).

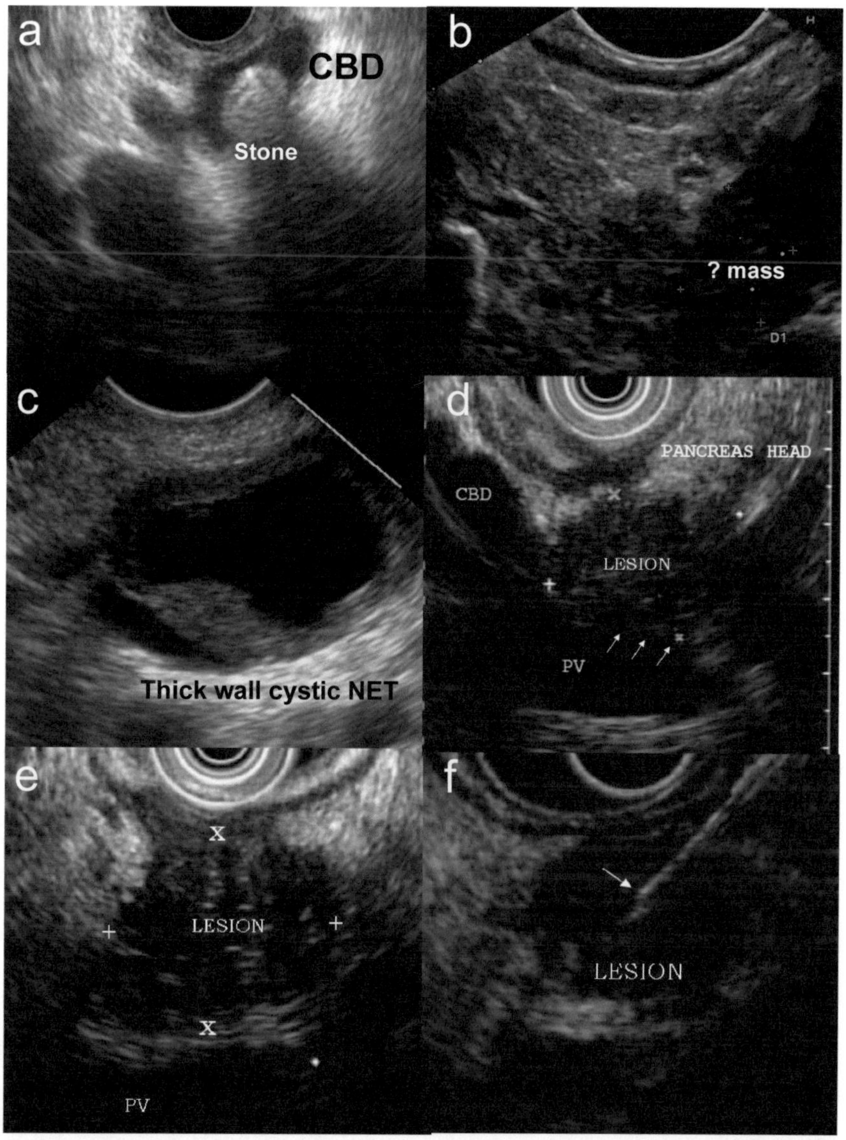

Fig. 3. EUS images demonstrating the presence of (a) a CBD stone, (b) a possible mass in a patient with pancreatic parenchymal changes consistent with chronic pancreatitis, (c) a cystic neuroendocrine tumor (NET), (d) a locally advanced pancreatic cancer invading the portal vein and (e & f) biopsy of a pancreatic lesion using EUS with fine-needle aspiration.

Currently, the procedure with the highest sensitivity for cancer is cytologic evaluation of fine-needle aspirates taken during endoscopic ultrasound (Figure 3f). In one randomized study in patients with suspected pancreatic cancer, rates for the detection of cancer in fine-needle aspirates were higher for specimens taken by endoscopic ultrasound (84%) than for specimens taken percutaneously under ultrasound or CT control (62%) (Horwhat et al., 2006). Similar results have been obtained for confirmation of bile duct cancer although the yield was significantly higher in distal cancer (81%) than in proximal cancer (59%) (Mohamadnejad et al., 2011).

2.7 Diagnostic cholangiopancreatoscopy

Although the first cholangioscope was developed over three decades ago, use of this technology was limited because of cost, endoscope fragility and the need for two experienced endoscopists to operate the "mother" and "daughter" scopes. However, interest in this technology has been reawakened by recent developments that include single-operator cholangiopancreatoscopy with facilities for forcep biopsy, the development of video endoscopes for cholangiopancreatoscopy and the development of balloon-facilitated ultrathin endoscopes that can be passed into the duct systems (Nguyen et al., 2009).

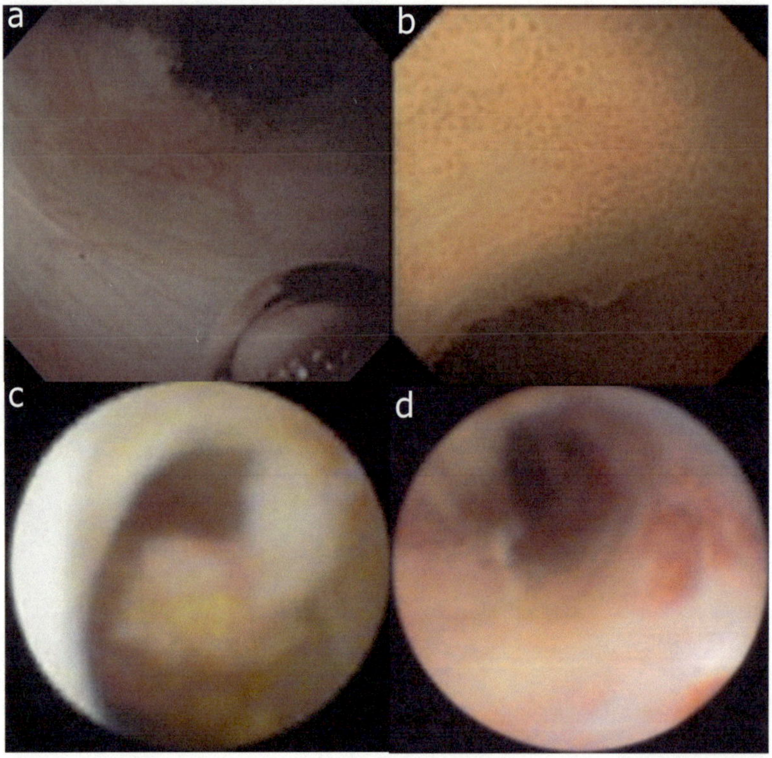

Fig. 4. Video (a & b) and SpyGlass (c & d) cholangiopancreatoscopy images showing (a) an early superficial papillary bile duct lesion, (b) the typical fish-egg like lesions of intraductal papillary mucinous neoplasia carpeting the bile duct, (c) an obstructing polypoid cholangiocarcinoma of the right hepatic duct and (d) occult malignancy in a patient with primary sclerosing cholangitis.

The aim of cholangiopancreatoscopy is the direct visualization of ductal strictures, particularly in the bile duct. The appearance of these strictures often facilitates the differentiation of benign from malignant disorders (Figure 4). Video ductal endoscopes provide images of high quality but, at present, do not permit endoscopic biopsy. In contrast, the SpyGlass system incorporates a fiberoptic probe with somewhat inferior images but, importantly, provides access for endoscopic biopsy. Histological confirmation of cancer can be achieved in 70-80% of patients (Nguyen et al., 2009).

3. Endoscopic interventions

3.1 Sphincterotomy and stone extraction

The contemporary technique of endoscopic sphincterotomy is remarkably similar to that described by Classen and Demling in 1974. The principles include selective cannulation of the bile duct with the papillotome, retraction of a diathermy wire to create a bow and passage of a current across the diathermy wire to make an endoscopic incision. This increases the diameter of the bile duct orifice from a pinhole to 2-5 mm. Prior to 1975, bile duct stones were initially left to pass spontaneously into the duodenum. However, within 2 years, stone extraction techniques had been described including the use of wire (Dormia) baskets and catheters with peripheral balloons (Figure 5, a-c).

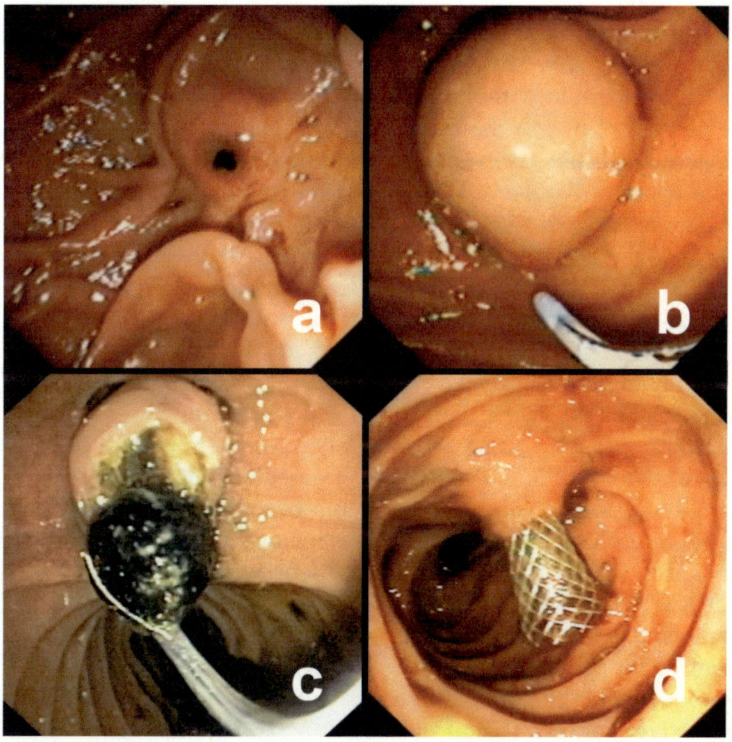

Fig. 5. Endoscopic features relevant to therapeutic endoscopy. (a) Impacted pigmented calculus in the orifice of the ampulla. (b) Bulbous papilla caused by an impacted calculus. (c) Extraction of a calculus after endoscopic sphincterotomy. (d) Metallic stent projecting into the duodenum in a patient with pancreatic cancer.

The above techniques have been remarkably successful when performed by experienced endoscopists. For example, most endoscopists now claim rates for successful extraction of stones of between 90 and 95% (Safrany, 1978; Roberts-Thomson, 1984). However, difficulties may arise with large stones, impacted stones, ampullary orifices located within duodenal diverticula and bile duct stones in patients who have previously been treated with a Billroth II gastrectomy. The management of large stones often includes fragmentation using reinforced crushing baskets. If endoscopic extraction of stones fails during the first attempt, one option is placement of a plastic stent around the stone (to minimize the risk of cholangitis) and a second attempt at stone extraction after 2-4 weeks. Another option is direct cholangioscopy with visualization of the stone and fragmentation with intraductal shockwave (electrohydraulic or laser) lithotripsy. In patients who have previously had a Billroth II gastrectomy, difficulties may arise with negotiation of the afferent loop, selective cannulation of the bile duct and appropriate orientation of the papillotome.

The complications of endoscopic sphincterotomy have been widely discussed and include pancreatitis (5%), significant bleeding from the margins of the incision (2%) and duodenal perforation (<1%). Mortality rates within 30 days are approximately 0.2% but only a minority of deaths are directly related to the procedure (Freeman et al., 1996; Cooper and Slivka, 2007).

3.2 Endoscopic stents

Options for patients with malignant strictures of the bile duct include radical surgery with the potential for cure, palliative surgery with a biliary bypass procedure and the endoscopic placement of a biliary stent. In patients scheduled for curative surgery, stents are sometimes used to relieve jaundice prior to the operation although this appears to be unnecessary in patients with a serum bilirubin of <250 μmol/l (van der Gaag et al., 2009). In patients who require palliative procedures, the choice of stent versus biliary bypass is often determined by factors such as age and perceived operative risk. For example, older patients with more complex medical problems are more likely to be treated with stents while younger patients with fewer operative risks are more likely to be treated by biliary bypass. An additional issue is the presence of malignant infiltration of the duodenum that may result in duodenal obstruction. In this setting, options include biliary and duodenal stents or a biliary bypass procedure with a gastroenterostomy.

The first endoscopic stents were composed of plastic and were 7F-8F in diameter. Subsequently, endoscopes with larger working-channels were introduced that permitted the insertion of larger stents (10F). Most patients treated with conventional 10F stents show improvement or resolution of jaundice but stents become obstructed by biofilms after 2-5 months. Attempts to prolong stent patency have included use of different plastic materials, changes in stent design and longer-term treatment with drugs such as antibiotics and ursodeoxycholic acid. These measures have been largely ineffective in clinical trials. Because of this, stents are usually changed electively at intervals of about 3 months in those patients who require stenting for prolonged periods.

Self-expanding metal stents (Figure 5d) are now widely used for palliation in patients with malignant obstructive jaundice (Chun et al., 2010). These stents expand to a diameter of approximately 30F (10 mm) and usually remain patent for 6-9 months. However, metal stents can still obstruct because of biofilms, the accumulation of biliary debris, tumor growth through the wire mesh or tumor growth above the stent. Additional issues are the higher cost of metallic stents and an inability to remove the stent if there are complications such as obstruction or cholangitis. However, these complications can usually be managed by insertion of a second metal stent or by the insertion of a plastic stent within the metal stent. Another approach that may delay tumor ingrowth is use of a "covered" metal stent although a potential problem is greater formation of biofilms. One practical approach is to use plastic stents in patients whose survival seems likely to be short and metal stents in patients with a predicted survival of more than 3-6 months.

3.3 EUS assisted therapeutic endoscopy

Access to the biliary system at ERCP can fail in 1-5% of patients. Reasons include large duodenal diverticula and a sphincter of Oddi that is either thickened or deformed. In this setting, one option is percutaneous cholangiography with passage of a guidewire into the duodenum. Another option is to use EUS to direct a 19F needle into the bile duct and then pass a guidewire into the duodenum. EUS with passage of a guidewire into the duodenum has also been used to facilitate cannulation of an obstructed main pancreatic duct. Success rates with these techniques are higher if ducts are dilated (Kim et al., 2010).

3.4 Cholangioscopy assisted therapeutic endoscopy

If difficulty is encountered with passage of a guidewire through a tight biliary stricture, it may be helpful to perform cholangioscopy with passage of a guidewire under direct vision. There are also reports of the use of cholangioscopes for the ablation of biliary tumors using either lasers or argon plasma coagulation (Nguyen et al., 2009).

3.5 Endoscopic ampullectomy

Neoplasms of the ampulla of Vater have traditionally been managed by laparotomy with local or more radical resections (Whipple's procedure). However, at least some neoplasms are now being managed by endoscopic resection, usually after staging by EUS. The technique of ampullectomy is similar to that for removal of larger polyps and includes elevation of the base with saline (with or without adrenaline) and resection using a polypectomy snare (Figure 6). In expert hands, successful eradication of adenomas has been reported in up to 85% of patients (Nguyen and Binmoeller, 2010). However, it may be inappropriate to attempt endoscopic resection for adenomas >4-5 cm in diameter because of higher risks for complications and higher rates of incomplete resection.

3.6 Endoscopic therapy for pancreatic pseudocysts, pancreatic necrosis and pancreatic ascites

Pancreatic pseudocysts can complicate both acute and chronic pancreatitis. The majority of pseudocysts are asymptomatic and resolve spontaneously. A drainage procedure is only indicated for pseudocysts that are symptomatic, infected, rapidly enlarging or causing obstruction of the gastrointestinal tract or neighbouring structures such as the biliary tract. An additional indication is the presence of cysts >10 cm in diameter because of the risk of spontaneous rupture or hemorrhage. Options for the drainage of pseudocysts include open or laparoscopic surgery, percutaneous drainage under US or CT guidance and endoscopic drainage with help from EUS. Unfortunately, these approaches have not been compared in randomized trials. Because of this, the choice of procedure is often determined by the availability of EUS and local expertise (Nguyen and Binmoeller, 2009). Percutaneous or endoscopic drainage is usually contraindicated for cysts that are multi-loculated or for cysts with solid components or other features suspicious of neoplasia.

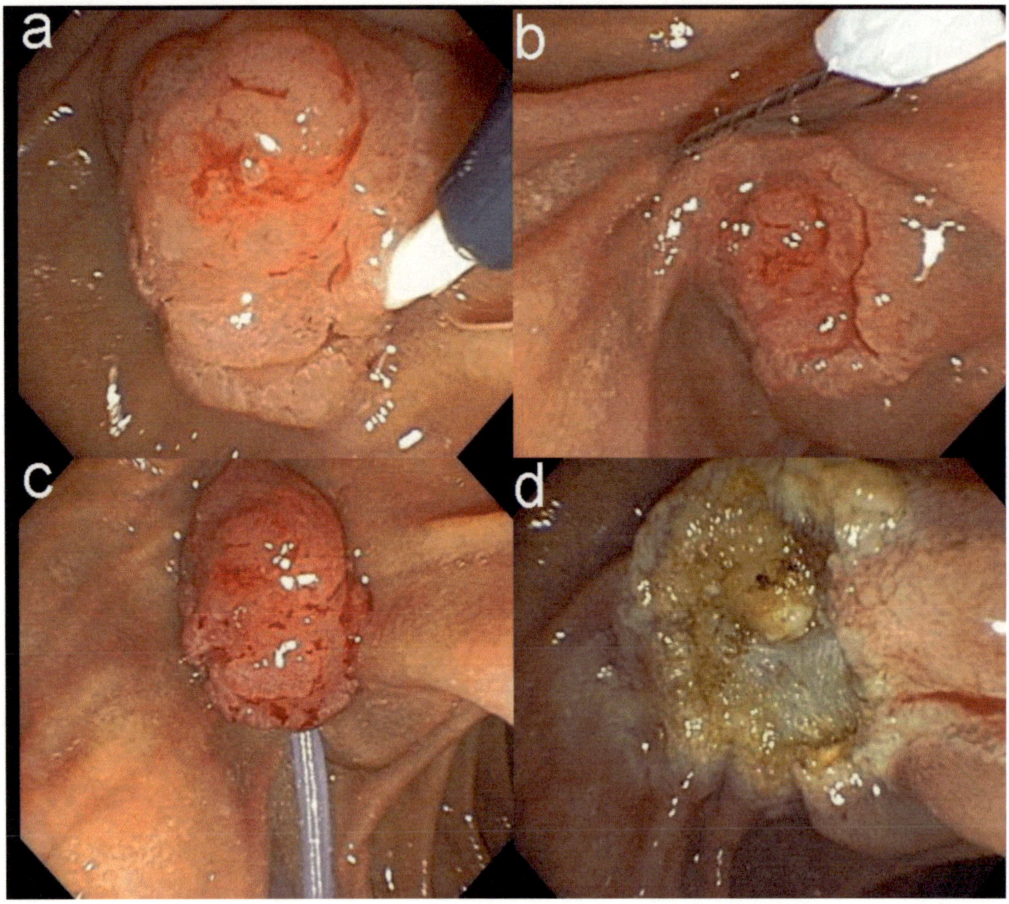

Fig. 6. *En bloc* endoscopic ampullectomy showing (a) an ampullary adenoma, (b & c) snaring of the adenoma in its entirety, (d) appearance of the area after resection.

Endoscopic approaches have also been used for the drainage of pancreatic fluid collections. These may develop because of severe pancreatitis or because of the development of pancreatic ascites. The latter is usually due to spontaneous rupture of a pseudocyst but, in a minority of cases, duct disruption can occur because of pancreatic necrosis. The endoscopic management of these patients needs to be individualized but may involve transpapillary drainage, transmural drainage or combined approaches. In this heterogeneous group, successful outcomes can be achieved in approximately 80% of patients although there are several potential complications including bleeding, perforation, infection and stent migration (Mergener and Kozarek, 2003).

3.7 Endoscopic therapy for chronic pancreatitis

Some patients with chronic pancreatitis have chronic pain or frequent episodes of pain that result in recurrent admissions to hospital or the use of escalating doses of narcotic analgesics. In this setting, management options include pancreatic surgery, endoscopic therapy and various measures for pain including a celiac plexus nerve block. At least one mechanism for pain is a degree of obstruction of the main pancreatic duct with elevated intraductal pressures. Because of this, some surgical and endoscopic approaches have endeavoured to relieve duct obstruction by removing stones or dilating or bypassing duct strictures. In calcific chronic pancreatitis, endoscopic removal of stones is difficult and many patients are treated by extracorporeal shockwave lithotripsy prior to endoscopic therapy. The latter usually involves biliary and pancreatic sphincterotomy, dilatation of strictures and extraction of stones in the main pancreatic duct. Responses to endoscopic therapy have been variable but most studies report improvement in pain in 30-70% of patients. Although these endoscopic results may be inferior to results from pancreatic surgery (Díte et al., 2003; Cahen et al., 2007), endoscopic therapy can be repeated with a relatively low risk for complications.

4. Future developments

Preliminary studies are evaluating the possibility of endoscopic therapy for solid and cystic neoplasms of the pancreas. One promising approach is EUS-guided ethanol lavage (with or without paclitaxel injections) for the treatment of cystic tumors of the pancreas (DeWitt et al., 2011; Oh et al., 2011). This appears to result in resolution of cysts in up to 70-80% of patients. Innovative approaches have also been taken for the treatment of locally advanced pancreatic cancer. These include EUS-guided injections of chemotherapeutic drugs and various immunomodulatory preparations including allogenic mixed lymphocyte cultures (Cytoimplants), adenovirus vectors carrying the tumor necrosis factor-alpha gene and attenuated adenoviruses that preferentially replicate in malignant cells. There are also on-going studies to evaluate local ablative therapies for cancer including therapies guided by EUS and therapies applied during direct visualization of ducts. Some of these therapies include radiofrequency ablation, photodynamic therapy and brachytherapy.

Other developments are likely to include endoscopes with multimodal features and endoscopic platforms that permit even more precise localization of lesions by combining information from radiological procedures in addition to EUS (Roberts-Thomson et al., 2010). It would also be helpful to have better endoscopic therapy for calcific chronic pancreatitis. One option is fragmentation of stones under direct vision using electrohydraulic lithotripsy or various lasers including the yttrium-aluminium-garnet (YAG) laser. There is also a need for more sensitive techniques for the diagnosis of biliary and pancreatic neoplasms that might include larger tissue samples or the identification of novel proteins or novel gene mutations.

5. Conclusion

The biliary tract and pancreas have now been explored with flexible endoscopes for 40 years. The era of diagnostic procedures using an injection of radiological contrast and fluoroscopy was soon followed by the therapeutic procedure of endoscopic sphincterotomy for bile duct stones. Subsequent developments included plastic and metallic stents for biliary obstruction and endoscopic therapy for chronic pancreatitis and pancreatic pseudocysts. More recently, direct visualization of biliary and pancreatic ducts has become possible using ultrathin endoscopes passed down the channel of conventional endoscopes. A complementary procedure is that of endoscopic ultrasound that facilitates biliary and pancreatic diagnoses, particularly when combined with fine-needle aspiration and tissue cytology. Future developments are likely to include various endoscopic therapies for cancer and the wider use of endoscopic procedures for complications of pancreatitis .

6. References

Cahen, D. L., D. J. Gouma, Y. Nio, E. A. Rauws, M. A. Boermeester, O. R. Busch, J. Stoker, J. S. Lameris, M. G. Dijkgraaf, K. Huibregtse and M. J. Bruno (2007). "Endoscopic versus surgical drainage of the pancreatic duct in chronic pancreatitis." N Engl J Med 356: 676-84.

Chun, H. J., E. S. Kim, J. J. Hyun, Y. D. Kwon, B. Keum and C. D. Kim (2010). "Gastrointestinal and biliary stents." J Gastroenterol Hepatol 25: 234-43.

Classen, M. and L. Demling (1974). "[Endoscopic sphincterotomy of the papilla of vater and extraction of stones from the choledochal duct (author's transl)]." Dtsch Med Wochenschr 99: 496-7.

Cooper, S. T. and A. Slivka (2007). "Incidence, risk factors, and prevention of post-ERCP pancreatitis." Gastroenterol Clin North Am 36: 259-76, vii-viii.

DeWitt, J., C. J. DiMaio and W. R. Brugge (2011). "Long-term follow-up of pancreatic cysts that resolve radiologically after EUS-guided ethanol ablation." Gastrointest Endosc 72: 862-6.

Díte, P., M. Ruzicka, V. Zboril and I. Novotny (2003). "A prospective, randomized trial comparing endoscopic and surgical therapy for chronic pancreatitis." Endoscopy 35: 553-8.

Freeman, M. L., D. B. Nelson, S. Sherman, G. B. Haber, M. E. Herman, P. J. Dorsher, J. P. Moore, M. B. Fennerty, M. E. Ryan, M. J. Shaw, J. D. Lande and A. M. Pheley (1996). "Complications of endoscopic biliary sphincterotomy." N Engl J Med 335: 909-18.

Gleeson, F. C. and M. Topazian (2007). "Endoscopic retrograde cholangiopancreatography and endoscopic ultrasound for diagnosis of chronic pancreatitis." Curr Gastroenterol Rep 9: 123-9.

Hochberger, J., S. Tex, J. Maiss and E. G. Hahn (2003). "Management of difficult common bile duct stones." Gastrointest Endosc Clin N Am 13: 623-34.

Horwhat, J. D., E. K. Paulson, K. McGrath, M. S. Branch, J. Baillie, D. Tyler, T. Pappas, R. Enns, G. Robuck, H. Stiffler and P. Jowell (2006). "A randomized comparison of EUS-guided FNA versus CT or US-guided FNA for the evaluation of pancreatic mass lesions." Gastrointest Endosc 63: 966-75.

Howell, D. A., W. G. Parsons, M. A. Jones, J. J. Bosco and B. L. Hanson (1996). "Complete tissue sampling of biliary strictures at ERCP using a new device." Gastrointest Endosc 43: 498-502.

Kawai, K., Y. Akasaka, K. Murakami, M. Tada and Y. Koli (1974). "Endoscopic sphincterotomy of the ampulla of Vater." Gastrointest Endosc 20: 148-51.

Kim, Y. S., K. Gupta, S. Mallery, R. Li, T. Kinney and M. L. Freeman (2010). "Endoscopic ultrasound rendezvous for bile duct access using a transduodenal approach: cumulative experience at a single center. A case series." Endoscopy 42: 496-502.

Kondo, S., H. Isayama, M. Akahane, N. Toda, N. Sasahira, Y. Nakai, N. Yamamoto, K. Hirano, Y. Komatsu, M. Tada, H. Yoshida, T. Kawabe, K. Ohtomo and M. Omata (2005). "Detection of common bile duct stones: comparison between endoscopic ultrasonography, magnetic resonance cholangiography, and helical-computed-tomographic cholangiography." Eur J Radiol 54: 271-5.

Lutz, H. and W. Rosch (1976). "Transgastroscopic ultrasonography." Endoscopy 8: 203-5.

McCune, W. S., P. E. Shorb and H. Moscovitz (1968). "Endoscopic cannulation of the ampulla of vater: a preliminary report." Ann Surg 167: 752-6.

Mergener, K. and R. A. Kozarek (2003). "Therapeutic pancreatic endoscopy." Endoscopy 35: 48-54.

Mohamadnejad, M., J. M. DeWitt, S. Sherman, J. K. LeBlanc, H. A. Pitt, M. G. House, K. J. Jones, E. L. Fogel, L. McHenry, J. L. Watkins, G. A. Cote, G. A. Lehman and M. A. Al-Haddad (2011). "Role of EUS for preoperative evaluation of cholangiocarcinoma: a large single-center experience." Gastrointest Endosc 73: 71-8.

Nguyen, N. and K. Binmoeller (2009). Endoscopic drainage of pancreatic fluid collections. Diagnostic and Therapeutic Procedures in Gastroenterology: An Illustrated Guide. A. Wu, and Varadarajulu, Humana Press: 211-221.

Nguyen, N. and K. Binmoeller (2010). "Endoscopic ampullectomy." Journal of Techniques in GI Endoscopy 12: 53-60.

Nguyen, N. Q., K. F. Binmoeller and J. N. Shah (2009). "Cholangioscopy and pancreatoscopy (with videos)." Gastrointest Endosc 70: 1200-10.

Oh, H. C., D. W. Seo, T. J. Song, S. H. Moon, H. Park do, S. Soo Lee, S. K. Lee, M. H. Kim and J. Kim (2011). "Endoscopic ultrasonography-guided ethanol lavage with paclitaxel injection treats patients with pancreatic cysts." Gastroenterology 140: 172-9.

Petersen, B. T. (2002). "ERCP outcomes: defining the operators, experience, and environments." Gastrointest Endosc 55: 953-8.

Roberts-Thomson, I. C. (1984). "Endoscopic sphincterotomy of the papilla of Vater: an analysis of 300 cases." Aust N Z J Med 14: 611-7.

Roberts-Thomson, I. C., R. Singh, E. Teo, N. Q. Nguyen and I. Lidums (2010). "The future of endoscopy." J Gastroenterol Hepatol 25: 1051-7.

Safrany, L. (1978). "Endoscopic treatment of biliary-tract diseases. An international study." Lancet 2: 983-5.

Soehendra, N. and V. Reynders-Frederix (1979). "[Palliative biliary duct drainage. A new method for endoscopic introduction of a new drain]." Dtsch Med Wochenschr 104: 206-7.

Takagi, K., S. Ikeda, Y. Nakagawa, N. Sakaguchi and T. Takahashi (1970). "Retrograde pancreatography and cholangiography by fiber duodenoscope." Gastroenterology 59: 445-52.

Tanaka, K. and M. Kida (2009). "Role of endoscopy in screening of early pancreatic cancer and bile duct cancer." Dig Endosc 21 Suppl 1: S97-S100.

van der Gaag, N. A., E. A. Rauws, C. H. van Eijck, M. J. Bruno, E. van der Harst, F. J. Kubben, J. J. Gerritsen, J. W. Greve, M. F. Gerhards, I. H. de Hingh, J. H. Klinkenbijl, C. Y. Nio, S. M. de Castro, O. R. Busch, T. M. van Gulik, P. M. Bossuyt and D. J. Gouma (2009). "Preoperative biliary drainage for cancer of the head of the pancreas." N Engl J Med 362: 129-37.

7

Endoscopic Management of Biliary Complications After Liver Transplantation

Firas Zahr ElDeen, Ching-Song Lee and Wei-Chen Lee
Chang-Gung Transplantation Institute, Chang-Gung Memorial Hospital, Chang-Gung University College of Medicine, Taoyuan, Taiwan

1. Introduction

Biliary reconstruction has been described 35 years ago by Sir Roy Calne as the technical 'Achilles heel' of orthotopic liver transplantation (OLT). The name "Achilles' heel" comes from Greek mythology, which is a metaphor of a single vulnerable spot. This is because the potential detrimental effects of biliary complications on graft and patient survival. Biliary complications, which "plagued" the early experience of liver transplantation occurring in nearly one of every three transplant recipients (Moser & Wall, 2001), have been reduced dramatically due to the improvements in organ selection, retrieval, preservation, and implantation techniques. However, biliary complications still remain a common source of morbidity and mortality (Greif et al., 1994). Additionally, they significantly affect the recipients' quality of life because they entail frequent readmissions, repeated imaging, invasive procedures, and even reoperation. All of them added to the financial and emotional toll suffer the patients (Sharma et al., 2008). Biliary leaks and strictures, either anastomotic or non-anastomotic, are the most frequent complications. Cystic duct obstruction due to mucocele, stones, sludge or casts, hemobilia and sphincter of Oddi dysfunction have also been recorded (Colonna et al., 1992; Greif et al., 1994). The surgical management used to be the standard of care for these conditions in earlier practice. However, the revolutionary progress in minimally invasive armamentarium, namely endoscopy and percutaneous radiologic interventional modalities, made it the current alternative first line of management displacing surgical intervention to be a second backup option (Sharma et al., 2008; Williams & Draganov, 2009). A living donor liver transplantation (LDLT) was first reported in 1988 by Raia in Brazil, followed by Nagasue in Japan in 1989. After the leading successful experience of right lobe living related liver transplantation (RL-LDLT) that has been reported by Hong Kong team in 1996, it rapidly evolved as a well-established practice in Asian countries. World wide organ shortage and promising results were alluring to other centers to consider (RL-LDLT) as a practical option. In this review we will shed more light on biliary complications related to right lobe living donor liver transplantation and their endoscopic management.

1.1 Incidence of biliary complications

Apparently, patients who were transplanted more recently are at increased risk of biliary complications. This could be explained by the awareness of this major problem, evolution of both invasive and non invasive diagnostic modalities, and more importantly, the marked increase in graft survival in the last decade since biliary problems such as strictures need some time to develop and become evident (Verdonk et al., 2006). The incidence of biliary complications is greatest in the first few months after transplantation. The frequency becomes very low after the first post transplantation year; however, occasionally appear after several years (Moser & Wall, 2001). The reported incidence of such complications differs considerably among centers which can be attributed to the wide variety of research methodologies as well as the different surgical techniques adopted. In a review article which included six studies over several years from various countries, the overall biliary complication rate in deceased donor liver transplantation (DDLT) averaged 17.3% (range, 9%-30%) with 6.8% (range, 0.3%-17%) bile leaks and 7.5% (range, 3%-13%) strictures (Dualilibi et al., 2010). While, overall biliary complication incidence in living donor liver transplantation (LDLT) was found to be 28.7% (range, 16.1%-33.3%) with 17.1% (range, 9.3%-23%) bile leaks and 15.2% (range, 9.3%-27%) strictures. These results were higher compared to those in other reviews. For instance, in a review article (Pascher & Neuhaus, 2005), 18.3% (8%-26.6%) was the reported incidence of biliary complications after right hepatic lobe grafting with 10.5% (range, 0%-26.6%) leakages and 9.1% (range, 3.3%-20%) strictures. Finally our results in right lobe LDLT show that rate of leakage and stricture were 14.4% and 18.9%, respectively (Lee et al., 2008). From the above figures, overall rate of biliary complications was lower in DDLT compared with LDLT; however, variables were poorly linked. Perhaps standardization of methodologies and large scale research could help us to discover correlations between complications and modalities of transplantation. Taken together, higher rates of biliary complications may suggest that the inherently sensitive nature of the biliary epithelium is more vulnerable to ischemic damage in comparison with hepatocytes and vascular endothelium (Sharma et al., 2008).

1.2 Etiology and classification of biliary complications after liver transplantation

The etiology of biliary complications is multifactorial. Risk factors implicated include elderly donor (Shah et al., 2007), gender mismatch with a female donor/male recipient (Verdonk et al., 2006), female recipient, age of recipient, severity of original disease, variations in the biliary tract anatomy, number and size of reconstructed bile dust(s), techniques in graft procurement and diseased liver removal, ischemic damage to bile duct (hepatic artery complication, warm and cold ischemia time, bile duct blood supply), method of biliary reconstruction (type, suture methods, suture material, stent, or T-tube use), immunological issues (ABO incompatibility, preformed antibody), infection (biliary sepsis, cytomegalovirus) (Todo et al., 2005). Moreover, Bile leakage after transplantation has been considered as a significant risk factor for the development of strictures (Lee et al., 2008; Shah et al., 2007; Verdonk et al., 2006). Other uncommon etiological factors that may present with biliary obstruction are post-transplantation lymphoproliferative disease and recurrent or de novo cancer (Wojcicki et al., 2008). In a review article published in 2005 (Todo et al., 2005), authors broadly classified the factors that must be considered while contemplating biliary complications, namely, biliary strictures after LDLT into two categories: anatomical and technical.

2. Anatomical factors

2.1 Bile duct anatomy

Clear understanding of biliary anatomy is crucial in living donor liver transplantation to ensure donor safety and to minimize complications in recipients. According to Couinaud's classification, patterns of the hepatic duct confluence fall into six groups: (A) typical anatomy (57%), (B) triple confluence (12%), (C) ectopic drainage of a right duct (anterior or posterior) into the common hepatic duct (20%), (D) ectopic drainage of a right duct (anterior or posterior) into the left hepatic duct (6%), (E) absence of the hepatic duct confluence (3%), and (F) absence of the right hepatic duct and ectopic drainage of the right posterior duct into the cystic duct (2%). These findings are comparable to those observed during hepatic resection and LDLT donor surgeries. Thanks to recent imaging modalities, particularly multiphase three-dimensional studies, that allowed us to identify invaluable preoperative information on the graft volume and the vascular structures. However, imaging studies of the biliary tree are still significantly less reliable. Therefore, it has been suggested to perform intraoperative cholangiography at every donor hepatpectomy in LDLT to confirm bile duct anatomy and the point of bile duct transection (Todo et al., 2005).

2.2 Blood supply of bile duct

Bile duct receives 60% its blood supply from axial branches arising from the posterior superior pancreaticoduodenal artery and the gastro-duodenal artery at 3 O'clock and 9 O'clock positions; while right and left hepatic arteries provides 38% of blood supply via a fine arterial plexus at the inferior aspect of the hilar plate nourishing the confluence and bilateral hepatic ducts. The remaining 2% of blood supply comes from the proper hepatic artery via transversal branches. Therefore, injury of the hilar plexus during donor or recipient hepatectomy may lead to leakage, stricture, or even necrosis due to bile duct ischemia (Todo et al., 2005).

3. Technical considerations

3.1 Donor hepatectomy (Graft harvesting)

Standard techniques and refinements in graft preparation have been described thoroughly in literature. Technical safeguards have been stressed upon based on biliary and arterial anatomical considerations including intraoperative cholangiography which has been advocated for safer intrahepatic bile duct division, leaving at least 2 mm stump from the confluence to secure safe closure, avoidance of dissection between hepatic duct and the hepatic artery beyond level of transection to maintain uninterrupted blood supply to bile ducts, avoidance of ischemic damage to the graft bile duct by excessive use of diathermy, and using fine suture ligation alternatively to control minor bleeding (Todo et al., 2005).

3.2 Recipient hepatectomy (Liver explantation)

By the same token, we should bear in mind biliary and arterial anatomical considerations in recipient hepatectomy. Preservation of uninterrupted blood supply to the biliary tract as high as possible in the hilum and leaving enough length for a tension-free biliary anastomosis are paramount. This has been fulfilled by a high hilar dissection method or intrahepatic Glissonian approach that proposed by Lee et al. and they showed good results in their series of adult duct to duct liver transplantation patients (Todo et al., 2005).

3.3 Graft implantation (Biliary reconstruction)

3.3.1 Type of biliary anastomosis

Early practice of utilizing gallbladder as a pedicle graft biliary conduit had been abandoned due to associated bile stasis with stone formation, frequent episodes of cholangitis and inferior outcomes. Roux-en-Y hepaticojejunostomy was the standard biliary reconstruction in living-donor liver transplantation and split liver transplantation. The growing evidence and experience in transplantation urged the surgeons to restore bilioenteric continuity through a duct-to-duct anastomosis which becomes the preferred choice of biliary reconstruction whenever possible and this for the following reasons: (i) technically faster, less number of anstomoses, (ii) preserved function of sphincter of Oddi as a defense against enteric reflux and ascending cholangitis, (iii) no need for intestinal manipulation, thus preventing possible intraoperative contamination and earlier oral feeding, (iv) the physiological bilio-enteric continuity enabling endoscopic access after right lobe-LDLT and (v) more treatment options for biliary complications including percutaneous approach, endoscopic approach, surgical revision, and surgical conversion to Roux-en-Y bilioenteric anastomosis (Yazumi & Chiba, 2005). Duct-to-duct anastomosis has been increasingly reported in right lobe living-donor transplants (Shah et al., 2007), in right lobe split transplants and also has been shown to be feasible in left lobe living-donor liver transplants. In earlier experience of living donor liver transplantation, duct-to-duct anastomosis has been only performed in presence of single biliary anastomosis. The use of the recipient right and left hepatic ducts as well as the cystic duct has been successfully utilized in later practice (Gondolesi et al., 2004). Having said that, Roux-en-Y reconstruction is still indispensable in pediatric LDLT, patients with bile duct diseases or prior biliary surgery, retransplantation (Todo et al., 2005), left lateral segment split liver grafts, left lateral segment and left lobe living donor grafts in presence of separate segmental II and III ducts, segment IV duct draining into the confluence, and the presence of multiple small bile ducts in grafts harvested with caudate lobe; and still an option in right lobe graft with multiple small bile ducts (Cuinaud's classification, types C-F). It is worth to mention that both duct-to-duct anastomosis and jujenal loop could be used in the same patient having a graft with multiple small ducts (Wojcicki et al., 2008). In an article published in 2005 (Yazumi & Chiba, 2005), the incidence of biliary complications has been reviewed and it had been shown the incidence of anatomotic leakage in right lobe living donor liver transplantation (RL-LDLT) with Roux-en-Y hepatico-jujonostomy (RYHJ) was higher than that with duct-to-duct anastomosis (12.4%- 18.2% and 4.7%-7.3%, respectively), while on the other side, the incidence of anastomotic stricture in RL-LDLT with RYHJ was found to be less than that with duct-to-duct anastomosis (8.3%-16.3% and 24.3%-31.7% , respectively) (Yazumi & Chiba, 2005). Although the superiority of either hepaticojejunostomy or duct-to-duct for biliary reconstruction in adult LDTT was debatable issue, it has been concluded that surgeons should follow the principle of tension-free, viable anastomosis, and be accustomed to both procedures at the forum of European Association for the Study of the Liver in 2005 annual meeting (Todo et al., 2005).

3.3.2 Stent or no stent

There is an ongoing hot debate regarding the use of a T tube for duct-to-duct anastomosis. Traditionally, proponents of using biliary stents argue that T tube aids to access biliary tree, monitor the quality and quantity of bile output, decrease the incidence of late anastomotic strictures, and lower the pressure in the biliary system which may be elevated as a result of anastomotic stricture or to sphincter of Oddi dysfunction (Rabkin et al., 1998). On the other hand, biliary drains were considered by opponents to increase complication rates as shown by frequent reports of biliary leak following bile drain removal, dislodgement, cholangitis and/or biliary obstruction (Greif et al., 1994; Scatton et al., 2001). The incidence of biliary drain related complications was found to range between 10 and 22% (Wojcicki et al., 2008), with bile leak after bile drain removal occurring in 5–15% of patients (Scatton et al., 2001; Vougas et al., 1996). The use of T tube in deceased-donor liver transplantation has been widely abandoned. This practice has been adopted after two prospective randomized trials (Scatton et al., 2001) showing that not using T tubes seems to be safe, efficacious, and cost-effective. Some have suggested that using 6 F double J ureteric as internal stents theoretically could eliminate possible complications associated with T tubes and offers the potential benefits of a splint. Yet, this has not shown uniformly reproducible results (Sharma et al., 2008). Stenting or no stenting of biliary reconstruction in living donor liver transplantation is still a debate that is far from being settled (Wojcicki et al., 2008).

3.3.3 Suturing technique and suture material

Using continuous or interrupted sutures, conventional or microscopic biliary reconstruction, absorbable or non absorbable sutures material in biliary anastomsis, is also a technical issue that has not been standardized. However, some authors recently advocated the use of microsurgical technique and synthetic non-absorbable sutures (Lin et al., 2009) for their feasibility, easier handling, supposedly less induction of the tissue reaction (Sharma et al., 2008) and theoretical durability in the early postoperative period especially with steroid based immunosuppressive regimen.

3.3.4 Implantation (vascular reconstruction)

Ischemic biliary problems are among the most troublesome complications both in early and late post transplantation periods. Two main broad categories are identified: hepatic artery thrombosis (HAT) and ischemic type biliary lesions (ITBL).

3.3.4.1 Hepatic artery thrombosis (HAT) or macroangiopathy

Hepatic artery thrombosis is generally divided into two categories: early and late hepatic artery thrombosis (eHAT and late HAT). Reports on eHAT are heterogeneous due to a lack of a commonly accepted definition. A systematic review by Bekker et al. from Netherlands that included all published work from 1990 to 2007 has provided us with valuable definitions. Early HAT is defined as a thromboembolic occlusion of the hepatic artery that occurrs within 2 months after liver transplantation (Bekker et al., 2009). The incidence of eHAT was found to be significantly higher in children (8.3%) than in adults (2.9%). eHAT presents with liver failure, hepatic necrosis, or bile duct necrosis in up to 58%of affected patients (Tzakis et al., 1985). Uncontrollable sepsis in the immunocompromised recipients and ultimately death are common scenarios after eHAT. Collaterals probably prevent similar ominous outcome in case of late HAT. Cholangiographic findings are characterized by confluent intraductal filling defects within irregular dilated or strictured bile ducts. These findings were reported in more than 80% of patients with hepatic artery thrombosis and were frequently associated with intrahepatic bile leak and biloma formation (Tzakis et al., 1985). In comparison, hepatic artery stenosis has a wide spectrum of presentations. Many patients only present with nonspecific elevation in liver enzyme levels, however abnormal cholangiograms can be present in up to 67% of patients with hepatic artery stenosis even in absence of any evident abnormality by Ultrasonorgraphy (Orons et al., 1995a). Early diagnosis is critical to avoid permanent allograft damage. Orons and coworkers found that the treatment of hepatic artery stenosis with balloon angioplasty was of limited benefit once significant allograft dysfunction had occurred (Orons et al., 1995b). The reported risk factors for eHAT are cytomegalovirus mismatch (seropositive donor liver in seronegative recipient), retransplantation, arterial conduits, prolonged operation time, low recipient weight, variant arterial anatomy, and low volume transplantation centers. However, the exact cause of eHAT remains debatable. Incidence of eHAT was found to be higher in low volume centers, while no difference in incidence of eHAT was found between studies reporting only on living donor liver transplantation versus studies reporting only on deceased donor liver transplantation; also no difference in incidence of eHAT in the living donor liver transplantation (LDLT) subgroup was found in centers using the operation microscope for the arterial anastomosis versus centers using loupe magnification. It has been found that revascularization attempt was performed in approximately half of the cases with a reported success rate of about 50%, therefore, early detection and urgent revascularization are paramount especially in centers that lack a back up system for urgent retransplanation (Bekker et al., 2009).

3.3.4.2 Ischemic type biliary lesions (ITBL) or microangiopathy

The incidence of ITLB varies between 5% and 15%. The exact pathophysiological mechanism of ITBL is still unclear, however, several risk factors have been identified and strongly suggested a multifactorial origin. Ischemia-reperfusion and preservation injury related variables are well-described risk factors for non-anastomotic strictures including prolonged cold ischemia time (>12 hours) or warm ischemia time (>60 minutes) and variables related to the efficacy of preservation of the peribiliary plexus, such as viscosity and perfusion pressure of the preservation fluid (Guichelaar et al., 2003; Verdonk et al., 2007). Generally speaking, as suggested by Buis et al., risk factors for ITBL can be divided into three categories: ischemia-related injury to the biliary epithelium, immunologically mediated injury, and cytotoxic injury induced by bile salts (Buis et al., 2006).

3.3.4.2.1 Cold ischemic and reperfusion injury

It has been shown by many studies that prolonged cold ischemia time (CIT) predisposes to ITBL. In an experimental study using cell cultures, it has been shown that biliary epithelial cells are more susceptible to reperfusion/re-oxygenation injury than hepatocytes. Moreover, clinical evidence was provided in a clinical study as reflected by postoperative peaks in serum aspartate aminotransferase and alanine aminotransferase (Buis et al., 2006).

3.3.4.2.2 Preservation injury

Preservation injury was found to increase the arterial resistance, leading to circulatory disturbances in the small capillaries of the biliary plexus (Buis et al., 2006).

3.3.4.2.3 Warm ischemic injury

Bile ducts, that are solely dependent on arterial blood supply for their nourishment, are exposed to warm ischemia during initial reperfusion via the portal vein alone. However, favorable effect of simultaneous arterial and portal reperfusion on the incidence of ITBL could not be clearly demonstrated. Moreover, the higher incidence of non-anastomotic strictures in liver transplantation from donors after cardiac death also strongly suggests an ischemia-related factor in its pathogenesis. Several studies have provided evidence for an immunological injury in the pathogenesis of ITBL such as ABO-incompatible liver transplantation and pre-existing diseases with a presumed autoimmune component, such as primary sclerosing cholangitis (PSC), autoimmune hepatitis (AIH), cytomegalovirus (CMV) infection, chronic rejection, and genetic polymorphism of chemokines (Buis et al., 2006).

4. Biliary complications in recipient

4.1 Biliary leak

Bile leaks are the second most common biliary tract complication in many series (Greif et al., 1994; Rerknimitr et al., 2002a). As we mentioned before, the incidence of anastomotic biliary leakage in right lobe live donor living transplants with bilioenteric anastomosis and that with duct-to-duct reconstruction were 12.4%-18.2% and 4.7%-7.3%, respectively. Remarkably, refractory biliary leakage was found to be associated with significant mortality in bilioenteric reconstruction patients and 12%-19.1% of the patients died from sepsis (Yazumi & Chiba, 2005). However, the incidence of early bile leak appears to be equal in patients with duct-to-duct anastomosis with or without a T-tube (Rabkin et al., 1998; Scatton et al., 2001). Generally, bile leakage could be divided into anastomotic and non-anastomotic in site. Non-anastomotic leaks could occur from the T tube exit site or tract, cystic duct stump, duct of Lushka or damaged accessory bile ducts or from the cut surface of the graft in LDLT (Greif et al., 1994; Rabkin et al., 1998; Thuluvath et al., 2005; Wojcicki et al., 2008). The diagonosis of bile leak was primarily evidenced by extravasation of contrast medium in retrograde endoscopic cholangiogram or bile-stained fluid in percutaneous drainage. Leaks could be categorized as early and late postoperative leaks (Thuluvath et al., 2005). As a general rule, the majority of bile leaks occurs early in the postoperative period and mandates intervention to avoid sepsis (Greif et al., 1994). However, bile leakage could be successfully managed either by endoscopic therapy as a first option, percutaneous transhepatic cholangiography-guided drainage, or surgical reconstruction. Bile leakage remains as a risk factor for subsequent development of anastomotic stricture. Endoscopic management seems to be the treatment of choice in biliary leakage as it offers excellent diagnostic and therapeutic results. It can treat over 90% of biliary tract leaks with minimal morbidity (Greif et al., 1994; Ostroff et al., 1990; Pfau et al., 2000; Thuluvath et al., 2005). By the same notion followed in management of biliary complications, percutaneous transhepatic approach or surgery should be reserved for patients in whom the endoscopic approach failed (Thuluvath et al., 2005).

4.1.1 Early postoperative leaks (within 4 weeks)

Early leaks usually occur from the anastomotic site, and most probably due to technical problems and/or local ischemia (Thuluvath et al., 2005; Wojcicki et al., 2008). These risk factors may include insufficient arterial supply to the biliary anastomosis, active bleeding from cut ends of bile ducts, denuding the bile ducts during harvesting, excessive tension on ductal anastomosis or excessive use of diathermy to control bleeding on the bile ducts (Thuluvath et al., 2005). Therefore, high index of suspicion should be maintained to exclude any hepatic artery thrombosis or any vascular compromise. In one report, cut surface biliary leakage developed in 8.3% patients (Gondolesi et al., 2004), and this may be explained by increased pressure of the intrahepatic bile duct (Pascher & Neuhaus, 2005). Double or triple hepaticojejunostomies were found to be significant risk factor for biliary leakage in patients with bilioenteric anastomosis (Kasahara et al., 2006). Welling et al. showed that warm ischemia was the only independent risk factor for a leakage, however, direct correlation of warm ishchemia to biliary stictures did not reach statistical significance in their study (Welling et al., 2008). In presence of T tube, leaks are easily diagnosed with a T tube cholangiogram and can be managed conservatively as leaks frequently is resolved on their own after a short course of unclamping of the T tube (Thuluvath et al., 2005; Wojcicki et al.,

2008). In the absence of a T tube, HIDA scanning or MRCP may be needed to diagnose bile leaks. However, if there is strong clinical suspicion or evidence like bile in drains, retrograde endoscopic stenting of the bile duct is preferable option, since endosocopy is both diagnostic and therapeutic and could identify the site of leaks in over 90% of patients (Pfau et al., 2000; Thuluvath et al., 2005). When leakage is suspected with a T−tube in situ and conservative management failed to control the leak, a 10 Fr biliary stent could be placed and then T tube should be removed. Although some reported success in sealing leaks within 6 weeks of stenting (Pfau et al., 2000), others recommended to leave the tube in place for approximately 2-3 months as healing is delayed probably due to immunosuppressive drug treatment and this approach is supported by the occurrence of bile leaks through the T tube exit site even with 3-4 months of T tube placement (Thuluvath et al., 2005).

Larger leaks, particularly those associated with bilioenteric anastomosis, tend to be less amenable to non-operative treatment. Immediate or early operative revision should be strongly considered as intestinal loop of the anastomosis increase the chance of intraabdominal abscess formation and sepsis. In case of bilioenteric anastomosis without a transanastomotic catheter in place, a bile leak could be diagnosed with ultrasound, computed tomography, magnetic resonance imaging, hepatobiliary scintigraphy and in selected cases with PTC, which was followed by non-surgical management of infection and leakage by systemic antibiotics. Percutaneous transhepatic biliary drainage and/or percutaneous transabdominal biloma and abscess drainage must be fully resolved before surgical reconstruction because regional sepsis and poor infection control can result in recurrent biliary leaks (Thuluvath et al., 2005). Non-surgical conservative treatment involves carrying out a PTC with placement of an internal-external drain that can be sequentially upsized for a total period of 3-6 months of stenting. However, surgical intervention may be required when conservative management fails or as a first line of treatment if there is evidence of HAT, or if the duct-to-duct anastomotic defect is too large. Traditionally, the duct-to-duct anastomosis is converted to a Roux-en-Y choledochojejunostomy which allows wide debridement of necrotic and infected tissue (Thuluvath et al., 2005).

4.1.2 Late postoperative bile leaks

Late postoperative bile duct leaks are nearly always related to elective or inadvertent removal of the T tube (Thuluvath et al., 2005). The incidence of late bile duct leakage is 7% (Scatton et al., 2001) with a mean time to presentation of 118 days after transplantation despite prolonged T tube placement (Thuluvath et al., 2005). Scatton et al. reported in their large randomized trial that the incidence of biliary fistula in DDLT was found to be 10% in the T-tube group and 2.2% in the group without a T tube (Scatton et al., 2001). Although the classical clinical picture of persistent abdominal discomfort or pain after T tube removal prompts the diagnosis of biliary leakage in most cases, the diagnosis is also suggested in a small subset of patients based on fluctuating cyclosporine levels, pneumoperitoneum or increased leakage through the T tube tract. Leaks resulting from T tubes are managed successfully by endoscopic placement of internal stents with resolution rate near to 100% (Pfau et al., 2000). In management of biliary leakage, several endoscopic strategies have also been described, such as biliary stents, nasobiliary drainage, sphincterotomy, or combination of the techniques. In the two large series, nasobiliary catheters were used successfully to treat post-transplant leaks (Ostroff et al., 1990). Other investigators have noted high closure rates with decompression by endoscopic sphincterotomy alone. It appears that any endoscopic technique significantly reduces or eliminates the pressure gradient between bile duct and duodenum will seal a biliary fistula (Rerknimitr et al., 2002a). Some reported that majority of patients could be discharged within 48 hours after endoscopic stenting (Thuluvath et al., 2005). Nasobiliary tube has some advantages that it allows cholangiographic follow–up every 3-5 days and is easily removed without the need for another endoscopic intervention. Sherman et al. reported symptomatic relief of patients within 12 hours of nasobiliary stenting, and closure of fistula at a mean of 6.3 days (Sherman et al., 1993). However, inconvenience due to nasal tube, prolonged hospital stay, in addition to alteration of cyclosporine bioavailability due to biliary diversion is considered among the disadvantages of this approach (Thuluvath et al., 2005).

4.2 Biliary strictures

Generally, biliary strictures could be classified into anastomotic strictures (AS) and non-anastomotic strictures (NAS). The former type is more frequent in living donor OLT as compared to recipients of deceased donor OLT (Tsujino et al., 2006; Yazumi et al., 2006). Strictures can present at any time after transplantation. The incidence is greatest in the first 5 to 8 months (range, 1 to 36 months) (Gondolesi et al., 2004; Yazumi & Chiba, 2005; Kasahara et al., 2006). Recently, it has been suggested that prevalence continues to increase with time after transplantation (Verdonk et al., 2006), and that NAS presents earlier than AS, with mean time 3.3-5.9 months (Graziadei et al., 2006; Guichelaar et al., 2003). Moreover, NAS secondary to ischemic causes was shown to present within 1 year of the transplant, whereas the occurrence after 1 year was more often secondary to immunological causes (Verdonk et al., 2007).

4.2.1 Diagnosis

Timely management of biliary complications is paramount to avoid unnecessary diagnostic procedures, improves graft survival, reduces morbidity, mortality and decreases the financial and psychological toll that patients suffer. High index of suspicion must be maintained for early diagnosis, and therefore, it would be desirable to have an easy and non-invasive diagnostic tool for differentiation between different causes of cholestasis. However, the exact diagnosis and localization of post transplant biliary strictures prior to endoscopic cholangiography are unfortunately difficult for the following reasons (Shastri et al., 2007; Zoepf et al., 2005): (1) Pain, a feature of Charcot's triad, may be absent in the transplant setting because of immunosuppression and hepatic denervation; (2) Derangements in biochemical profile may be misleading as it could be due to recurrence of the underlying pretransplant liver illnesses or graft rejection; (3) Clinical symptoms like fever, anorexia are non-specific; (4) Epithelial casts may fill the biliary system rendering it difficult to be visualized by indirect radiological imaging; and (5) Dilatation of the biliary system in allografts may develop slower (Thuluvath et al., 2005; Verdonk et al., 2006; Williams & Draganov, 2009).

4.2.1.1 Value of biochemical and laboratory parameters

There are diverse results about the value of biochemical parameters either in prediction or follow up of biliary complications. Some reported that they are not reliable enough (Thuluvath et al., 2005) or just could provide a hint to detect biliary complications post transplantation (Zoepf et al., 2005). While others concluded that Gamma glutamyl transferase (GGT) and serum alkaline phosphatase (AP) (Shastri et al., 2007), but not serum bilirubin, to be early, non-invasive and inexpensive diagnostic markers. Moreover, they could be of great help during follow up and to correlate with adequacy of endoscopic therapy in patients presenting with early onset biliary complications after transplantation. However, others found that elevated serum bilirubin level >1.5 mg/dL is highly sensitive tool with negative predictive value of 100% and its decline is well correlated with clinical and radiographic improvement (Venu et al., 2007).

4.2.1.2 Value of radiological modalities in diagnosis of biliary strictures

Ultrasonography (US) with Doppler examination of hepatic vessels is usually the first imaging modality of choice when a biliary complication is suspected, followed by biliary imaging and may be biopsy depending on the pattern of liver test abnormalities. However, in post–transplant patients, the interpretation of histological findings due to ischemia, recurrence of liver disease or rejection can sometimes be misleading. Retrograde endoscopic cholangiography (ERC) can directly show the patency of biliary tree or the stenosis of biliary stree and show the site of stenosis/stricture. Definitely, ERC is the better diagnostic option than other modalities. Hepatic angiography may be indicated if hepatic vascular abnormality was suspected (Thuluvath et al., 2005). US may have low sensitivity (close to 50%) to detect biliary dilatation in patients who received transplantation (Graziadei et al., 2006; Zoepf et al., 2005) and not accurate enough to diagnose or localize biliary strictures either because the true diameter of cast filled bile ducts could not be properly determined, acute obstruction may not result in a prompt dilatation of the prestenotic bile ducts (Zoepf et al., 2005) or because dilatation of the biliary system in allografts may develop slower (Shastri et al., 2007). Different studies reported variable results for helical computed tomography and magnetic resonance imaging. However, exact data were not available, questionable or not applicable due to low accuracy in localizing stricture site (Zoepf et al., 2005). While Scintigraphy of the hepatobiliary tract is rarely performed when biliary stricture is suspected but still remains an excellent test to detect biliary leaks. Magnetic resonance cholangiography (MRC) was shown to have a sensitivity of 95%, a positive predictive value of 98% and an overall accuracy of 95% compared to ERCP as the reference standard (Valls et al., 2005). Due to the progressive advancement in its computation modes, it is suggested that MRC becomes the most promising future diagnostic tool before referral to endoscopic intervention. Recently, a hepatocyte-specific contrast agent gadolinium ethoxybenzyl diethylenetriamine pentaacetic acid (Gd-EOB-DTPA)–enhanced MR cholangiography has been utilized in evaluation of biliary anatomy, differentiation of biliary from extrabiliary lesions, assessment of bile duct obstruction, detection of bile duct injury including leakage and stricture, evaluation of biliary-enteric anastomoses, post-procedure evaluation, differentiation of biloma from other pathologic conditions, and evaluation of sphincter of Oddi dysfunction, and was found to be effective. However, the clinical applications of this imaging technique have not yet been fully explored. Moreover, the chief disadvantage of MRC in general, beyond lack of availability, is the lack of its therapeutic ability (Williams & Draganov, 2009). Currently, cumulative results confirm that none of the indirect imaging modalities could replace direct cholangiography for diagnosis of post transplantation biliary strictures (Pascher & Neuhaus, 2006; Pfau et al., 2000; Rerknimitr et al., 2002; Thuluvath et al., 2005; Zoepf et al., 2005).

4.2.2 Anastomotic strictures (AS)

Incidence of anastomotic strictures reported is around 5%-10% of transplanted patients. AS is usually isolated, short in length, and resulted from fibrotic changes within the first year after transplantation (Greif et al., 1994; Verdonk et al., 2006). Surgical technical issues seem to be the most important etiological factors in the early post transplant period, and may include improper techniques, small diameter of the bile ducts, size mismatch between the donor and recipient bile ducts, tension at the anastomosis, excessive use of electrocauterization for control of bile duct bleeding, infection and bile leakage which has been found to be an independent risk factor for AS (Lee et al., 2008; Welling et al. 2008). Later onset anastomotic stricture is most likely to indicate fibrotic changes due to ischemia either of donor or recipient bile duct (Verdonk et al., 2007; Pascher & Neuhaus, 2006).

4.2.2.1 Management of AS

The trend in management of AS has changed over the past 20 years from predominantly surgical to primarily endoscopic, namely endoscopic regtrograde cholangiography (ERC). ERC is considered as the gold standard, most physiological, least invasive diagnostic and therapeutic interventional option that carries good long term results in terms of graft and patient survival. ERC has an overall success rate in the range of 70%-100% in deceased donor liver transplantation (DDLT) (Graziadei et al., 2006; Morelli et al., 2003; Thuluvath et al., 2005; Williams & Draganov, 2009) and 60-75% in living donor liver transplantation (LDLT) (Hisatsune et al., 2003; Tsujino et al., 2006; Yazumi & Chiba, 2006). Percutaneous transhepatic cholangiography (PTC), although it has high success rate (50%-75%), is most often spared as a second line option for patients with Roux-en-Y bilioenteric reconstruction or failed ERC; and this is because the possible associated morbidities of PTC like hemorrhage and bile leak ((Sharma et al., 2008; Williams & Draganov, 2009). In high volume centers with experienced endoscopists, newer approaches of ERC have been described using the variable stiffness pediatric colonoscope, double balloon enteroscope, single balloon enteroscope, and spiral overtube. Moreover, both techniques could be combined by "rendezvous" endoscopy when endoscopic access to the anastomotic stricture can not be obtained. It is worth to mention that using ERCP or PTC is not only dependent on the type of biliary reconstruction, but also on the possibility of therapeutic intervention and the available expertise (Williams & Draganov, 2009). Therapeutic ERCP whether is successful or ultimately unsuccessful and necessitating surgical intervention does not negatively affect survival. Therefore, in the majority of patients with biliary complications, a trial of endoscopic therapy should be performed to delay or defer a post-OLT surgical procedure (Pfau et al., 2000). Surgical revision is now only reserved for patients who have failed the endoscopic and transhepatic percutaneous measures. Surgical revision in the form of Roux-en-Y bilio-enteric reconstruction is usually the operation of choice in patients with duct-to-duct anastomosis. In those who already have a Roux-en-Y bilioenteric anastomosis, repositioning the graft bile duct to a better vascularized area may be required (Verdonk et al., 2007), while retransplantation could be the last resort when all else fail (Graziadei et al., 2006; Williams & Draganov, 2009).

4.2.2.2 Deceased donor liver transplantation (DDLT)

Factors found to be associated with poor outcome and/or higher recurrence following endoscopic treatment or stent removal include delayed initial presentation (more than 6 months after transplantation), presence of tight strictures (Alazmi et al., 2006; Verdonk et al., 2007), presence of bile leaks, and use of T tubes (Sharma et al., 2008; Alazmi et al., 2006). The conventional method of endoscopic treatment comprises of stricture localization followed by guidewire cannulation, balloon dilatation, and subsequent placement of plastic stents. It has been reported that success rate of balloon dilation is approximately 40% (Shwartz et al.,

2000); however, additional stent placement seems to have more successful and durable outcomes in 75% of patients (Shwartz et al., 2000; Zoepf et al., 2005). Dual or multiple stents placed side by side further improves outcomes in up to 80-90% of patients (Morelli et al., 2003; Graziadei et al., 2006). The stents are generally replaced by larger stents every 3 months (Shwartz et al., 2000; Morelli et al., 2003) to prevent the complication of clogging, cholangitis, or stone formation (Sharma et al., 2008). The majority of patients with anastomotic strictures will require several endoscopic interventions every 3 months with a mean of 3 to 5 sessions, using balloon dilation of 6-10 mm and multiple stents of 7 Fr to 10 Fr repeated for 12-24 months (Morelli et al., 2003; Thuluvath et al., 2005). The long-term success rates were in the range of 70%-100% (Alazmi et al., 2006; Morelli et al., 2003; Rerknimitr et al., 2002; Verdonk et al., 2006). A small group of patients, with transient anastomotic narrowing during the first 1-2 month post transplant, presumably due to postoperative edema, may respond with a single session of endoscopic balloon dilatation and plastic stent placement with no need for further intervention (Verdonk et al., 2006). An "aggressive approach" has been advocated by Pasha et al., which they defined as combination of maximal dilation and placement of maximum number of stents. Temporary placement of covered self-expanding metal stents has been tried to reduce the need for repeated stent exchanges, however, the data are limited (Williams & Draganov, 2009). Another protocol proposed an accelerated dilation every 2 weeks and a shortened stenting period of an average of 3.6 months. The results were encouraging with a high success rate 87%. Generally, it seems that shorter intervals in between treatments may ultimately reduce the time needed for successful long term outcomes (Williams & Draganov, 2009).
Significantly, more recurrences were seen in the patients who developed AS after more than 6 months after orthotopic liver transplantation compared to those with AS in the first 6 months (Verdonk et al., 2006). Recurrence rate of post-anastomotic biliary strictures was reported by Alzami et al. to be relatively small (18%) over a follow-up period of almost 3 years (Alazmi et al., 2006), while others reported to be around 10%-13% (Morelli et al., 2003). They concluded that recurrence could be effectively diagnosed and treated by endosopic approach requiring between one and four additional sessions. However, they did not identify any clinical or endoscopic parameters that predicted recurrence of anastomotic biliary strictures in post-OLT patients.

4.2.2.3 Living donor liver transplantation

However, the results of endoscopic intervention for biliary strictures in DDLT is excellent, but cannot be extrapolated to right-lobe LDLT. Inability to cannulate the stricture (Yazumi & Chiba, 2006; Tashiro et al., 2007) and difficulty to place a stent (Tsujino et al., 2006) were found to be the most common reasons for the failure of endoscopic treatment in this group of patients. The difference in outcome might be explained by the presence of multiple ductal anastomosis, smaller size, peripheral location, and increased risk of devascularization (Sharma et al., 2008). However, as in DDLT, the combination of balloon dilatation and stenting was superior to either modality alone (Tashiro et al., 2007). Kyoto group classified the strictures in living donor liver transplants into four types: unbranched, fork-shaped, trident-shaped, and multibranched (Hisatsune et al., 2003). Moreover, they were the first to describe the "crane neck deformity", in which the biliary anastomosis was located at a point that was far below the highest portion of the recipient duct. This event was probably related to compensatory hypertrophy of the graft that resulted in sharp angulation of the bile duct rendering it extremely difficult to be managed endoscopically (Yazumi & Chiba, 2006). Generally, it is recommended to start with endosocpic therapy as the first approach while percutaneous therapy should be spared for rescue therapy for following reasons (Chang et al., 2010). First, although the rates of successful interventions and patency do not differ for percutaneous or endoscopic therapy, the numbers of necessary interventions are higher for percutaneous therapy; second, the inconvenience of the percutaneous drain catheter cannot be ignored which significantly affects quality of life of those patients. Lastly but not the least, percutaneous drain related complications, such as leakage, pain, infection, and accidental removal of the drain are not uncommon. Other reported complications of percutatneous approach include portal vein injury, hepatic artery injury, and death (Yazumi & Chiba, 2005). In other studies, PTBD resulted in hemobilia, cholangitis, and a hemothorax (Schwartz et al., 2000). The patients in whom the endoscopic treatment is unsuccessful are rescued with a percutaneous transhepatic biliary drainage. The procedure could be summarized as follows: under fluoroscopic guidance, the right intrahepatic duct is punctured with a 21G Chiba needle and then few ml of bile is aspirated. After insertion of 0.018-inch hairwire, a yellow sheath followed by a 0.035-inch guide wire is introduced. After confirmation of anastomotic stricture, dilatation of biliary stricture with balloon catheters is performed. An 8 F pigtail catheter is inserted over the wire with its tip placed within the common bile duct or duodenum, and tubogram is then obtained. The catheter is anchored to the skin with anchoring device (Chang et al., 2010). If primary or rescue percutaneous approach is successfully performed, subsequent insertion of endoscopic retrograde biliary stents is recommended. Consequently, percutaneous drain catheter could be removed earlier and its related complications can be reduced. If the insertion of stents is expected to be difficult because of sharp or twisted angle of the anastomosis or for other reasons, endoscopic approach can be successfully performed with the "rendezvous" method, which could be generally described as, insertion of 0.035-inch or (0.025-inch) guidewire through the catheter into the intrahepatic bile duct proximal to the site of biliary stricture; then dilatation using a bougination catheter (7 F-11.5 F), a stent retriever (7 F-11.5 F) or a balloon catheter (6 or 8 mm in diameter) according to the indications. After stricture dilatation and minor sphincterotomy, stents as many and as big as possible, are endoscopically placed. The proximal side of the stent is located sufficiently over the stricture and the distal side of the stent is passed 1-2 cm outside the major papilla (Chang et al., 2010). Sphincterotomy is usually required during endoscopic stenting to avoid acute pancreatitis as a result of compression of pancreatic duct orifice by the duodenal end of stents. However, this procedure could be associated with cholangitis. Other theoretically possible long term complications in patients who underwent endoscopic sphicterotomy for choledocholithiasis unrelated to transplantation might be reported in transplant patients. When longer term results are more available in the future, these complications include recurrent stones (12.3%), biliary carcinoma (2.0%), and liver abscess (1.2%) (Tanaka et al., 1998). There was a successful trial by Koyoto group (Hisatsune et al., 2003; Yazumi et al., 2006) with endoscopic stenting of biliary strictures without sphincterotomy. Placing the inside stent above the papilla of Vater apparently has two clinical benefits. First, the inside stents are not directly exposed to digested food and this may reduce the possibility of being occluded. The average patency of the inside stent was found to be 450 days, exceeding the median patency of the conventional endoscopic biliary stent (about 3 months); Secondly, more stents could be placed because the orifice of the pancreatic duct is not compressed by the distal ends of these stents. Magnetic compression anastomosis (MCA) is revolutionary method of performing choledochocholedochostomy in patients with biliary obstruction after LDLT (Itoi et al., 2010). Endoscopically, a samarium-cobalt (Sm-Co) rare-earth magnet is placed at the superior site of obstruction via the percutaneous transhepatic biliary drainage route, and another Sm-Co magnet is also placed at the inferior site of obstruction with the aid of an endoscope.

4.2.3 Non anastomotic stricutes (NAS)

NAS after liver transplantation is not just single disease but rather an array of biliary abnormalities with different pathogenesis and variations in anatomical localization and severity, ranging from slight, localized mucosal irregularity to extensive and diffuse biliary strictures (Verdonk et al., 2007). Non-anastomotic strictures account for 10%-25% of all stricture complications after OLT with an incidence of 1%-19%. These strictures are often multiple, longer, proximal to the anastomosis in the extra- or intra-hepatic bile ducts and occur earlier than anastomotic strictures with a mean time to stricture development of 3-6 months (Graziadei et al., 2006; Guichelaar et al., 2003; Williams & Draganov, 2009). Verdonk et al. reported that more than 50% of the cases presented within the first year post transplantation. However, long-term follow-up revealed gradual increase in incidence up to 12 years after transplantation, resulting in steep initial rise of the cumulative incidence curve of NAS during the first year after OLT and followed by a smaller increment beyond the first year. The cumulative incidence was 14%, 15%, and 16% at 3, 5, and 10 years after OLT, respectively (Verdonk et al., 2007). As we discussed before, the risk factors could be broadly classified as macroangiopathic due to hepatic artery thrombosis (HAT) or microantiopathic which also known as ischemic type biliary lesions (ITBL). ITBL could be divided into three categories: ischemia-related injury to the biliary epithelium; imunologically mediated injury; and cytotoxic injury induced by bile salts. Groningen team reported that ischemia-related injury represented around 80% of NAS cases. Non-anastomotic strictures secondary to ischemic causes presented within 1 year of transplant and found around the bifurcation and the common bile duct had severer course and higher risk of progression. Whereas, the occurrence of NAS after 1 year was more often related to immunological causes as the risk factors identified more frequently in the periphery of the liver and represented around 20% of NAS cases. Groningen team also showed that cold and warm ischemia times were significantly longer for the group with early NAS compared to the group with late NAS. Anastomotic bile leak which is generally associated with local bile duct ischemia is observed in the group with early NAS. Moreover, higher incidence of NAS in liver transplantation from donors after cardiac death (non–heart-beating donors) also strongly suggests an ischemia-related factor in the pathogenesis of NAS. The critical relevance of arterial blood supply for the viability of the larger and extrahepatic bile ducts is well described. This part of the biliary tree in the graft becomes entirely dependent on arterial blood from the hepatic artery, making them more prone to hypoperfusion and ischemia. This may explain the central localization of NAS presenting early after transplantation (Buis et al., 2007; Verdonk et al., 2007). They also analyzed the risk factors in relation to the outcome and concluded that patients with following criteria: hepaticojejunostomy as biliary reconstruction and early diagnosis of NAS, NAS presenting at the level of the peripheral branches of the biliary tree were at risk for the development of recurrent cholangitis, radiological progression, development of cirrhosis, and eventually retransplantation (Verdonk et al., 2007).

4.2.3.1 Management of NAS

NAS secondary to early HAT usually requires urgent revascularization or retransplantation, whereas NAS due to late HAT or any other etiological risk factor could be salvaged by endoscopic means (Sharma et al., 2008). Compared to AS, non-anastomotic strictures are more difficult to treat with more complications and less favorable overall outcomes including increased graft loss and death (Williams & Draganov, 2009). It is reported that only 50%-75% of DDLT patients had a long term response to endoscopic therapy and the median time of response was 185 days; on the other hand, long term response in patients with anastomotic strictures was 70%-100% and the median time of response was 67 days (Graziadei et al., 2006; Pfau et al., 2000; Rerknimitr et al., 2002; Thuluvath et al., 2005). The results of endoscopic approaches in the context of NAS in LDLT are even more disappointing, as the average success rate varies from 25% to 33%(Todo et al., 2005; Tsujino et al., 2006; Yazumi et al., 2006), which is way below the success rate seen with NAS in DDLT. Non-anastomotic strictures required an increased number of interventions, and also did not result in significant long term improvement (Graziadei et al., 2006) as it is complicated by the development of repeated episodes of cholangitis, biliary cirrhosis, atrophy of the involved lobe and graft failure (Sharma et al., 2008). It did not appear that the poor response of non-anastomotic treatment varied with etiology (Guichelaar et al., 2003). In patients with changes located primarily in the extrahepatic bile duct and the duct bifurcation, complex surgical reconstruction with resection of the bifurcation and Roux-en-Y hepaticojejunostomy could be an option. Ultimately, up to 30-50% of the patients with NAS either required retransplantation or died as a consequence of these complications despite endoscopic or percutaneous therapy (Graziadei et al., 2006; Guichelaar et al., 2003; Pascher & Neuhaus, 2006; Shah et al., 2007; Thuluvath et al., 2005). Generally, endoscopic therapy of NAS is challenging and comprises of extraction of the biliary sludge and casts, balloon dilation of all accessible strictures and placement of plastic stents which are replaced every 3 months. However, dilatation of all strictures is not possible due to their multifocal distribution, involvement of the smaller and peripheral intrahepatic ducts, and rapid stent occlusion by biliary sludge and casts (Williams & Draganov, 2009). Although endoscopic therapy is considered as first line in management of non-anastomotic strictures and may occasionally be a definite solution in selected patients, it requires lifelong surveillance since strictures are likely to recur, and more importantly, it seems to play a prominent role as a bridge to liver retransplantation. A stricture that is too tight precluding successful cannulation of biliary system by the guidewire is the commonest cause of endoscopic failure in management of biliary strictures after LDLT (Tashiro et al., 2007; Verdonk et al., 2007). However, once a stricture is cannulated, the reported success for this procedure is about 80%-90%, which highlights the importance of cannulation of the stricture as a critical event in predicting the success or failure of the endoscopic treatment. Sharma et al. used the Spyglass direct visualization system as the guidance system for the passage of the guidewire through very tight strictures in this subset of patients where conventional ERCP failed. However, definitive answers on the best treatment modality for NAS should come from multicenter, prospective, randomized studies (Sharma et al., 2008).

4.3 Other indications of endoscopy in recipients

4.3.1 Sphincter of Oddi Dysfunction (SOD)

Also termed ampullary dysfunction occurs in from 0-7% of liver transplant recipients with duct to duct anastomosis. Its pathophysiology in the post-transplant setting is poorly understood (Thuluvath et al., 2005), but it is probably related to denervation of the ampullary region of the native duct, resulting in abnormal ampullary relaxation and increased intraductal biliary pressure (Clavien et al., 1995). However, distal bile duct obstruction in the post transplant setting might be due to a combination of SOD, edema, or inflammatory stricturing due to long term stenting with a T tube or internal stent when the distal end protrudes into the sphincter. CMV and other opportunistic infections may also play a pathological role in post-transplant sphincter of Oddi dysfunction (Thuluvath et al., 2005). It is usually suspected clinically by persistently elevated liver enzymes in an obstructive/cholestatic pattern, dilation of the native duct to a diameter greater than 10 mm (Pfau et al., 2000), improvements in liver tests with T tube unclamping, delayed drainage of contrast (> 15 min) in a cholangiography that fails to show any evident cause of obstruction (Greif et al., 1994). Hepatobiliary scintigraphy and sphincter or T tube manometry could also be diagnostic (Thuluvath et al., 2005). Endoscopic sphincterotomy and/or biliary stenting is usually a successful treatment. Some reported 100% response to sphincterotomy without stenting (Pfau et al., 2000; Thuluvath et al., 2005; Wojcicki et al., 2008). Therefore, manometric studies, although diagnostic, are not performed in most cases because evidence to support this approach has been largely anecdotal and remains controversial (Pfau et al., 2000). A study reported that conversion to a hepaticojejunostomy may occasionally be required to resolve the dysfunction (Greif et al., 1994).

4.3.2 Biliary stones

The incidence of biliary stones after liver transplantation is quite variable in different reports. For instance, Riknimitir et al. reported the occurrence of biliary stones in 38% of their patients (Rerknimitr et al., 2002), while others reported an incidence of 4-18% of post liver transplant patients (de la Mora-Levy & Baron, 2005).The exact etiology is unclear, however, this could be explained theoretically by increased lithogenicity of the bile or as a result of cyclosporine inhibitory effect on bile acid production and bile flow. However, post transplant calculi formation is most likely the result of mechanical obstruction mainly strictures (de la Mora-Levy & Baron, 2005; Thuluvath et al., 2005), biliary tract infection, biliary reflux and biliary mucosal inflammation. The stones or debris can be removed successfully after sphincterotomy in almost all cases, and patients with strictures require dilation of the strictures before stone removal (de la Mora-Levy & Baron, 2005; Pfau et al., 2000; Thuluvath et al., 2005).

4.3.3 Biliary cast syndrome

Biliary cast syndrome is an ill-defined entity that includes a number of pathophysiologies that share similar cholangiographic findings. Biliary casts, rare in nontransplant patients, are associated with morbidity, graft failure, need for retransplantation, and mortality. Biliary cast syndrome describes the cholangiographic findings of multiple fixed filling defects in the intrahepatic or extrahepatic biliary tree that conform to the luminal dimensions of the segment of bile duct. Cast material may be hard or soft, may adhere to the bile duct wall, and may have a "staghorn" configuration. Theories as to the etiology include sloughed biliary epithelium due to prolonged cold storage time or transient or ongoing ischemia, chronic rejection, infection, bile stasis, and alteration of the bile milieu (Pfau et al., 2000); and are often accompanied by strictures including diffuse stricturing of the hilum. Evidence suggests that endoscopic therapy will fail to treat multiple biliary casts and many patients may be better managed with the percutaneous approach. Ursodeoxycholic acid might delay new formation of sludge and stones. Although enough data are not available, most patients may require retransplantation (Pfau et al., 2000; Thuluvath et al., 2005).

4.3.4 Mucocele

It is a very rare complication after liver transplantion. It can develop when the outflow end of the blind donor cystic duct remnant is incorporated into the suture line of a biliary anastomosis (Koneru et al., 1989). This creates the blind mucosa-lined sac which can later on become distended by accumulated mucus and leads to bile duct obstruction by extrinsic compression (Osroff et al., 1990; Wojcicki et al., 2008). Computed tomography and ultrasonography will reveal the mucocele as a fluid collection in the porta hepatis and should be differentiated from other conditions, including hepatic artery pseudoaneurysm, biloma, loculated ascites, abscess, liquefied hematoma, tumor, adenopathy, and a fluid filled Roux−en−Y loop of jejunum. Surgical excision or drainage of the cystic duct remnant by enteric anastomosis is curative (Koneru et al., 1989; Thuluvath et al., 2005).

4.3.5 Posttransplant lymphoproliferative disease and opportunistic infection

Posttransplant lymphoproliferative disease is generally associated with over-mmunosuppression in the setting of Epstein-Barr virus infection and may respond to lowering of immunosuppression and antiviral therapy. Bile duct obstruction may occur at the hilum and can be relieved with temporary endoscopic biliary stent placement. However, if the disease progresses to lymphoma, long-term biliary stent placement may be necessary (de la Mora-Levy & Baron, 2005). Chronic CMV infection can cause chronic cholangitis and lead to multiple strictures mimicking PSC.

4.3.6 Recurrence of the primary sclerosing cholangitis

Primary sclerosing cholangitis recurs after OLT in 5–20% of patients, and the risk seems to be increased in males and in recipients who have not undergone colectomy before transplantation. The recurrence may be difficult to distinguish from ischemic-type biliary lesions (Wojcicki et al., 2008). The diagnosis is usually based on preoperative diagnosis of primary sclerosing cholangitis. Cholangiographic findings inculde non-anastomotic biliary strictures of the intrahepatic and/or extrahepatic biliary tree with beading and irregularity occurring more than 90 days after transplantation (Graziadei et al., 2006; Wojcicki et al., 2008). Differential diagnosis includes wide spectrum of factors such as hepatic artery thrombosis or stenosis and ischemic-type biliary lesions of other etiology. However, it seems that patient and graft survival are not negatively affected in the intermediate term of follow-up. An increased incidence of biliary strictures and reduced graft and patient survival are observed in patients with duct-to-duct anastomosis, as compared to those undergoing hepaticojejunostomy reconstructions. Therefore, Roux loop has been preferentially performed aiming at reducing the risk of disease recurrence. However, some authors reported that duct-to-duct anastomosis in these patients could be performed if the disease was not involving the distal duct, and the results in terms of the rates of biliary complications and patient and graft survival were comparable (Wojcicki et al., 2008).

5. Biliary complications in donor

The incidence of biliary complications in donors tends to be about 5% based on recent publications. Bile leakage and biliary strictures are the most common biliary complications. Most bile leakages occurred from cut surfaces, and others may originate from biliary radicles draining the caudate lobe (Yuan & Gotoh, 2010). When strictures develop, they tend to occur at the hilum. The same endoscopic treatments previously described are used.

Specifically for the cut surface of the liver, endoscopic biliary drainage could be successfully used as demonstrated in patients undergoing liver resection for other causes (Hasegawa et al., 2003).

6. Conclusion

ERCP has become an established procedure in the management of post-transplantation biliary complications both in recipients and donors with a comprehensive body of literature published for more than 20 years to support its use. In addition to the formentioned indications, it also has diagnostic and/ therapeutic role in management of hemobilia, necrosis of the bile duct, bile duct redundancy/kinking, and retained surgical stents. In genereal, therapeutic ERC, whether successful or ultimately unsuccessful and necessitating surgical intervention, does not negatively affect survival. Therefore, in the majority of patients with biliary complications, a trial of endoscopic therapy should be performed to delay or defer a post-OLT surgical procedure.

7. References

Alazmi, W. M., E. L. Fogel, Watkins, J.L, McHenry, L., Tector, J.A., Fridell, J., Mosler, P., Sherman, S. & Lehman, G.A. (2006). "Recurrence rate of anastomotic biliary strictures in patients who have had previous successful endoscopic therapy for anastomotic narrowing after orthotopic liver transplantation." *Endoscopy* 38(6): 571-574, ISSN 0013-726X.

Bekker, J., Ploem, S. & de Jong, K.P. (2009). "Early hepatic artery thrombosis after liver transplantation: a systematic review of the incidence, outcome and risk factors." *Am J Transplant* 9(4): 746-757, ISSN 1600-6143.

Buis, C. I., Hoekstra, H., Verdonk, R.C., & Porte, R.J. (2006). "Causes and consequences of ischemic-type biliary lesions after liver transplantation." *J Hepatobiliary Pancreat Surg* 13(6): 517-524, ISSN 0944-1166 .

Buis, C. I., Verdonk, R.C., Van der Jagt, E.J, Van der Hilst, C.S., Sloof, M.J., Haagsma, E.B. & Porte, R.J. (2007). "Nonanastomotic biliary strictures after liver transplantation, part 1: Radiological features and risk factors for early vs. late presentation." *Liver Transpl* 13(5): 708-718.

Chang, J. H., Lee, I.S., Choi, J.Y., Yoon, S.K., Kim, D.G., You, Y.K., Chun, H.J., Lee, D.K., Choi, M.G & Chung, I.S. (2010). "Biliary Stricture after Adult Right-Lobe Living-Donor Liver Transplantation with Duct-to-Duct Anastomosis: Long-Term Outcome and Its Related Factors after Endoscopic Treatment." *Gut Liver* 4(2): 226-233, ISSN 1976-2283 .

Clavien, P. A., Camargo, C.A., Jr., Baillie, J. & Fitz, J.G. (1995). "Sphincter of Oddi dysfunction after liver transplantation." *Dig Dis Sci* 40(1): 73-74, ISSN 0163-2116.

Colonna, J. O., 2nd, Shaked, A., Gomes, A.S., Coloquhoun, S.D., Jurim, O., McDiarmid, S.V., Millis, J.M., Goldstein, L.I., & Busuttil, R.W. (1992). "Biliary strictures complicating liver transplantation. Incidence, pathogenesis, management, and outcome." *Ann Surg* 216(3): 344-350; discussion 350-342, ISSN 0003-4932 .

de la Mora-Levy, J. G. & Baron, T.H. (2005). "Endoscopic management of the liver transplant patient." *Liver Transpl* 11(9): 1007-1021, ISSN 1527-6465 .

Duailibi, D. F. & Ribeiro, M.A., Jr. (2010). "Biliary complications following deceased and living donor liver transplantation: a review." *Transplant Proc* 42(2): 517-520, ISSN 0041-1345.

Gondolesi, G. E., Varotti, G., Florman, S.S., Munoz, L., Fishbein, T.M., Erme, S.H., Schwartz, M.E. & Miller, C. (2004). "Biliary complications in 96 consecutive right lobe living donor transplant recipients." *Transplantation* 77(12): 1842-1848, ISSN 0041-1337.

Graziadei, I. W., Schwaighofer, H., Kock, R., Nachbaur, K., Koenigsrainer, A., Margreiter, R. & Vogel, W. (2006). "Long-term outcome of endoscopic treatment of biliary strictures after liver transplantation." *Liver Transpl* 12(5): 718-725 ISSN 1527-6465.

Graziadei, I. W., Wiesner, R. H., Batts, K.P., Marotta, P.J., LaRusso, N.F., Parayko, M.K., Hay, J. E.., Gores, G. J., Charlton, M. R., Ludwig, J., Poterucha, J. J., Steers, J. L., & Krom, R. A. (1999). "Recurrence of primary sclerosing cholangitis following liver transplantation." *Hepatology* 29(4): 1050-1056, ISSN0270-9139 .

Greif, F., O. L. Bronsther, et al. (1994). "The incidence, timing, and management of biliary tract complications after orthotopic liver transplantation." Ann Surg 219(1): 40-45.

Guichelaar, M. M., Benson, J. T., Malinchoc, M., Krom, R. A., Wiesner, R. H. & Charlton, M. R. (2003). "Risk factors for and clinical course of non-anastomotic biliary strictures after liver transplantation." *Am J Transplant* 3(7): 885-890, ISSN 1600-6135 .

Hasegawa, K., Yazumi, S., Egawa, H., Tamaki, H., Asada, M., Kodama, Y., Hisatsune, H., Okazaki, K., Tanaka, K. & Chiba, T. (2003). "Endoscopic management of postoperative biliary complications in donors for living donor liver transplantation." *Clin Gastroenterol Hepatol* 1(3): 183-188, ISSN 1542-3565.

Hisatsune, H., Yazumi, S., Egawa, H., Asada, M., Hasegawa, K., Kodama, Y., Okazaki, K., Itoh, K., Takakuwa, H., Tanaka, K. & Chiba, T. (2003). "Endoscopic management of biliary strictures after duct-to-duct biliary reconstruction in right-lobe living-donor liver transplantation." *Transplantation* 76(5): 810-815 ISSN 0041-1337.

Itoi, T., Yamanouchi, E., Ikeuchi, N., Kasuya, K., Iwamoto, H. & Tsuchida, A. (2010). "Magnetic Compression Duct-to-duct Anastomosis for Biliary Obstruction in a Patient with Living Donor Liver Transplantation." *Gut Liver* 4 Suppl 1: S96-98, ISSN 1976-2283 .

Kasahara, M., Egawa, H., Takada, Y., Oike, F., Sakamoto, S., Kiuchi, T., Yazumi, S., Shibata, T. & Tanaka, K. (2006). "Biliary reconstruction in right lobe living-donor liver transplantation: Comparison of different techniques in 321 recipients." *Ann Surg* 243(4): 559-566, ISSN 0003-4932.

Koneru, B., Zajko, A. B., Sher, L., Marsh, J. W., Tzakis, A. G., Iwatsuki, S. & Starzl, T. E. (1989). "Obstructing mucocele of the cystic duct after transplantation of the liver." *Surg Gynecol Obstet* 168(5): 394-396, ISSN 0039-6087.

Lee, C. S., Liu, N. J., Lee, C. F., Chou, H. S., Wu, T. J., Pan, K. T., Chu, S. Y. & Lee, W. C. (2008). "Endoscopic management of biliary complications after adult right-lobe living donor liver transplantation without initial biliary decompression." *Transplant Proc* 40(8): 2542-2545, ISSN 0041-1345 .

Lin, T. S., Concejero, A. M., Chen, C. L., Chiang, Y. C., Wang, C. C., Wang, S. H., Liu, Y. W., Yang, C. H., Yong, C. C., Jawan, B. & Cheng, Y. F. (2009). "Routine microsurgical biliary reconstruction decreases early anastomotic complications in living donor liver transplantation." *Liver Transpl* 15(12): 1766-1775, ISSN 1527-6465.

Morelli, J., Mulcahy, H. E., Willner, I. R., Cunningham, J. T. & Draganov, P. (2003). "Long-term outcomes for patients with post-liver transplant anastomotic biliary strictures treated by endoscopic stent placement." *Gastrointest Endosc* 58(3): 374-379, ISSN 0016-5107.

Moser, M. A. & Wall, W. J. (2001). "Management of biliary problems after liver transplantation." *Liver Transpl* 7(11 Suppl 1): S46-52, ISSN 1527-6465.

Orons, P. D., Sheng, R. & Zajko, A. B. (1995a). "Hepatic artery stenosis in liver transplant recipients: prevalence and cholangiographic appearance of associated biliary complications." *AJR Am J Roentgenol* 165(5): 1145-1149, ISSN 0361-803X.

Orons, P. D., Zajko, A. B., Bron, K. M., Trecha, G. T., Selby, R. R. & Fung, J. J. (1995b). "Hepatic artery angioplasty after liver transplantation: experience in 21 allografts." *J Vasc Interv Radiol* 6(4): 523-529, ISSN 1051-0443 .

Ostroff, J. W., Roberts, J. P., Gordon, R. L., Ring, E. J. & Ascher, N. L. (1990). "The management of T tube leaks in orthotopic liver transplant recipients with endoscopically placed nasobiliary catheters." *Transplantation* 49(5): 922-924, ISSN 0041-1337.

Pascher, A. & Neuhaus, P. (2005). "Bile duct complications after liver transplantation." *Transpl Int* 18(6): 627-642, ISSN 0934-0874 .

Pascher, A. & Neuhaus, P. (2006). "Biliary complications after deceased-donor orthotopic liver transplantation." *J Hepatobiliary Pancreat Surg* 13(6): 487-496, ISSN 0944-1166.

Pasha, S. F., Harrison, M. E., Das, A., Nguyen, C. C., Vargas, H. E., Balan, V., Byrne, T. J., Douglas, D. D. & Mulligan, D. C. (2007). "Endoscopic treatment of anastomotic biliary strictures after deceased donor liver transplantation: outcomes after maximal stent therapy." *Gastrointest Endosc* 66(1): 44-51, ISSN 0016-5107 .

Pfau, P. R., Kochman, M. L., Lewis, J. D., Long, W. B., Lucey, M. R., Olthoff, K., Shaked, A. & Ginsberg, G. G. (2000). "Endoscopic management of postoperative biliary complications in orthotopic liver transplantation." *Gastrointest Endosc* 52(1): 55-63, ISSN 0016-5107.

Rabkin, J. M., Orloff, S. L., Reed, M. H., Wheeler, L. J., Corless, C. L., Benner, K. G., Flora, K. D., Rosen, H. R. & Olyaei, A. J. (1998). "Biliary tract complications of side-to-side without T tube versus end-to-end with or without T tube choledochocholedochostomy in liver transplant recipients." *Transplantation* 65(2): 193-199, ISSN 0041-1337 .

Rerknimitr, R., Sherman, S., Fogel, E. L., Kalayci, C., Lumeng, L., Chalasani, N. Kwo, P. & Lehman, G. A. (2002). "Biliary tract complications after orthotopic liver transplantation with choledochocholedochostomy anastomosis: endoscopic findings and results of therapy." *Gastrointest Endosc* 55(2): 224-231, ISSN 0016-5107.

Scatton, O., Meunier, B., Cherqui, D., Boillot, O., Sauvanet, A., Boudjema, K., Launois, B., Fagniez, P. L., Belghiti, J., Wolff, P., Houssin, D. & Soubrane, O. (2001). "Randomized trial of choledochocholedochostomy with or without a T tube in orthotopic liver transplantation." *Ann Surg* 233(3): 432-437, ISSN 0003-4932.

Schwartz, D. A., Petersen, B. T., Poterucha, J. J. & Gostout, C. J. (2000). "Endoscopic therapy of anastomotic bile duct strictures occurring after liver transplantation." *Gastrointest Endosc* 51(2): 169-174, ISSN 0016-5107 .

Shah, S. A., Grant, D. R., McGilvray, I. D., Greig, P. D., Selzner, M., Lilly, L. B., Girgrah, N., Levy, G. A. & Cattral, M. S. (2007). "Biliary strictures in 130 consecutive right lobe living donor liver transplant recipients: results of a Western center." *Am J Transplant* 7(1): 161-167, ISSN 1600-6135.

Sharma, S., Gurakar, A. & Jabbour, N. (2008). "Biliary strictures following liver transplantation: past, present and preventive strategies." *Liver Transpl* 14(6): 759-769,ISSN 1527-6465 .

Shastri, Y. M., Hoepffner, N. M., Akoglu, B., Zapletal, C., Bechstein, W. O., Caspary, W. F. & Faust, D. (2007). "Liver biochemistry profile, significance and endoscopic management of biliary tract complications post orthotopic liver transplantation." *World J Gastroenterol* 13(20): 2819-2825, ISSN 1007-9327.

Sherman, S., Shaked, A., Cryer, H. M., Goldstein, L.I. & Busuttil , R.w. (1993). "Endoscopic management of biliary fistulas complicating liver transplantation and other hepatobiliary operations." *Ann Surg* 218(2): 167-175, ISSN 0003-4932.

Tanaka, M., Takahata, S., Konomi, H., Matsunaga, H., Yokohata, K., Takeda, T., Utsunomiya, N. & Ikeda, S. (1998). "Long-term consequence of endoscopic sphincterotomy for bile duct stones." *Gastrointest Endosc* 48(5): 465-469, ISSN 0016-5107.

Tashiro, H., Itamoto, T., Sasaki, T., Ohdan, H., Fudaba, Y., Amano, H., Fukuda, S., Nakahara, H., Ishiyama, K., Ohshita, A., Kohashi, T., Mitsuta, H., Chayama, K. & Asahara, T. (2007). "Biliary complications after duct-to-duct biliary reconstruction in living-donor liver transplantation: causes and treatment." *World J Surg* 31(11): 2222-2229, ISSN 0364-2313.

Thuluvath, P. J., Pfau, P. R., Kimmey, M. B. & Ginsberg, G. G. (2005). "Biliary complications after liver transplantation: the role of endoscopy." *Endoscopy* 37(9): 857-863, ISSN 0013-726X.

Todo, S., Furukawa, H. & Kamiyama, T. (2005). "How to prevent and manage biliary complications in living donor liver transplantation?" *J Hepatol* 43(1): 22-27, ISSN 0168-8278 .

Tsujino, T., Isayama, H., Sugawara, Y. Sasaki, T. Kogure, H. Nakai, Y.,Yamamoto, N., Sasahira, N., Tada, M., Yoshida, H., Kokudo, N., Kawabe, T., Makuuchi, M. & Omata, M. (2006). "Endoscopic management of biliary complications after adult living donor liver transplantation." *Am J Gastroenterol* 101(10): 2230-2236, ISSN 0002-9270.

Tzakis, A. G., Gordon, R. D., Shaw, B. W., Jr., Iwatsuki, S. & Starzl, T. E. (1985). "Clinical presentation of hepatic artery thrombosis after liver transplantation in the cyclosporine era." *Transplantation* 40(6): 667-671, ISSN 0041-1337 .

Valls, C., Alba, E., Cruz, M., Figueras, J., Andia, E., Sanchez, A., Llado, L. & Serrano, T. (2005). "Biliary complications after liver transplantation: diagnosis with MR cholangiopancreatography." *AJR Am J Roentgenol* 184(3): 812-820, ISSN 0361-803X.

Venu, M., Brown, R. D., Lepe, R., Berkes, J., Cotler, S. J., Benedetti, E., Testa, G. & Venu, R. P.(2007). "Laboratory diagnosis and nonoperative management of biliary complications in living donor liver transplant patients." *J Clin Gastroenterol* 41(5): 501-506, ISSN 0192-0790.

Vera, A., Moledina, S., Gunson, B., Hubscher, S., Mirza, D., Olliff, S. & Neuberger, J. (2002). "Risk factors for recurrence of primary sclerosing cholangitis of liver allograft." *Lancet* 360(9349): 1943-1944, ISSN 0140-6736.

Verdonk, R. C., Buis, C. I., Porte, R. J., van der Jagt, E. J., Limburg, A. J., van den Berg, A. P., Slooff, M. J., Peeters, P. M., de Jong, K. P., Kleibeuker, J. H. & Haagsma, E. B. (2006). "Anastomotic biliary strictures after liver transplantation: causes and consequences." *Liver Transpl* 12(5): 726-735, ISSN 1527-6465 .

Verdonk, R. C., Buis, C. I., van der Jagt, E. J., Gouw, A. S., Limburg, A. J., Slooff, M. J., Kleibeuker, J. H., Porte, R. J. & Haagsma, E. B. (2007). "Nonanastomotic biliary strictures after liver transplantation, part 2: Management, outcome, and risk factors for disease progression." *Liver Transpl* 13(5): 725-732, ISSN 1527-6465.

Vougas, V., Rela, M., Gane, E., Muiesan, P., Melendez, H. V., Williams, R. & Heaton, N. D. (1996). "A prospective randomised trial of bile duct reconstruction at liver transplantation: T tube or no T tube?" *Transpl Int* 9(4): 392-395, ISSN0934-0874 .

Welling, T. H., Heidt, D. G., Englesbe, M. J., Magee, J. C., Sung, R. S., Campbell, D. A., Punch, J. D. & Pelletier, S. J. (2008). "Biliary complications following liver transplantation in the model for end-stage liver disease era: effect of donor, recipient, and technical factors." *Liver Transpl* 14(1): 73-80, ISSN 1527-6465.

Williams, E. D. and Draganov P. V. (2009). "Endoscopic management of biliary strictures after liver transplantation." *World J Gastroenterol* 15(30): 3725-3733, ISSN1007-9327 .

Wojcicki, M., Milkiewicz, P. & Silva, M. (2008). "Biliary tract complications after liver transplantation: a review." *Dig Surg* 25(4): 245-257, ISSN 0253-4886.

Yazumi, S. & Chiba, T. (2005). "Biliary complications after a right-lobe living donor liver transplantation." *J Gastroenterol* 40(9): 861-865, ISSN 0944-1174.

Yazumi, S. & Chiba, T. (2006). "Endoscopic management of biliary stricture after right-lobe living-donor liver transplantation with biliary anastomosis." *Clin Gastroenterol Hepatol* 4(10): 1296; author reply 1296, ISSN 1542-3565 .

Yazumi, S., Yoshimoto, T., Hisatsune, H., Hasegawa, K., Kida, M., Tada, S., Uenoyama, Y., Yamauchi, J., Shio, S., Kasahara, M., Ogawa, K., Egawa, H., Tanaka, K. & Chiba, T. (2006). "Endoscopic treatment of biliary complications after right-lobe living-donor liver transplantation with duct-to-duct biliary anastomosis." *J Hepatobiliary Pancreat Surg* 13(6): 502-510, ISSN 0944-1166 .

Yuan, Y. & Gotoh M. (2010). "Biliary complications in living liver donors." *Surg Today* 40(5): 411-417, ISSN 0941-1291 .

Zoepf, T., Maldonado-Lopez, E. J., Hilgard, P., Dechene, A., Malago, M., Broelsch, C. E., Schlaak, J. & Gerken, G. (2005). "Diagnosis of biliary strictures after liver transplantation: which is the best tool?" *World J Gastroenterol* 11(19): 2945-2948, ISSN 1007-9327.

8

Stents in Gastrointestinal Endoscopy

Michael Pavlides and David A Gorard
Wycombe Hospital, High Wycombe,
United Kingdom

1. Introduction

Advanced endoscopy can be used to insert stents (hollow tubes) into various sites of the gastrointestinal tract and this has proved to be a major therapeutic advance. Stents can hold open strictured areas in the oesophagus, the biliary tree, the colon and the gastroduodenal region. Stents are usually positioned in order to overcome stricturing associated with cancerous tumours. They are used as definitive treatment, as a bridge to surgery, and for palliation of obstructive symptoms. In the setting of incurable gastrointestinal cancer, the endoscopic placement of such stents allows palliation of symptoms non-invasively, and is an attractive alternative to surgery. Stents can also be used in benign disease of the gastrointestinal tract.

The basic principles of stent insertion involve the initial placement of a guidewire, (and sometimes an overrunning introducing catheter) across the region to be stented, using endoscopic vision and often fluoroscopic guidance too. The stent is advanced over the guidewire until it traverses the area to be stented. In the case of self-expanding stents, the restraining mechanism is then released to deploy the stent.

Gastrointestinal stent insertion is not the sole domain of the endoscopist. Gastrointestinal stents are also placed non-endoscopically by radiologists. For example, interventional radiologists use fluoroscopic guidance to position oesophageal stents in the oesophagus, or can use a combination of sonography and percutaneous transhepatic cholangiography to place biliary stents in the biliary tree. The route of stent insertion may be influenced by local expertise, but the indications for stent insertion are usually those benefitting from a multidisciplinary approach involving endoscopists, surgeons, interventional radiologists and oncologists. Gastrointestinal stent insertion is an area of medicine where the territorial boundaries of interventional endoscopists, minimally invasive surgeons and interventional radiologists are increasingly blurred.

2. Technology of stents

2.1 Simple plastic stents

Initially endoscopic stents were solely plastic. Up until the 1990s, rigid plastic stents were used to stent stricturing oesophageal cancers. However the development of safer Self-Expanding Metal Stents (SEMS) has rendered these rigid plastic oesophageal stents obsolete. Today plastic stents are mainly confined to use in the biliary tree and pancreas. These plastic stents are usually composed of one of three polymers - polyethylene, polyurethane or Teflon. Plastic stents used in the biliary tree and pancreas may be straight with anchoring side-flaps to prevent migration. Alternatively, pigtailed stents may be used in the biliary tree. The curled end of a pigtail stent is straightened over the guidewire during positioning and the pigtail resumes its shape once the guidewire has been removed. The pigtail anchors the stent in position. The diameter of a plastic stent is usually described in terms of the French scale, where 1 French (Fr) is 0.33 mm. Thus a 6 Fr stent has a diameter of 2 mm. The maximum diameter of a simple plastic stent is limited by the maximum size of an endoscope's operating channel size at 12 Fr or 4 mm.

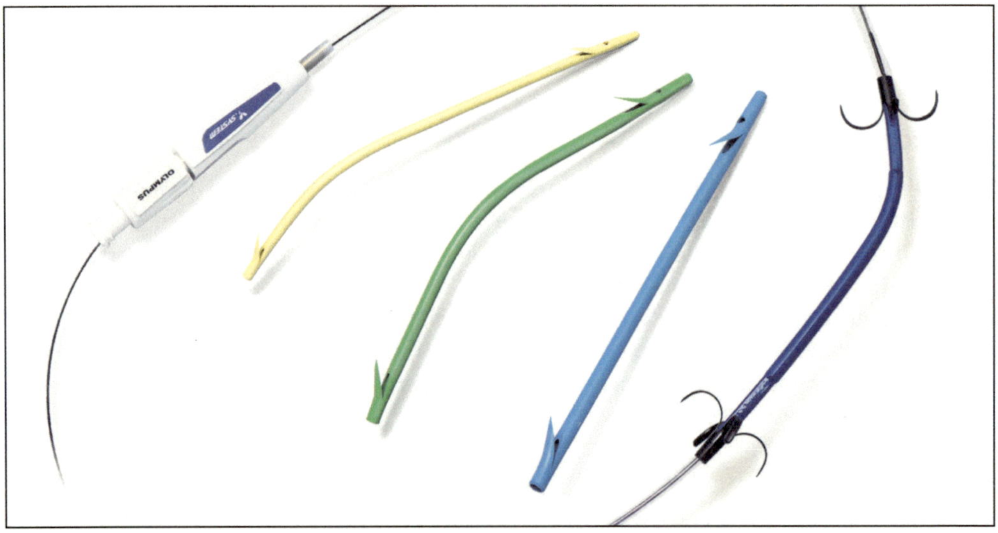

Fig. 1. Straight plastic stents used for biliary and pancreatic stenting

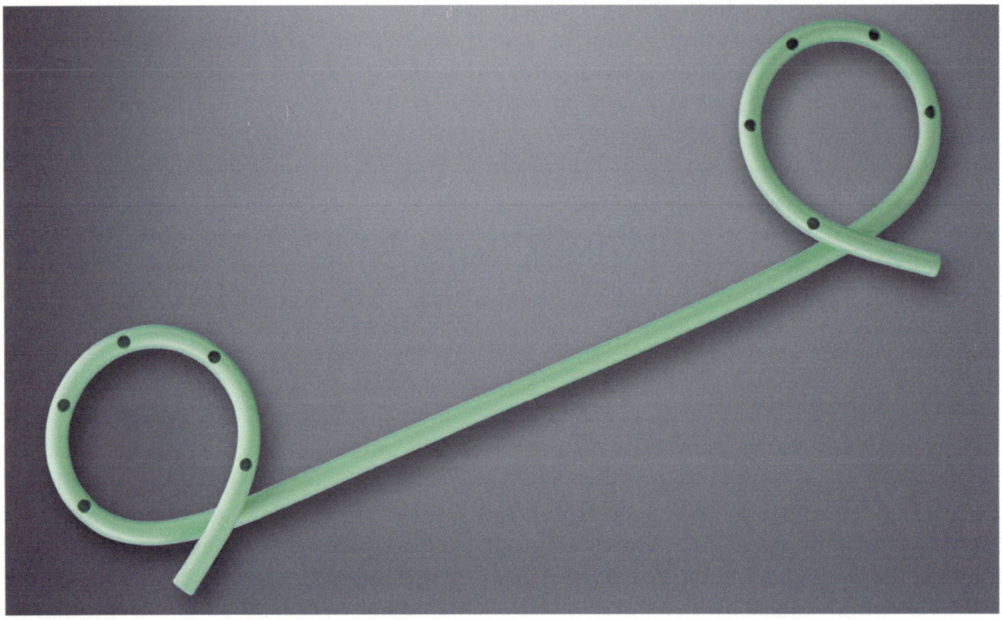

Fig. 2. Pigtail stent used for biliary stenting

2.2 Self-expanding stents

Although simple plastic stents still have a role in biliary and pancreatic stenting, technological improvements have led to the development of smarter stents. Self-Expanding Metal Stents (SEMS) are positioned while collapsed, using a small calibre introducer. Insertion of SEMS is easier, safer, with a reduced risk of perforation, and much reduced need for prior stricture dilatation.

Metals in SEMS need to be biocompatible i.e. biologically innocuous when functioning in patients. Shape memory alloys are 'intelligent', possessing the ability to recover a previously defined length or shape when deployed in the patient (Tarnita et al., 2009). There are several types and sizes of SEMS on the market. Each has its own characteristics in terms of radial forces exerted, foreshortening on deployment, and flexibility. SEMS can be made from stainless steel e.g. *Z-stent*® (Cook Medical, Bloomington, IN, USA) or from alloys. Nitinol is an alloy of nickel and titanium used in *Ultraflex*® stent (Boston Scientific, Natick, MA, USA) and *Alimaxx E*® stent (Alveolus, Charlotte, NC, USA). Elgiloy, a cobalt /chromium /nickel alloy, is used in *Wallstent*® (Boston Scientific).

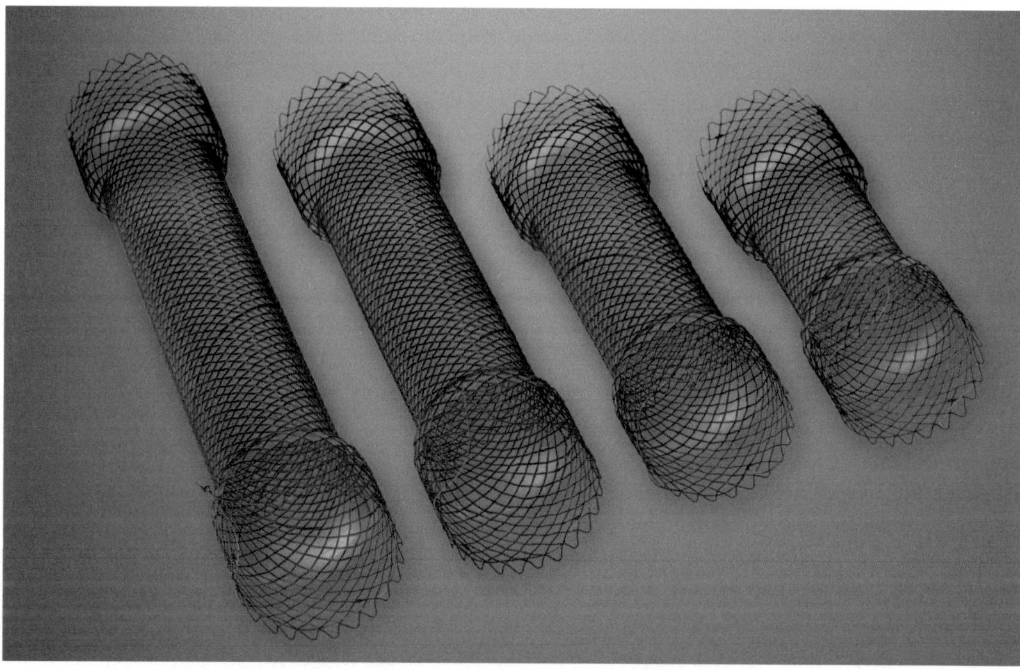

Fig. 3. Different sizes of Self-Expanding Metal Stents used in oesophageal stenting

SEMs should be fluoroscopically opaque to aid positioning, and should be easily deployable via a small calibre introducer. They are introduced in a collapsed position, being run over a guidewire positioned through the region to be stented. Once in position the constraining mechanism is released and the stent expands, exerting radial forces on any stricturing lesion thus increasing the lumen of the area being stented. SEMS are designed to expand to a diameter of more than 20mm. The bare metal strands of an uncovered stent may embed in the underlying tumour and serve to anchor the stent in position. Through pressure necrosis, the struts of the stent migrate into the mucosa and submucosa of the gut wall. A fibrous reaction with chronic lymphocytic infiltration occurs, as the stent becomes embedded in collagen and fibrous tissue. A chronic lymphocytic reaction occurs in the normal tissue underlying the proximal and distal ends of the stent (Bethge et al.,1996). Once *in situ* the stent should be MRI compatible.

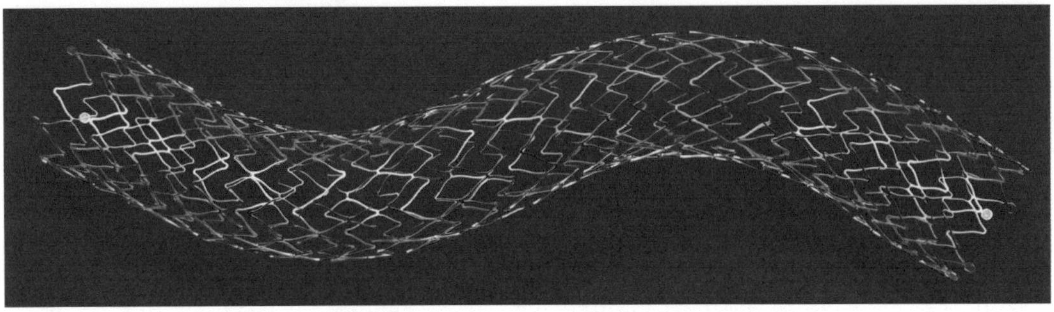

Fig. 4. Uncovered Self-Expanding Metal Stent used in biliary stenting

SEMS may be covered with a silicone membrane to reduce the risk of tumour in-growth and to seal fistulas. However fully covered stents are less likely to embed in the underlying tissues, and have an increased risk of stent migration compared to uncovered stents. Therefore, partially covered stents have been developed with flared uncovered segments at both ends to anchor on to the tissue. Fully covered SEMS are also increasingly used in benign oesophageal disease, such as non-malignant strictures and anastomotic leaks. The *Polyflex* ® stent (Boston Scientific, Natick, MA, USA) is a removable self-expanding plastic stent for use in the management of benign and malignant oesophageal strictures. Such a removable self-expanding plastic stent allows temporary stent insertion for benign oesophageal disease and for patients undergoing neoadjuvant chemotherapy prior to oesophagectomy. Recently biodegradable stents have been developed which slowly break down over time, e.g. the *SX-Ella Esophageal Degradable BD stent*®, (ELLA-CS, Hradec-Kralove, Czech Republic) made from the biodegradable polymer poly-dioxanon, and the *Tanaka-Marui stent* (Marui Textile Machinery Co., Osaka, Japan) composed of biodegradable poly-L-lactic acid monofilaments.
Potential complications of SEMS insertion include perforation, tumour overgrowth or ingrowth, and stent migration. Newer stents are being developed with the aim of increasing technical and clinical success rates, while reducing complication rates. Other areas of development include radioactive or drug-eluting stents for malignant disease.

3. Oesophageal stents for malignant oesophageal obstruction

Patients with oesophageal cancer experience progressive dysphagia and weight loss. Radical surgery in the form of oesophagectomy offers the only chance of cure. Unfortunately, patients often present late with inoperable tumours, or are too frail to be considered for surgery which itself caries significant morbidity and mortality. Dysphagia is a distressing and unpleasant symptom. Relief of dysphagia, so that patients can swallow again, is very important in the treatment of oesophageal cancer. Oesophageal stents are an excellent option for the palliation of dysphagia. In contrast to other treatment modalities like endoscopic laser or brachytherapy, stents are widely available and are not restricted to specialised centres. They can be inserted under endoscopic or fluoroscopic guidance or a combination of both. They rapidly relieve dysphagia, and can be used in

patients with advanced inoperable disease or in patients too frail to have chemotherapy or radiotherapy.
The first stents used in malignant dysphagia were rigid plastic stents. Placing such rigid stents, and the necessary prior stricture dilatation carried a substantial risk of perforation. SEMS were developed in the early 1990s. Their design allows them to be preloaded onto a delivery mechanism typically measuring 5-10mm in diameter. Consequently little or no dilatation is needed prior to stent insertion. Oesophageal SEMS are deployed over a guidewire after delineating the margins of the stricture endoscopically. Although the stents are usually deployed under fluoroscopic guidance, increasingly many endoscopists deploy them under direct endoscopic vision with the endoscope positioned alongside the guidewire–stent assembly. The diameter of most fully deployed oesophageal SEMS varies between 16 and 24 mm and their length varies between 7 and 15 cm. SEMS are usually partially or fully covered with a membrane to prevent tumour ingrowth through the metal mesh.
Early studies comparing traditional rigid plastic stents and SEMS demonstrated the superiority of the latter in several domains. Knyrim et al (1993) compared the two types of stents and showed SEMS and rigid plastic stents to be equivalent in their improvement of dysphagia, 30 day mortality and re-intervention rates. However, metal stents were associated with fewer complications, shorter hospitalisation after stent placement and superior cost effectiveness (Knyrim et al., 1993). Subsequent randomised studies and a retrospective review produced similar results (De Palma et al., 1996; Roseveare et al., 1998; Eickhoff et al., 2005). Furthermore, the perforation rates and early mortality rates were lower in those patients receiving SEMS. Rigid plastic stents are no longer used in oesophageal cancer.
Although the procedure-related complication rates are lower with SEMS, these devices are still subject to late complications including stent migration and stent occlusion due to food bolus or tumour overgrowth. One study has suggested that such late complications are more common with SEMS compared to rigid plastic stents (Kozarek et al., 1996). In a retrospective study of SEMS for malignant dysphagia, repeat endoscopy to address complications was needed in 46 of 97 patients, and in 10 of these a further stent had to be inserted (Ross et al., 2007). Acid reflux frequently occurs when stents are placed across, and thus hold open, the gastro-oesophageal junction. Patients with stents traversing the gastro-oesophageal junction should experience fewer reflux symptoms if they take acid suppressive drugs to decrease gastric acid production, prokinetic drugs to hasten stomach emptying, avoid eating within 2-3 hours of bed-time, and elevate the head of the bed. Despite these measures patients can still experience significant reflux symptoms and consequently stents with inherent anti-reflux mechanisms have been developed e.g. the *Oesophageal Z stent with Dua anti-reflux valve* ®, (Cook Medical, Bloomington, USA), and the *FerX-ELLA Esophageal Stent – Boubella* ®, (ELLA-CS, Hradec-Kralove, Czech Republic).

3.1 Types of expandable oesophageal stents used for oesophageal cancer

The majority of commercially available oesophageal SEMS are made of nitinol or stainless steel. Covered stents are less prone to tumour ingrowth, but more prone to migration. Consequently partially covered stents have been developed. These have a central covered portion which is placed across the oesophageal tumour with the two ends left uncovered to allow embedding and anchoring into the adjacent tissue. Patients with partially covered stents have less tumour ingrowth and fewer interventions for recurrent dysphagia than patients with bare metal stents (Vakil et al; 2001; Saranovic et al., 2005). Studies comparing different commercially available covered stents have shown all the studied stents to have similar efficacy and complication rates (May et al., 1996; Sabharawal et al., 2003; Siersema et al., 2001).

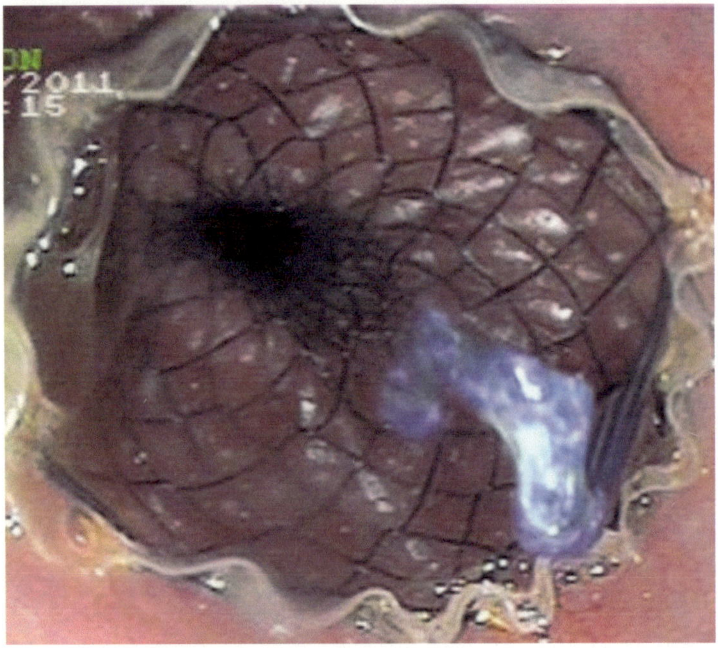

Fig. 5. Endoscopic view immediately after deployment of a SEMS for oesophageal cancer

In addition to SEMS, an self-expanding plastic stent made of polyester and covered with silicone (*Polyflex®*, Boston Scientific, Natick, MA, USA) has become available. Randomised controlled studies have shown that it can be successfully placed in the majority of cases and produces similar improvements in dysphagia when compared to SEMS (Conio et al., 2007; Verschuur et al., 2008). However, self-expanding plastic stents are associated with more complications, in particular stent migration (Conio et al., 2007), and for this reason are not routinely used for the treatment of malignant oesophageal obstruction.

3.2 Effect of oesophageal stenting on symptom palliation and quality of life

SEMS improve swallowing in malignant dysphagia. When formally studied, SEMS have consistently been shown to improve dysphagia scores (Knyrim et al., 1993). Oesophageal SEMS enable patients to ingest semi-solids but rarely improve dysphagia to the point of taking a completely normal diet. Patients with SEMS run the risk of causing food bolus obstruction if they attempt to take an unrestricted diet. Roast meats and crusty bread are particular culprits in blocking stents. In addition to the symptomatic improvement some studies have documented a benefit in the overall quality of life (Diamantis et al., 2011). Karnofsky scores were shown to significantly improve from a median of 40 before SEMS insertion to a median of 65 after SEMS insertion (Knyrim et al., 1993). Other advantages of SEMS include nutritional benefits, with patients receiving SEMS enjoying food more and maintaining their weight longer compared to patient receiving rigid plastic stents (Roseveare et al., 1998).

3.3 Comparison of stenting with other palliative treatments in malignant dysphagia

Alternative treatments for malignant dysphagia include endoscopic laser and brachytherapy. A multi-centre randomised trial found that SEMS improved dysphagia quicker than single dose brachytherapy, but brachytherapy was associated with better long term improvements in dysphagia, fewer complications and better quality of life scores (Homs et al., 2004). A Belgian centre retrospectively compared 125 patients with malignant dysphagia treated with endoscopic laser, rigid plastic stents and SEMS. Dysphagia improved significantly in all 3 groups but the rate of complications was significantly higher in both stent groups, compared to endoscopic laser (Gevers et al., 1998). In a prospective comparison, SEMS insertion was as safe and effective as laser combined with radiotherapy for inoperable oesophageal cancer (Königsrainer et al., 2000). SEMS insertion seems to be the preferred option for treating malignant dysphagia, since SEMS are widely available, relatively easy to place endoscopically or under fluoroscopic guidance, and provide rapid symptom relief. Brachytherapy, although efficacious remains a treatment that is not widely available.

3.4 Stents for benign oesophageal peptic strictures

Benign oesophageal strictures are most commonly caused by chronic reflux of gastric acid into the distal oesophagus. Such benign peptic strictures can lead to significant dysphagia. They are normally readily treated by endoscopic dilatation and acid suppression therapy. Rarely, the stricture repeatedly recurs within a few weeks. In these patients alternative treatments to repeated dilatation and acid suppressants may be needed. Although surgery is the mainstay of treatment in these refractory cases, oesophageal stenting should be considered in those less suitable for surgery. The ideal oesophageal stent for use in benign disease should, as with malignant disease, be easy to place, use a small calibre delivery mechanism and have a low rate of migration. However it should also be easy to retrieve, easy to reposition, and have low rates of insertion and removal related complications (Sharma & Kozarek, 2010).

Data on the use of SEMS in benign oesophageal strictures come from case reports and case series. These reports show that SEMS are associated with high rates of complications. The most commonly reported are stent migration occurring in 12.5-31%, new stricture formation in 20-100% and fistula formation in 6-33% of patients (Sandha & Marcon, 1999; Fiorini et al., 2000; Ackroyd et al., 2001; Wadhwa et al., 2003). Stent migration is more likely to occur with covered stents while uncovered stents or partially covered stents become embedded in the tissue making their removal difficult and traumatic. These complications rates are generally felt to be too high to justify in the treatment of benign disease. Therefore SEMS are best avoided in benign oesophageal strictures (Sharma & Kozarek, 2010).

In distinction to metal stents, expandable plastic stents such as the removable *Polyflex®* stent have been increasingly studied in benign oesophageal strictures that do not respond to conventional treatments. A recent meta-analysis of fully covered self-expanding metal and plastic stents has shown that the improvement in dysphagia was significantly better in patients receiving a *Polyflex®* stent (55.3%) compared to those receiving a nitinol stent (21.8%) (Thomas et al., 2011).

A more exciting prospect in the treatment of benign oesophageal conditions has been the recent development of biodegradable stents. Such stents are designed to stay in place for a few weeks before disintegrating. This avoids the need for further procedures to remove the stent. Some small series have now reported on their efficacy in benign strictures (Saito et al., 2007; Repici et al., 2010).

3.5 Stents for malignant tracheo-oesophageal fistulas

Malignant tracheo-oesophageal fistulas may arise from infiltration of oesophageal cancers into the respiratory tract, or cancers of the trachea and bronchi infiltrating into the oesophagus. These life-threatening connections between the digestive tract and the airways are usually difficult to treat and are associated with poor prognosis. Patients receiving best supportive treatment survive a median of 22 days (Burt et al., 1991).There are no randomised controlled data on the use of SEMS in these patients. However, several case series have demonstrated that covered SEMS can lead to fistula occlusion in 70-100% of patients (May & Ell, 1998). A retrospective study has shown covered SEMS to be more successful at fistula occlusion compared to rigid plastic stents, 92% vs. 77% (Low & Kozarek, 1998). Furthermore, successful occlusion of the fistula was associated with improved 30 day survival, 90% vs. 25% (Dumonceau et al., 1999) and overall survival, 15.1 vs. 6.2 weeks (Shin et al., 2004).

3.6 Stents for oesophageal perforations and leaks

Spontaneous and iatrogenic perforations of the oesophagus also carry a very high mortality and morbidity. Early diagnosis and prompt treatment are essential to achieve a good outcome.

Spontaneous oesophageal perforation as a result of vomiting (Boerhaave's syndrome) is a surgical emergency, requiring surgical intervention within hours of the perforation. Rarely, patients present late and there have been a handful of reports of oesophageal SEMS being used in the treatment of spontaneous oesophageal perforations if the patient has presented late (Eubanks et al., 1999; Chung et al., 2001).

Iatrogenic perforations of the oesophagus are more common than spontaneous perforations. They usually occur at endoscopy, most frequently when malignant stricture dilatation is undertaken. The diagnosis of perforation is usually obvious and rapid. Although iatrogenic oesophageal perforation is life-threatening, contamination of the mediastinum and pleural space with stomach contents is less problematic compared to spontaneous perforation, since the patient is fasted. Small case series have shown that insertion of a covered SEMS, together with thoracostomy tube drainage of the pleural space and antibiotic administration is a successful strategy in sealing off iatrogenic perforations (Siersema et al., 2003). Prompt stent insertion (average delay 45 minutes) after iatrogenic oesophageal perforation leads to minimal morbidity compared to delayed treatment, and produces results similar to surgical treatment (Fischer et al., 2006). It has to be emphasised that the clinical state of patients may individualise therapy for oesophageal perforations; although most centres consider surgery as first-line therapy (Keeling et al., 2010; Kiernan et al., 2010), endoscopic stenting is an option in many patients (Johnsson et al., 2005; van Heel et al., 2010).

3.7 Oesophageal stenting for anastomotic leaks

Post-operative anastomotic leaks are another area where oesophageal stents are increasingly used. Case series of anastomotic leaks following upper gastrointestinal surgery have demonstrated high success and low complications rates, with patients returning to eating 2 days after stent insertion.

3.8 Stenting for bleeding oesophageal varices

Oesophageal stents have recently been used to arrest bleeding from oesophageal varices in patients with portal hypertension. Bleeding from oesophageal varices has a high mortality, especially in patients with advanced liver disease. Bleeding is usually controlled by endoscopic band ligation of the varices, and vasopressor medication to decrease portal pressure. If these measures fail, the bleeding can be controlled with the insertion of a Sengstaken-Blakemore tube which tamponades the varices. Balloon tamponade is a temporary measure often used as a bridge to treatment with a transjugular intrahepatic portosystemic stent shunt (TIPSS).

A covered self-expanding oesophageal stent (*SX-Ella Stent Danis®*,ELLA-CS, Hradec-Kralove, Czech Republic) has recently been developed as another treatment option in variceal bleeding. It is an alternative to balloon tamponade in patients who are not suitable for TIPSS or in whom Sengstaken-Blakemore tube insertion is not possible, has failed or is complicated by oesophageal perforation. The *SX-Ella Stent Danis®* delivery mechanism is inserted over a guidewire that has been endoscopically placed in the stomach. The endoscope is then withdrawn and the delivery mechanism advanced through the oesophagus into the stomach. A balloon located at the stent's distal end is then inflated, and the whole mechanism is withdrawn until the balloon reaches the cardia and resistance is felt. The stent, now positioned in the distal oesophagus can be deployed, followed by balloon deflation and removal of the delivery mechanism. The stent can also be placed without prior endoscopy in emergency situations. Once deployed, the tamponading stent permits ongoing oral nutrition, unlike balloon tamponade. Case series show that such stents are efficacious in bleeding oesophageal varices. They can be successfully placed in the majority of patients and are removed within 14 days of insertion. The only complication that has been reported is of oesophageal ulceration (Hubmann et al., 2006; Zehetner et al., 2008; Wright et al., 2010).

4. Gastroduodenal stents

Recurrent and distressing vomiting due to gastric outlet obstruction occurs in some patients with pancreatic cancer, distal gastric cancer, duodenal cancer and some metastatic cancers. Most of these patients have advanced and inoperable disease, and only a few months of life remaining. Until recently the only treatment to prevent relentless vomiting and allow oral nutrition was the fashioning of a surgical gastroenterostomy to bypass the antro-pyloro-duodenal region. Even though such surgery can now often be done laparoscopically, complications are not uncommon in such patients who are often malnourished and frequently have comorbidities. The development of gastroduodenal stent insertion offers a noninvasive means of palliating vomiting without surgery (Martin & Laasch, 2004; Lowe et al., 2007; Kim et al., 2007).

Gastroduodenal stents are of the SEMS variety and are positioned under direct endoscopic vision, and with fluoroscopic guidance. Before stent placement is attempted, a period of gastric drainage using a wide-bore nasogastric tube is recommended. Drainage of gastric contents will improve endoscopic views and reduce the risk of vomiting and aspiration during the procedure. At endoscopy, the stricture's proximal anatomy is assessed but usually the endoscope's diameter is too large to allow safe negotiation through the stricture. The stricture can be outlined by fluoroscopy after the injection of a contrast agent. A guidewire is then passed down the operating channel of a therapeutic endoscope and advanced through the stricture. The stent assembly is then passed over the wire and positioned so that its ends overlap the ends of the stricture. Once fluoroscopy confirms a satisfactory position, the SEMS is deployed. An alternative method of gastroduodenal stent insertion involves a radiologist placing the stent via the oral route using fluoroscopy alone.

Once a gastroduodenal stent has been sited, patients can resume oral intake without vomiting. Patients should be advised to chew all foods well, and initially a soft diet is recommended. Patients who remain on a semi-solid diet are less likely to experience food impaction in their stent, but many patients are able to tolerate all food consistencies. Following gastroduodenal stent insertion, potential early complications include bleeding and perforation. Late complications include distal stent migration, and stent obstruction by tumour ingrowth, reactive tissue hyperplasia, tumor overgrowth, and food impaction.

4.1 Endoscopic stenting *v.* gastrojejunostomy in malignant gastric outlet obstruction

Most comparisons of gastroduodenal stent insertion with surgical gastrojejunostomy in malignant outlet obstruction have been retrospective. There is little in the way of large randomised trial data prospectively comparing these two palliative procedures. Despite the limitations of studies to date, some conclusions can be drawn (Gaidos & Draganov, 2009; Ly et al., 2010). Compared to surgical gastrojejunostomy, gastroduodenal stent insertion is associated with a shorter hospital stay, fewer costs (Johnsson et al., 2004) and fewer complications at the time of intervention. Stent insertion also leads to faster resumption of oral food intake than surgical gastrojejunostomy (Maettani et al., 2004; Ly et al., 2010). However, in the longer term there may be stent migration or obstruction, and long term results are better with surgery (Jeurnink et al., 2010).

4.2 Combined biliary and gastric outlet obstruction

By the time an inoperable pancreatic cancer causes gastric outlet obstruction, there has often already been biliary obstruction. Endoscopic access to the duodenal papilla is important for biliary stenting and jaundice relief (see below). A gastroduodenal stent will cover the duodenal papilla, but with an uncovered stent some endoscopic access to the papilla can be achieved through the holes in the metal mesh. However it is technically very difficult to perform biliary stenting though the mesh of an uncovered metal duodenal stent, and biliary stent insertion or exchange is more readily achieved percutaneously via the transhepatic cholangiographic route once a gastroduodenal stent is present. Covered gastroduodenal stents will further confound endoscopic access to the duodenal papilla and impede percutaneous biliary stent placement, as well as being more likely to migrate. Consequently uncovered gastroduodenal stents are most frequently used in gastric outlet obstruction due to pancreatic head cancers.

Simultaneous biliary and gastroduodenal metal stenting can be done in patients with inoperable pancreatic cancers causing obstructive jaundice and gastric outlet obstructive symptoms (Kaw et al., 2003; Mutignani et al., 2007). Whenever a gastroduodenal stent is to be inserted in a pancreatic cancer patient, consideration should be given to initially stenting the bile duct. A pre-existing plastic biliary stent can be changed for a wider biliary SEMS before the gastroduodenal stent is placed. If the duodenal obstruction does not allow passage of the duodenoscope to reach the ampullary region, then transhepatic insertion of a biliary SEMS should be considered prior to placing the gastroduodenal stent.

5. Biliary stents

5.1 Biliary strictures

Biliary stents are inserted at Endoscopic Retrograde Cholangio-Pancreatography (ERCP) in the setting of malignant bile duct strictures (pancreatic head cancers and cholangiocarcinomas). At ERCP, biliary stents are positioned through a side-viewing duodenoscope under direct endoscopic vision, and with fluoroscopic guidance. Despite advances in healthcare, most patients with malignant biliary strictures are not surgically curable. The obstructive jaundice and pruritus arising from blockage to the flow of bile into the duodenum can be very distressing. Endoscopic biliary stenting at ERCP provides relief from obstructive jaundice and pruritus, with associated improvement in quality of life (Ballinger et al., 1994). Stents used can be plastic or SEMS. Prior to the development of endoscopic stenting, relief of obstructive jaundice in unresectable malignant disease required a surgical biliary bypass operation. The first endoscopic transpapillary biliary stent insertion was performed in 1979 (Soehendra et al., 1980).

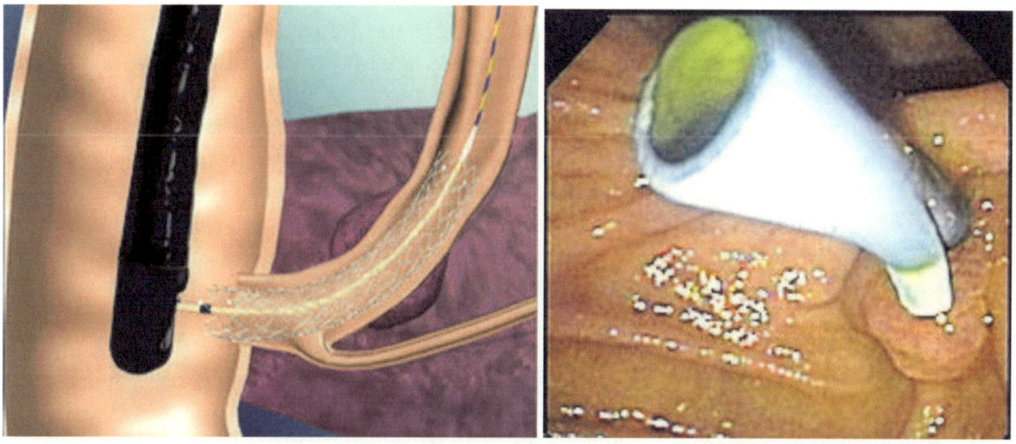

Fig. 6. Diagram of a SEMS deployed in distal bile duct at ERCP (left panel), and endoscopic view of a plastic biliary stent protruding from the duodenal ampulla in a patient with pancreatic cancer (right panel)

5.1.1 Role of stenting in obstructive jaundice due to operable pancreatic head carcinoma

Approximately 20% of patients with pancreatic cancer have localised disease making a surgical resection technically possible. Surgical candidates for the required pancreaticoduodenectomy (Whipple's procedure) may require preoperative biliary stenting to improve symptoms of obstructive jaundice while awaiting surgery. Furthermore, traditional surgical teaching has stated that operating in the presence of obstructive jaundice is linked to increased postoperative complications, and that the biochemical correction of jaundice preoperatively is linked to fewer surgical complications. However there are now increasing data indicating that preoperative biliary drainage using plastic stents may not actually be beneficial but may even be associated with more complications, particularly from cholangitis (van der Gaag et al., 2010). Therefore, if there is no time delay to surgical resection, preoperative biliary drainage using endoscopic stenting is best avoided.

5.1.2 Biliary stenting v. surgery for jaundice in unresectable pancreatic head carcinoma

Most (80%) patients with pancreatic head cancers and consequent biliary tract obstruction are not candidates for surgical resection. This is because of locally advanced disease (particularly infiltration of the major mesenteric vessels) or distant metastases, or patient frailty/comorbidities. Until the advent of biliary stenting, obstructive jaundice and pruritus could only be relieved by a palliative surgical biliary bypass procedure (cholecystojejunostomy or choledochojejunostomy). The introduction of plastic biliary stent placement at ERCP has allowed a non-invasive means of palliating jaundice and pruritus. Comparative trials of plastic stent placement with biliary bypass operations have shown similar survival outcomes, but stenting is associated with fewer complications, less use of resources and a shorter period of hospitalisation (Shepherd et al., 1988; Andersen et al., 1989; Smith et al., 1994; Moss et al., 2007). However plastic biliary stenting is associated with a higher risk of recurrent biliary obstruction than surgery. There have been no direct prospective trials comparing SEMS with biliary bypass surgery.

5.1.3 Plastic stents v. SEMS in unresectable pancreatic head carcinoma

Plastic stents tend to become blocked with biliary sludge and bacterial biofilm formation. A standard plastic 10 Fr stent may only last 3-5 months. A blocked stent will lead to a recurrence of jaundice and frequently cholangitis too. In the setting of inoperable pancreatic head cancer, the short life-span of the plastic stent is often greater than the life expectancy of the patient. Therefore although there is no doubt that modern biliary SEMS are less likely to become blocked (Davids et al., 1992; Moss et al., 2007; Weber et al., 2009), their superior patency over plastic stents will not become manifest in pancreatic head cancer patients with short life expectancy (Moss et al., 2006; Gronroos et al., 2010).

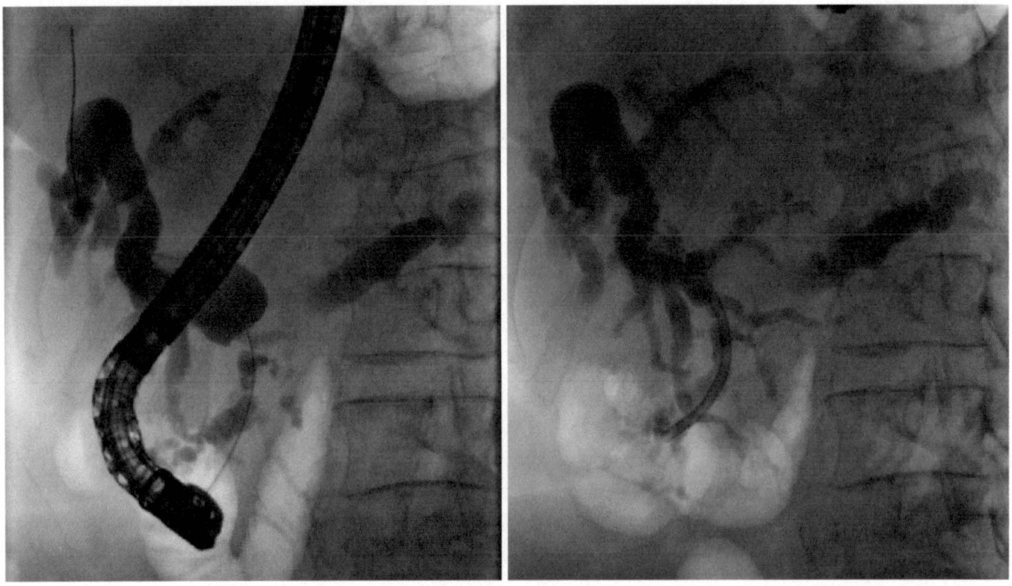

Fig. 7. ERCP images in a patient with carcinoma of head of pancreas. A wire has been placed across a stricture of the distal common bile duct into the dilated obstructed biliary system above (left hand image). Following insertion of a plastic stent (right hand image).

Wider plastic stents will remain patent for longer, but 12 Fr currently represents the maximum diameter of a plastic biliary stent since it is limited by the diameter of the duodenoscope's operating channel. Biliary stents, whether plastic or metal, traverse the Sphincter of Oddi which is the physiological barrier preventing bacteria from the duodenum refluxing into the biliary system. Since occlusion of biliary stents is in part due to bacterial biofilm formation, consideration has been given to prolonging stent patency by impregnating stents with antimicrobial agents or coating them with silver or hydrophilic polymer which reduce bacterial adhesion. However these approaches are based on *in vitro* observations and have not been translated into clinical advantage (Schilling et al., 2003; Donelli et al., 2007). Similarly administering oral antibiotics or using the choleretic agent ursodeoxycholic acid does not reliably lead to prolongation of plastic stent patency (Galandi et al., 2002).

For patients with inoperable pancreatic head cancer whose survival is predicted to be several months or longer, and for patients who cannot undergo resective surgery for distal common bile duct cholangiocarcinomas or ampullary tumours (both slower growing than pancreatic cancers), SEMS placement is superior to plastic stent placement. Biliary SEMS remain patent for longer periods than plastic stents (Moss et al., 2006). At least in part this is due to the fact that the diameter of a biliary SEMS is three times that of plastic stent. Biliary SEMS are far more costly than plastic stents, but their use is justified in patients whose survival is predicted to be more than 6 months since a repeat endoscopic procedure to replace an occluded plastic stent is likely to be needed by then. Although SEMS undoubtedly have greater patency, tumour tissue may grow through the gaps in the metal mesh leading to subsequent occlusion. The stent can be unblocked by trawling a balloon through its lumen, by using diathermy devices or by placing another (metal or plastic) stent within it. Tumour ingrowth can be offset by using silicone-covered biliary stents, but as with all covered stents these are more likely to migrate, compared to uncovered bare metal stents.

In the constant quest to improve stent design, a biliary SEMS incorporating a novel antireflux device has been developed with the hope that preventing reflux of duodenal contents into the biliary tract will aid stent patency (Hu et al., 2011).

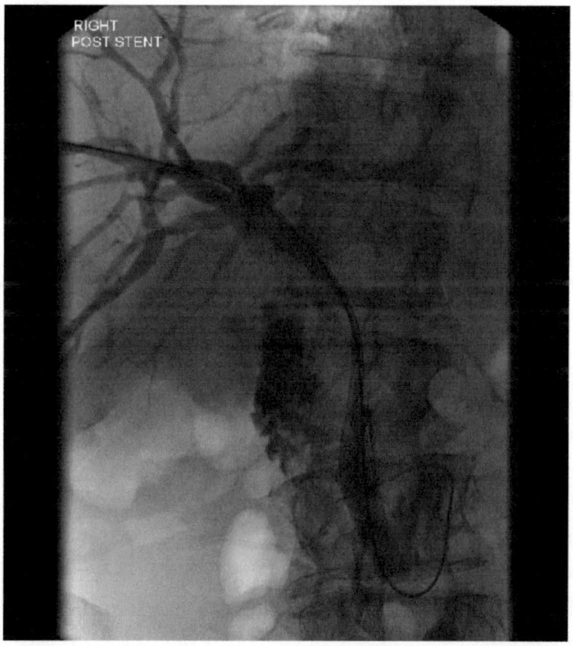

Fig. 8. SEMS being deployed across a malignant stricture of the common bile duct at transhepatic cholangiography

5.1.4 Biliary stenting in obstructive jaundice due to unresectable hilar malignancies

Malignant biliary obstruction at the liver hilum is usually due to cholangiocarcinoma, a primary cancer originating from the biliary ductal system (Aljiffry et al., 2009). Metastatic cancer infiltrating lymph nodes at the liver hilum can also cause stricturing at this site. While the most proximal cholangiocarcinomas originate from either the right or the left intrahepatic ductal system, cholangiocarcinomas more commonly involve the confluence of the two ductal systems where they join to form the common hepatic duct and are then known as hilar tumours. These intrahepatic and hilar chlangiocarcinomas often cause obstructive jaundice and pruritus. The only chance of a cure is a hepatic resection, but for many patients this is not an option due to advanced disease or due to frailty/comorbidities. In unresectable disease, palliation of jaundice and pruritus may be achieved by biliary stenting.

Stenting across malignant hilar strictures can be technically challenging at ERCP. Prior imaging of the biliary ductal system using Magnetic Resonance Cholangio-Pancreatography (MRCP) provides invaluable information before stenting is attempted. Strictures at the liver hilum may be complex and it may not be possible to drain obstructed liver segments at ERCP. There is a significant risk of causing cholangitis by injecting contrast medium into undrained ductal segments, therefore drainage of contrast-filled obstructed biliary branches is crucial. There has been much debate about the importance of establishing drainage of both liver lobes in malignant hilar obstruction. Although the right hepatic duct drains a greater volume of liver than the left hepatic duct, successful stenting of either side achieves a similar symptomatic and biochemical improvement (Polydoru et al., 1989). A randomised trial comparing the insertion of a single plastic stent to drain one side of the liver with placing two plastic stents to drain both sides, found that there was no advantage in placing two stents. Attempts to place two stents were associated with more complications, particularly cholangitis (de Palma et al., 2001). Extrapolating from this, it would seem that that if endoscopic stenting is to be performed for malignant hilar strictures, then a single SEMS is the best strategy. As with distal biliary strictures SEMS are less likely than plastic stents to occlude (Perdue at al., 2008).

Satisfactory biliary drainage of hilar strictures may not be possible at ERCP. Percutaneous hepatic drainage and stenting can be performed by an interventional radiologist if initial ERCP is unsuccessful, or if following endoscopic stenting there are undrained hepatic segments requiring treatment. Percutaneous stenting is performed using local anaesthetic and with intravenous sedation. Initial percutaneous transhepatic cholangiography will delineate the strictured area at the hilum and, usually after a period of external biliary drainage, a stent can be positioned at a second percutaneous transhepatic biliary procedure. ERCP and percutaneous transhepatic biliary radiology are thus complimentary interventions in the approach to proximal obstructive biliary strictures. There are few data comparing endoscopic and percutaneous stenting for hilar strictures. One retrospective study concluded that biliary decompression using SEMS was more likely to be successful if the SEMS was inserted via the percutaneous transhepatic route than if inserted via the endoscopic route (Paik et al., 2009).

5.2 Biliary stenting for common bile duct stones (choledocholithiasis)

Choledocholithiasis can lead to pain, obstructive jaundice, acute pancreatitis and cholangitis. Endoscopic removal of stones at ERCP is safer than open surgical exploration of the common bile duct. Common bile duct stone extraction at ERCP is usually successful using balloon catheters, baskets or lithotripsy after performing endoscopic sphincterotomy or sphincteroplasty (Williams et al., 2008). However it is not always possible to clear the common bile duct of stones, particularly large stones. The insertion of a stent to splint residual stone(s) is a reasonable temporary strategy, although it is preferable to clear the duct completely at a later procedure. Biliary stents used to splint common bile duct stone(s) are typically of the plastic pigtail variety. They are usually of smaller calibre, typically 7 Fr and inserted over a guidewire. The pigtail stent splints the stone within the bile duct, allowing bile to drain around it, and does not rely solely on the stent remaining patent. Stent placement for choledocholithiasis is a good temporising intervention in the setting of common bile duct stone(s) causing jaundice and/or cholangitis (Cairns et al., 1989; Maxton et al., 1995). Previously nasobiliary drainage was used as an emergency intervention in patients with life-threatening supporative cholangitis but the placement of a plastic stent provides as effective biliary drainage in this acute emergency (Sharma et al., 2005; Park et al., 2008).

If intervention at the index ERCP does not clear common bile duct stones and a stent is left *in situ* to provide drainage, then a follow up ERCP or surgical exploration of the common bile duct will be necessary (Williams et al., 2008). A second therapeutic ERCP after an interval is often successful at clearing the common bile duct (Maxton et al., 1995; Horiuchi et al., 2010). Clearing the bile duct is the preferred management course since the retention of common bile duct stones and ongoing presence of a plastic splinting stent makes a bout of future cholangitis more likely (Bergman et al., 1995; Chopra et al., 1996). Only patients who have limited life expectancy, or who have significant comorbidity should have plastic biliary stents left as sole therapy for their retained common bile duct stones (van Steenbergen et al., 1992; Williams et al., 2008).

5.3 Stenting for biliary leaks following cholecystectomy

Biliary leaks are not uncommon after cholecystectomy (Lau et al., 2010), and the advent of the laparoscopic approach to cholecystectomy has, if anything, made this surgical complication more common. Biliary leaks usually become evident in the early post-operative period, and may arise from an inadvertent intraoperative bile duct injury, or from the clips on the transected cystic duct becoming displaced. Once it is evident that a biliary leak with consequent biliary peritonitis is occurring, endoscopic treatment at ERCP is the preferred intervention (Tzovaras et al., 2001; Sandha et al., 2004; Agarwal et al., 2006). Endoscopic sphincterotomy alone will reduce pressure in the biliary system by equating it with intraduodenal pressure. The elimination or reduction in pressure gradient promotes preferential flow of bile from the common bile duct into the duodenum instead of extravasation via the leak. This allows a more proximal bile duct leak or cystic duct stump leak to heal spontaneously. However many endoscopists prefer to insert a temporary plastic stent. This can be a short stent across the Sphincter of Oddi, again effectively reducing pressure in the biliary system, so that the defect can heal spontaneously (Bjorkman et al., 1995). Alternatively a longer stent can be placed to cover the leak. For example in the case of a leaking cystic duct stump, a long straight plastic stent might be positioned with the proximal end above the junction of the cystic duct and bile duct. Endoscopically-placed plastic stents can be removed after approximately 6 weeks, by which time the biliary leak will have healed.

5.4 Stenting of biliary strictures caused by cholecystectomy or liver transplant

Bile duct stricturing may complicate bile duct injury at cholecystectomy. Traditionally a hepaticojejunostomy has been the definitive treatment for such stricturing after

cholecystectomy. However endoscopic access to the common bile duct at ERCP allows balloon dilatation and the insertion of a plastic biliary stent across the stricture. If plastic stents are routinely changed (to avoid clogging) every 3 months, then after approximately one year, stents can then be removed and in most cases the stricturing will not recur (de Palma et al., 2003; Vitale et al., 2008).
Biliary stricturing remains a common problem after orthotopic liver transplantation (Ayoub et al., 2010). The two usual types of bile duct reconstruction performed at the time of transplantation are duct-to-duct (choledocho-choledochostomy) and hepatico-jejunostomy. Duct-to-duct biliary reconstructions allow endoscopic access to the reconstructed bile duct. Strictures of the biliary anastomosis are characteristically localised and short. They respond well to endoscopic treatment with balloon dilatation and plastic biliary stenting (Seo et al., 2009). However transplant recipients may also experience non-anastomotic strictures which are a consequence of ischaemia or immunological reaction. These non-anastomotic strictures may be more diffuse and longer. They respond less well to endoscopic therapy with repeated dilatations and stenting (Williams & Draganov, 2009).

6. Pancreatic stents

Stenting of the pancreatic duct at ERCP is used in chronic pancreatitis, pancreatic duct leaks and the prevention of ERCP-induced pancreatitis. Invariably plastic stents are used in these settings. The pancreatic duct is much narrower than the biliary ductal system, and stents in the pancreatic duct can induce fibrosis and stricturing.

6.1 Chronic pancreatitis

Refractory pain in chronic pancreatitis may be associated with an obstructed pancreatic duct. In patients suffering ongoing pain due to chronic pancreatitis, pancreatic stenting helps relieve pressure in a pancreatic duct obstructed by an inflammatory stricture or stone, often with subsequent pain relief (Wilcox & Varadarajulu, 2006, Weber et al., 2007, Nguyen-Tang & Dumonceau, 2010). Patients with a dominant pancreatic duct stricture in the pancreatic head seem to derive most benefit from such transpapillary stent placement. However well-performed prospective controlled studies of pancreatic endoscopic therapy for chronic pancreatitis are lacking. Furthermore, pancreatic duct stenting is inferior to surgical drainage in relieving pain associated with an obstructed pancreatic duct (Cahen et al,, 2007). When pancreatic stents are used in chronic pancreatitis, endoscopists typically use stent calibres ranging from 7 Fr to 11.5 Fr, and elective stent changes are needed every 2-3 months. Smaller calibre stents will occlude more easily and need more frequent changing.

6.2 Pancreatic duct fistulae

The pancreatic duct can be disrupted by an attack of acute pancreatitis or following surgery. Subsequent pancreatic duct leaks with/without pseudocyst formation can be treated by the insertion of a transpapillary pancreatic duct stent (Cicek et al,, 2006). Any discrete connection between the pancreatic duct and a pancreatic pseudocyst can be sealed off by the insertion of a pancreatic stent.

6.3 Preventing ERCP-induced pancreatitis

Acute pancreatitis is a recognised complication of ERCP, occurring in up to approximately 5% of therapeutic ERCPs (Freeman et al., 1996; Arata et al., 2010). The risk of pancreatitis is greater in some patient categories (Cheng et al., 2006), and may be as great as 20-30% in women with Sphincter of Oddi dysfunction. Pancreatic stent placement decreases the risk of post-ERCP pancreatitis in high-risk patients (Arata et al., 2010; Choudhary et al., 2011). Typically 5 Fr or 3 Fr gauge straight stents are used. Unflanged stents are advantageous in this setting since they are more likely to spontaneously dislodge, and a second endoscopic procedure to remove the stent is avoided.

7. Colorectal stents

Colorectal cancer is usually treated by planned surgery, but many patients present as an emergency with acute colonic obstruction. Colorectal SEMS can be used in the treatment of acute malignant colonic obstruction as a bridge to definitive surgery. Secondly, some patients with colonic cancers which are starting to produce obstructive symptoms may not be surgical candidates due to metastatic disease or frailty/comorbidities. These patients can be electively palliated using SEMS.

Colonic SEMSs are usually uncovered and can be inserted with a combination of endoscopy and fluoroscopic guidance. Typically an endoscope is used to identify the obstructing cancer, and a wire is passed through the stricture and into the proximal bowel. The endoscope is then withdrawn and the stent delivery mechanism is fed over the wire. The endoscope can be reinserted alongside the stent delivery mechanism and together with fluoroscopy can be used to guide the deployment of the stent across the obstructing lesion. For obstructing cancers in the proximal colon, stent placement is best achieved using a "through the scope" delivery mechanism. The stent delivery mechanism is delivered over a guidewire through the working channel of a colonoscope and deployed without removing the colonoscope.

7.1 Colorectal SEMS for acute colonic obstruction

Up to 20% of patients with colon cancer initially present with symptoms of acute colonic obstruction. Obstruction is more common in the distal colon, which has a smaller calibre than the proximal colon. Emergency surgery plays a major role in the management of these patients. However, emergency decompressive surgery on the unprepared and obstructed bowel, in patients who are often very sick, carries a significant risk of morbidity (32%-64%) and mortality (15%-34%) (McLoughlin & Byrne, 2008).

Emergency surgical decompression invariably involves colostomy formation, since primary anastomosis in the setting of an unprepared and obstructed bowel is likely to break down. Operations range from a loop colostomy, a Hartmann's procedure or sometimes a subtotal colectomy. Following such emergency surgery, a patient with a potentially resectable cancer will then require a planned second operation at a later stage. However, in up to 40% patients the colostomy becomes permanent and will not be closed because of metastatic disease or frailty.

Placement of a colonic SEMS to relieve the malignant obstruction in the emergency setting will spare the patient emergency surgery and colostomy formation. Stenting allows time for the patient to recover from acute symptoms, and undergo appropriate cancer staging investigations. In patients whose staging investigations confirm operable cancer, stenting as a bridge to a definitive resection allows better preparation for the surgery which is less likely to then involve stoma formation. In these situations the stent is removed together with the resected tumour. In patients whose staging investigations reveal inoperable cancer, the stent provides palliation.

Early studies showed that colorectal stents inserted under a combination of endoscopic and fluoroscopic (Baron et al., 1998) or fluoroscopic guidance alone (Mainar et al., 1996) are safe and effective in the treatment of acute malignant colonic obstruction. A randomised study of 48 patients with obstructing left distal colonic cancers compared SEMS placement followed by definitive laparoscopic-assisted colonic resection and conventional emergency open surgery. Patients in the SEMS / laparoscopic surgery group were more likely to have a successful single stage operation (67% vs 38%), less likely to have a permanent stoma (0% vs 25%), and less likely to have complications than the emergency surgery group (Cheung et al., 2009). In another prospective randomised study, obstructed patients who were stented prior to surgery were also more likely to have a primary anastomosis compared to those who had emergency surgery (85% vs 41%). They also had fewer complications, re-interventions and a reduced total hospital and ITU stay (Martinez-Santos et al., 2002). In a meta-analysis that included non randomised and somewhat heterogeneous studies comparing SEMS and open surgery for malignant large bowel obstruction, mortality was 5.7% in those undergoing SEMS compared to 12.1% in those having emergency surgery (Tilney et al., 2007).

7.2 Colorectal SEMS for palliation of incurable colonic cancer

SEMS are also used electively for palliation of symptoms in patients who are frail and not fit for surgery, or in cases of advanced cancer. Two small randomised controlled trials have compared SEMS to colostomy for the palliation of malignant obstruction (Fiori et al., 2004; Xinopoulos et al., 2004). They found that patients who were treated with SEMS spent less time in hospital and had a shorter time to oral intake and restoration of bowel function. A recent retrospective study from a single centre also showed a high technical and clinical success rate for SEMS insertion, with few complications up to 30 days after stent insertion. However complications (mainly stent re-obstruction and stent migration necessitating the placement of a second stent) after 30 days were higher in patients treated with SEMS than in those treated with surgery (Lee et al., 2011).

7.3 Technical success and complications associated with colorectal SEMS

Colonic stents have now been used in malignant colorectal obstruction for two decades. Two systematic reviews of non randomised studies (Khot et al., 2002; Sebastian et al., 2004) conclude that colonic stents can be successfully placed in the majority of cases (92% and 94%) with a good clinical result (88% and 91%). Complications in these reviews included perforation in about 4%, stent migration in 10% and re-obstruction in 10% of patients. Stent related mortality is approximately 1%. Based on the available data, the World Society of Emergency Surgery and the Peritoneum and Surgery Society advocate the use of colorectal stents in preference to colostomy in cases where palliation is needed, and endorse their use as a bridge to surgery in cases of acute malignant colonic obstruction (Ansaloni et al., 2010)
SEMS insertion for benign diseases of the colon is somewhat controversial. The role for SEMS in treating benign colonic strictures has yet to be established.

8. Summary

Advances in endoscopy and in stent technology in the past 20 years have allowed non-invasive palliation of obstructive symptoms within the gastrointestinal tract using stents. In many clinical scenarios, stent placement has proved advantageous over surgery.

9. Acknowledgments

Figures of *in vitro* stents are reproduced with permission from Cook Medical and Olympus.

10. References

Ackroyd, R., Watson, D. I., Devitt, P. G. & Jamieson, G. G. (2001). Expandable metallic stents should not be used in the treatment of benign esophageal strictures. *J Gastroenterol Hepatol*, 16, 484-7.

Agarwal, N., Sharma, B. C., Garg, S., Kumar, R. & Sarin, S. K. (2006). Endoscopic management of postoperative bile leaks. *Hepatobiliary Pancreatic Dis Int*, 5, 273-7.

Aljiffry, M., Walsh, M. J. & Molinari, M. (2009). Advances in diagnosis, treatment and palliation of cholangiocarcinoma: 1990-2009. *World J Gastroenterol*, 15, 4240-62.

Andersen, J. R., Sørensen, S. M., Kruse, A., Rokkjaer, M. & Matzen, P. (1989). Randomised trial of endoscopic endoprosthesis versus operative bypass in malignant obstructive jaundice. *Gut*, 30, 1132-5.

Ansaloni, L., Andersson, R. E., Bazzoli, F., Catena, F., Cennamo, V., Di Saverio, S., Fuccio, L., Jeekel, H., Leppäniemi, A., Moore, E., Pinna, A. D., Pisano, M., Repici, A., Sugarbaker, P. H. & Tuech, J. J. (2010). Guidelines in the management of obstructing cancer of the left colon: consensus conference of the world society of emergency surgery (WSES) and peritoneum and surgery (PnS) society, *World J Emerg Surg*, 28, 29.

Arata, S., Takada, T., Hirata, K., Yoshida, M., Mayumi, T., Hirota, M., Yokoe, M., Hirota, M., Kiriyama, S., Sekimoto, M., Amano, H., Wada, K., Kimura, Y., Gabata, T., Takeda, K., Kataoka, K., Ito, T. & Tanaka, M. (2010). Post-ERCP pancreatitis. *J Hepatobiliary Pancreat Sci*, 17, 70-8.

Ayoub, W. S., Esquivel, C. O. & Martin, P. (2010). Biliary complications following liver transplantation. *Dig Dis Sci*, 55, 1540-6.

Ballinger, A. B., McHugh, M., Catnach, S. M., Alstead, E. M. & Clark, M. L. (1994). Symptom relief and quality of life after stenting for malignant bile duct obstruction. *Gut*, 35, 467-70.

Baron, T. H., Dean, P. A., Yates 3rd, M. R., Canon, C. & Koehler, R. E. (1998). Expandable metal stents for the treatment of colonic obstruction: techniques and outcomes, *Gastrointest Endosc*, 47, 277-86.

Bergman, J. J., Rauws, E. A., Tijssen, J. G., Tytgat, G. N. & Huibregtse, K. (1995). Biliary endoprostheses in elderly patients with endoscopically irretrievable common bile duct stones: report on 117 patients. *Gastrointest Endosc*, 42, 195-201.

Bethge, N., Sommer, A., Gross, U., von Kleist, D. & Vakil, N. (1996). Human tissue responses to metal stents implanted in vivo for the palliation of malignant stenoses. *Gastrointest Endosc*, 43, 596-602.

Bjorkman, D. J., Carr-Locke, D. L., Lichtenstein, D. R., Ferrari, A. P., Slivka, A., Van Dam, J. & Brooks, D. C. (1995). Postsurgical bile leaks: endoscopic obliteration of the transpapillary pressure gradient is enough. *Am J Gastroenterol*, 90, 2128-33.

Burt, M., Diehl, W., Martini, N., Bains, M. S., Ginsberg, R. J., McCormack, P. M. & Rusch, V. W. (1991). Malignant esophagorespiratory fistula: management options and survival. *Ann Thorac Surg*, 52, 1222-8.

Cahen, D. L., Gouma, D. J., Nio, Y., Rauws, E. A., Boermeester, M. A., Busch, O. R., Stoker, J., Laméris, J. S., Dijkgraaf, M. G., Huibregtse, K. & Bruno, M. J. (2007). Endoscopic versus surgical drainage of the pancreatic duct in chronic pancreatitis. *N Engl J Med*, 356, 676-84.

Cairns, S. R., Dias, L., Cotton, P. B., Salmon, P. R. & Russell, R. C. (1989). Additional endoscopic procedures instead of urgent surgery for retained common bile duct stones. *Gut*, 30, 535-40.

Cheng, C. L., Sherman, S., Watkins, J. L., Barnett, J., Freeman, M., Geenen, J., Ryan, M., Parker, H., Frakes, J. T., Fogel, E. L., Silverman, W. B., Dua, K. S., Aliperti, G., Yakshe, P., Uzer, M., Jones, W., Goff, J., Lazzell-Pannell, L., Rashdan, A., Temkit, M. & Lehman, G. A. (2006). Risk factors for post-ERCP pancreatitis: a prospective multicenter study. *Am J Gastroenterol*, 101, 139-47.

Cheung, H. Y., Chung, C. C., Tsang, W. W., Wong, J. C., Yau, K. K. & Li, M. K. (2009). Endolaparoscopic approach vs conventional open surgery in the treatment of obstructing left-sided colon cancer: a randomized controlled trial. *Arch Surg*, 144, 1127-32.

Chopra, K. B., Peters, R. A., O'Toole, P. A., Williams, S. G., Gimson, A. E., Lombard, M. G. & Westaby, D. (1996). Randomised study of endoscopic biliary endoprosthesis versus duct clearance for bile duct stones in high-risk patients. *Lancet*, 348, 791-3.

Choudhary, A., Bechtold, M. L., Arif, M., Szary, N. M., Puli, S. R., Othman, M. O., Pais, W. P., Antillon, M. R. & Roy, P. K. (2011). Pancreatic stents for prophylaxis against post-ERCP pancreatitis: a meta-analysis and systematic review. *Gastrointest Endosc*, 73, 275-82.

Chung, M. G., Kang, D. H., Park, D. K., Park, J. J., Park, H. C. & Kim, J. H.(2001). Successful treatment of Boerhaave's syndrome with endoscopic insertion of a self-expandable metallic stent: report of three cases and a review of the literature. *Endoscopy*, 33, 894-7.

Cicek, B., Parlak, E., Oguz, D., Disibeyaz, S., Koksal, A. S. & Sahin, B. (2006). Endoscopic treatment of pancreatic fistulas. *Surg Endosc*, 20, 1706-12.

Conio, M., Repici, A., Battaglia, G., De Pretis, G., Ghezzo, L., Bittinger, M., Messmann, H., Demarquay, J. F., Blanchi, S., Togni, M., Conigliaro, R. & Filiberti, R. (2007). A randomized prospective comparison of self-expandable plastic stents and partially covered self-expandable metal stents in the palliation of malignant esophageal dysphagia. *Am J Gastroenterol*, 102, 2667-77.

Davids, P. H. P., Groen, A. K., Rauws, E. A. J., Tytgat, G. N. & Huibregtse, K. (1992). Randomized trial of self-expanding metal stents versus polyethylene stents for distal malignant biliary obstruction. *Lancet*, 340, 1488-92.

De Palma, G. D., di Matteo, E., Romano, G., Fimmano, A., Rondinone, G. & Catanzano, C. (1996). Plastic prosthesis versus expandable metal stents for palliation of inoperable esophageal thoracic carcinoma: a controlled prospective study. *Gastrointest Endosc*, 43, 478-82.

De Palma, G. D., Galloro, G., Siciliano, S., Iovino, P. & Catanzano, C. (2001). Unilateral versus bilateral endoscopic hepatic duct drainage in patients with malignant hilar biliary obstruction: results of a prospective, randomized, and controlled study. *Gastrointest Endosc*, 53, 547-53.

De Palma, G. D., Galloro, G., Romano, G., Sottile, R., Puzziello, A., Persico, F., Masone, S., Labianca, O. & Persico, G. (2003). Long-term follow-up after endoscopic biliary stent placement for bile duct strictures from laparoscopic cholecystectomy. *Hepatogastroenterology*, 50, 1229-31.

Diamantis, G., Scarpa, M., Bocus, P., Realdon, S., Castoro, C., Ancona, E. & Battaglia, G. (2011). Quality of life in patients with esophageal stenting for the palliation of malignant dysphagia. *World J Gastroenterol*, 17, 144-50.

Donelli, G., Guaglianone, E., Di Rosa, R., Fiocca, F. & Basoli, A. (2007). Plastic biliary stent occlusion: factors involved and possible preventive approaches. *Clin Med Res*, 5, 53-60.

Dumonceau, J. M., Cremer, M., Lalmand, B. & Devière, J. (1999). Esophageal fistula sealing: choice of stent, practical management, and cost. *Gastrointest Endosc*, 49, 70-8.

Eickhoff, A., Knoll, M., Jakobs, R., Weickert, U., Hartmann, D., Schilling, D., Eickhoff, J. C. & Riemann, J. F. (2005). Self-expanding metal stents versus plastic prostheses in the palliation of malignant dysphagia: long-term outcome of 153 consecutive patients. *J Clin Gastroenterol*, 39, 877-85.

Eubanks, P. J., Hu, E., Nguyen, D., Procaccino, F., Eysselein, V. E. & Klein, S. R. (1999). Case of Boerhaave's syndrome successfully treated with a self-expandable metallic stent. *Gastrointest Endosc*, 49, 780-3.

Fiori, E., Lamazza, A., De Cesare, A., Bononi, M., Volpino, P., Schillaci, A., Cavallaro, A. & Cangemi, V. (2004). Palliative management of malignant rectosigmoidal obstruction. Colostomy vs. endoscopic stenting. A randomized prospective trial. *Anticancer Res*, 24, 265-8.

Fiorini, A., Fleischer, D., Valero, J., Israeli, E., Wengrower, D. & Goldin, E. (2000). Self-expandable metal coil stents in the treatment of benign esophageal strictures refractory to conventional therapy: a case series. *Gastrointest Endosc*, 52, 259-62.

Fischer, A., Thomusch, O., Benz, S., von Dobschuetz, E., Baier, P., Hopt, U. T. (2006). Nonoperative treatment of 15 benign esophageal perforations with self-expandable covered metal stents. *Ann Thorac Surg*, 81, 467-72.

Freeman, M. L., Nelson, D. B., Sherman, S., Haber, G. B., Herman, M. E., Dorsher, P. J., Moore, J. P., Fennerty, M. B., Ryan, M. E., Shaw, M. J., Lande, J. D. & Pheley, A. M. (1996). Complications of endoscopic biliary sphincterotomy. *N Engl J Med*, 335, 909-18.

Gaidos, J. K. & Draganov, P. V. (2009). Treatment of malignant gastric outlet obstruction with endoscopically placed self-expandable metal stents. *World J Gastroenterol*, 15, 4365–4371.

Galandi, D., Schwarzer, G., Bassler, D. & Allgaier, H. P. (2002). Ursodeoxycholic acid and/or antibiotics for prevention of biliary stent occlusion. *Cochrane Database of Systematic Reviews*, 3, (2002), CD003043.

Gevers, A. M., Macken, E., Hiele, M. & Rutgeerts, P. (1998). A comparison of laser therapy, plastic stents, and expandable metal stents for palliation of malignant dysphagia in patients without a fistula. *Gastrointest Endosc*, 84, 383-8.

Grönroos, J. M., Gullichsen, R., Laine, S. & Salminen, P. (2010). Endoscopic palliation of malignant obstructive jaundice in extremely elderly patients: plastic stent is enough. *Minim Invasive Ther Allied Technol*, 19, 122-4.

Homs, M. Y., Steyerberg, E. W., Eijkenboom, W. M., Tilanus, H. W., Stalpers, L. J., Bartelsman, J. F., van Lanschot, J. J, Wijrdeman, H. K., Mulder, C. J., Reinders, J. G., Boot, H., Aleman, B. M., Kuipers, E. J. & Siersema, P. D. (2004). Single-dose brachytherapy versus metal stent placement for the palliation of dysphagia from oesophageal cancer: multicentre randomised trial. *Lancet*, 364, 1497-504.

Horiuchi, A., Nakayama, Y., Kajiyama, M., Kato, N., Kamijima, T., Graham, D. Y. & Tanaka, N. (2010). Biliary stenting in the management of large or multiple common bile duct stones. *Gastrointest Endosc*, 71, 1200-1203.

Hu, B., Wang, T.,T., Shi, Z. M., Wang, S. Z., Lu, R., Pan, Y. M., Huang, H. & Wang, S.P.(2011). A novel antireflux metal stent for the palliation of biliary malignancies: a pilot feasibility study (with video). *Gastrointest Endosc*, 73, 143-8.

Hubmann, R., Bodlaj, G., Czompo, M., Benkö, L., Pichler, P., Al-Kathib, S., Kiblböck, P., Shamyieh, A. & Biesenbach, G. (2006). The use of self-expanding metal stents to treat acute esophageal variceal bleeding. *Endoscopy*, 38, 896-901.

Jeurnink, S. M., Steyerberg, E. W., van Hooft, J. E., van Eijck, C. H., Schwartz, M. P., Vleggaar, F. P., Kuipers, E. J. & Siersema, P. D for the Dutch SUSTENT Study Group. (2010). Surgical gastrojejunostomy or endoscopic stent placement for the palliation of malignant gastric outlet obstruction (SUSTENT study): a multicenter randomized trial. *Gastrointest Endosc*, 71, 490-9.

Johnsson, E., Thune, A. & Liedman, B. (2004). Palliation of malignant gastroduodenal obstruction with open surgical bypass or endoscopic stenting: clinical outcome and health economic evaluation. *World J Surg*, 28, 812-7.

Johnsson, E., Lundell, L. & Liedman, B. (2005). Sealing of esophageal perforation or ruptures with expandable metallic stents: a prospective controlled study on treatment efficacy and limitations. *Dis Esophagus*, 18, 262-6.

Kaw, M., Singh, S. & Gagneja, H. (2003). Clinical outcome of simultaneous self-expandable metal stents for palliation of malignant biliary and duodenal obstruction. *Surg Endosc*, 17, 457-61.

Keeling, W. B., Miller, D. L., Lam, G. T., Kilgo, P., Miller, J. I., Mansour, K. A. & Force, S. D. (2010). Low mortality after treatment for esophageal perforation: a single-center experience. *Ann Thorac Surg*, 90, 1669-73.

Khot, U. P., Lang, A. W., Murali, K. & Parker, M. C. (2002). Systematic review of the efficacy and safety of colorectal stents, *Br J Surg*, 89, 1096-102.

Kiernan, P. D., Khandhar, S. J., Fortes, D. L., Sheridan, M. J. & Hetrick, V. (2010) Thoracic esophageal perforations. *Am Surg*, 76, 1355-62.

Kim, J. H., Song, H. Y., Shin, J. H., Choi, E., Kim, T. W., Jung, H. Y., Lee, G. H., Lee, S. K., Kim, M. H., Ryu, M. H., Kang, Y. K., Kim, B. S. & Yook, J. H. (2007). Metallic stent placement in the palliative treatment of malignant gastroduodenal obstructions: prospective evaluation of results and factors influencing outcome in 213 patients. *Gastrointest Endosc*, 66, 256-64.

Knyrim, K., Wagner, H. J., Bethge, N., Keymling, M. & Vakil, N. (1993). A controlled trial of an expansile metal stent for palliation of esophageal obstruction due to inoperable cancer. *N Engl J Med*, 329, 1302-7.

Königsrainer, A., Riedmann, B., De Vries, A., Ofner, D., Spechtenhauser, B., Aigner, F., Fritsch, E. & Margreiter, R. (2000). Expandable metal stents versus laser combined with radiotherapy for palliation of unresectable esophageal cancer: a prospective randomized trial. *Hepatogastroenterology*, 47, 724-7.

Kozarek, R. A., Ball, T. J., Brandabur, J. J., Patterson, D. J., Low, D., Hill, L. & Raltz, S. (1996). Expandable versus conventional esophageal prostheses: easier insertion may not preclude subsequent stent-related problems. *Gastrointest Endosc*, 43, 204-8.

Lau, W. Y., Lai, E. C. & Lau, S. H. (2010). Management of bile duct injury after laparoscopic cholecystectomy: a review. *ANZ J Surg*, 80, 75-81.

Lee, H. J., Hong, S. P., Cheon, J. H., Kim, T. I., Min, B. S., Kim, N. K. & Kim, W. H. (2011). Long-term outcome of palliative therapy for malignant colorectal obstruction in patients with unresectable metastatic colorectal cancers: endoscopic stenting versus surgery. *Gastrointest Endosc*, 73, 535-42.

Low, D. E. & Kozarek, R. A. (1998). Comparison of conventional and wire mesh expandable prostheses and surgical bypass in patients with malignant esophagorespiratory fistulas. *Ann Thorac Surg*, 65, 919-23.

Lowe, A. S., Beckett, C. G., Jowett, S., May, J., Stephenson, S., Scally, A., Tam, E. & Kay, C. L. (2007). Self-expandable metal stent placement for the palliation of malignant gastroduodenal obstruction: experience in a large, single, UK centre. *Clin Radiol*, 62, 738-44.

Ly, J., O'Grady, G., Mittal, A., Plank, L. & Windsor, J. A. (2010). A systematic review of methods to palliate malignant gastric outlet obstruction. *Surg Endosc*, 24, 290-7.

Maetani, I., Tada, T., Ukita, T., Inoue, H., Sakai, Y. & Nagao, J. (2004). Comparison of duodenal stent placement with surgical gastrojejunostomy for palliation in patients with duodenal obstructions caused by pancreaticobiliary malignancies. *Endoscopy*, 36, 73-8.

Mainar, A., De Gregorio Ariza, M. A., Tejero, E., Tobío, R., Alfonso, E., Pinto, I., Herrera, M. & Fernández, J. A. (1996). Acute colorectal obstruction: treatment with self-expandable metallic stents before scheduled surgery--results of a multicenter study, *Radiology*, 210, 65-9.

Martin , D. F. & Laasch, H. U. (2004). Gastroduodenal stenting. *Semin Intervent Radio*l, 21, 167-79.

Martinez-Santos, C., Lobato, R. F., Fradejas, J. M., Pinto, I., Ortega-Deballón, P. & Moreno-Azcoita, M. (2002). Self-expandable stent before elective surgery vs. emergency surgery for the treatment of malignant colorectal obstructions: comparison of primary anastomosis and morbidity rates, *Dis Colon Rectum*, 45, 401-6.

Maxton, D. G., Tweedle, D. E. & Martin, D. F. (1995). Retained common bile duct stones after endoscopic sphincterotomy: temporary and longterm treatment with biliary stenting. *Gut*, 36, 446-9.

May, A., Hahn, E. G. & Ell, C. (1996). Self-expanding metal stents for palliation of malignant obstruction in the upper gastrointestinal tract. Comparative assessment of three stent types implemented in 96 implantations. *J Clin Gastroenterol*, 22, 261-6.

May, A. & Ell, C. (1998). Palliative treatment of malignant esophagorespiratory fistulas with Gianturco-Z stents. A prospective clinical trial and review of the literature on covered metal stents. *Am J Gastroenterol*, 93, 532-5.

McLoughlin, M.T., & Byrne, M.F. (2008). Endoscopic stenting: where are we now and where can we go?, *World J of Gastroenterol*, 14, 3798-803.

Moss, A. C., Morris, E. & Mac Mathuna, P. (2006). Palliative biliary stents for obstructing pancreatic carcinoma. *Cochrane Database Systematic Reviews*, 19, 2, (April 2006), CD004200.

Moss, A. C., Morris, E., Leyden, J. & MacMathuna, P. (2007). Malignant distal biliary obstruction: a systematic review and meta-analysis of endoscopic and surgical bypass results. *Cancer Treat Rev*, 33, 213-21

Mutignani, M., Tringali, A., Shah, S. G., Perri, V., Familiari, P., Iacopini, F., Spada, C. & Costamagna, G. (2007). Combined endoscopic stent insertion in malignant biliary and duodenal obstruction. *Endoscopy*, 39, 440-7.

Nguyen-Tang, T. & Dumonceau, J. M. (2010). Endoscopic treatment in chronic pancreatitis, timing, duration and type of intervention. *Best Pract Res Clin Gastroenterol*, 24, 281-98.

Paik,W. H., Park, Y. S., Hwang, J. H., Lee, S. H., Yoon, C. J., Kang, S. G., Lee, J. K., Ryu, J. K., Kim, Y. T. & Yoon, Y. B. (2009). Palliative treatment with self-expandable metallic stents in patients with advanced type III or IV hilar cholangiocarcinoma: a percutaneous versus endoscopic approach. *Gastrointest Endosc*, 69, 55-62.

Park, S. Y., Park, C. H., Cho, S. B., Yoon, K. W., Lee, W. S., Kim, H. S., Choi, S.K. & Rew, J. S. (2008). The safety and effectiveness of endoscopic biliary decompression by plastic stent placement in acute suppurative cholangitis compared with nasobiliary drainage. *Gastrointest Endosc*, 68, 1076-80.

Perdue, D. G., Freeman, M. L., DiSario, J. A., Nelson, D. B., Fennerty, M. B., Lee, J. G., Overby, C. S., Ryan, M. E., Bochna, G. S., Snady, H. W. & Moore, J. P. (2008). Plastic versus self-expanding metallic stents for malignant hilar biliary obstruction: a prospective multicenter observational cohort study. *J Clin Gastroenterol*, 42, 1040-6.

Polydorou, A. A., Chisholm, E. M., Romanos, A. A., Dowsett, J. F., Cotton, P. B., Hatfield, A. R. & Russell, R. C. (1989). A comparison of right versus left hepatic duct endoprosthesis insertion in malignant hilar biliary obstruction. *Endoscopy*, 21, 266-71.

Repici, A., Vleggaar, F. P., Hassan, C., van Boeckel, P. G., Romeo, F., Pagano, N., Malesci, A. & Siersema, P. D. (2010). Efficacy and safety of biodegradable stents for refractory benign esophageal strictures: the BEST (Biodegradable Esophageal Stent) study. *Gastrointest Endosc*, 72, 927-34.

Roseveare, C. D., Patel, P., Simmonds, N., Goggin, P. M., Kimble, J. & Shepherd, H. A. (1998). Metal stents improve dysphagia, nutrition and survival in malignant oesophageal stenosis: a randomized controlled trial comparing modified Gianturco Z-stents with plastic Atkinson tubes. *Eur J Gastroenterol Hepatol*, 10, 653-7.

Ross, W. A., Alkassab, F., Lynch, P. M., Ayers, G. D., Ajani, J., Lee, J. H. & Bismar, M. (2007). Evolving role of self-expanding metal stents in the treatment of malignant dysphagia and fistulas. *Gastrointest Endosc*, 65, 70-6.

Sabharwal, T., Hamady, M. S., Chui, S., Atkinson, S., Mason, R. & Adam, A. (2003). A randomised prospective comparison of the Flamingo Wallstent and Ultraflex stent for palliation of dysphagia associated with lower third oesophageal carcinoma. *Gut*, 52, 922-6.

Saito, Y., Tanaka, T., Andoh, A., Minematsu, H., Hata, K., Tsujikawa, T., Nitta, N., Murata, K. & Fujiyama, Y. (2007). Usefulness of biodegradable stents constructed of poly-l-lactic acid monofilaments in patients with benign esophageal stenosis. *World J Gastroenterol*, 13, 3977-80.

Sandha, G. S. & Marcon, N. E. (1999). Expandable metal stents for benign esophageal obstruction. *Gastrointest Endosc Clin North Am*, 9, 437-46.

Sandha, G. S., Bourke, M. J., Haber, G. B. & Kortan, P. P. (2004). Endoscopic therapy for bile leak based on a new classification: results in 207 patients. *Gastrointest Endosc*, 60, 567-74.

Saranovic, D., Djuric-Stefanovic, A., Ivanovic, A., Masulovic, D. & Pesko, P. (2005). Fluoroscopically guided insertion of self-expandable metal esophageal stents for palliative treatment of patients with malignant stenosis of esophagus and cardia: comparison of uncovered and covered stent types. *Dis Esophagus*, 18, 230-8.

Schilling, D., Rink, G., Arnold, J. C., Benz, C., Adamek, H. E., Jakobs, R. & Riemann, J. F. (2003). Prospective, randomized, single-center trial comparing 3 different 10F plastic stents in malignant mid and distal bile duct strictures. *Gastrointest Endosc*, 58, 54-8.

Sebastian, S., Johnston, S., Geoghegan, T., Torreggiani, W. & Buckley, M. (2004). Pooled analysis of the efficacy and safety of self-expanding metal stenting in malignant colorectal obstruction, *Am J Gastroenterol*, 99, 2051-7.

Seo, J. K., Ryu, J. K., Lee, S. H., Park, J. K., Yang, K. Y., Kim, Y. T., Yoon, Y. B., Lee, H. W., Yi, N. J. & Suh, K. S. (2009). Endoscopic treatment for biliary stricture after adult living donor liver transplantation. *Liver Transpl*, 15, 4, 369-80.

Sharma, B. C., Kumar, R., Agarwal, N. & Sarin, S. K. (2005). Endoscopic biliary drainage by nasobiliary drain or by stent placement in patients with acute cholangitis. *Endoscopy*, 37, 439-43.

Sharma, P. & Kozarek, R. (2010). Role of esophageal stents in benign and malignant diseases. *Am J Gastroenterol*, 105, 258-73.

Shepherd, H. A., Royle, G., Ross, A. P., Diba, A., Arthur, M. & Colin-Jones, D. (1988). Endoscopic biliary endoprosthesis in the palliation of malignant obstruction of the distal common bile duct: a randomized trial. *Br J Surg*, 75, 1166-8.

Shin, J. H., Song, H. Y., Ko, G. Y., Lim, J. O., Yoon, H. K. & Sung, K.B. (2004) Esophagorespiratory fistula: long-term results of palliative treatment with covered expandable metallic stents in 61 patients. *Radiology*, 232, 252-9.

Siersema, P. D., Hop, W. C., van Blankenstein, M., van Tilburg, A. J., Bac, D. J., Homs, M. Y. & Kuipers, E. J. (2001), A comparison of 3 types of covered metal stents for the palliation of patients with dysphagia caused by esophagogastric carcinoma: a prospective, randomized study. *Gastrointest Endosc*, 54, 145-53.

Siersema, P. D., Homs, M. Y., Haringsma, J., Tilanus, H. W. & Kuipers, E. J. (2003). Use of large-diameter metallic stents to seal traumatic nonmalignant perforations of the esophagus. *Gastrointest Endosc*, 58, 356-61.

Smith, A. C., Dowsett, J. F., Russell, R. C., Hatfield, A. R. & Cotton, P. B. (1994). Randomised trial of endoscopic stenting versus surgical bypass in malignant low bile duct obstruction. *Lancet*, 344, 1655-60.

Soehendra, N. & Reynders-Frederix, V. (1980). Palliative bile duct drainage - a new endoscopic method of introducing a transpapillary drain. *Endoscopy*, 12, 8-11.

Tarnasky, P. R. (2003). Mechanical prevention of post-ERCP pancreatitis by pancreatic stents: results, techniques, and indications. *JOP*, 4, 58-67.

Tarniţă, D., Tarniţă, D. N., Bîzdoacă, N., Mîndrilă, I. & Vasilescu, M. (2009). Properties and medical applications of shape memory alloys. *Rom J Morphol Embryol*, 50, 15-21.

Thomas, T., Abrams, K. R., Subramanian, V., Mannath, J. & Ragunath, K. (2011) Esophageal stents for benign refractory strictures: a meta-analysis. *Endoscopy*, (in press).

Tilney, H. S., Lovegrove, R. E., Purkayastha, S., Sains, P. S., Weston-Petrides, G. K, Darzi, A. W., Tekkis, P. P. & Heriot, A. G. (2007). Comparison of colonic stenting and open surgery for malignant large bowel obstruction, *Surg Endosc*, 21, 225-33.

Tzovaras, G., Peyser, P., Kow, L., Wilson, T., Padbury, R. & Toouli, J. (2001). Minimally invasive management of bile leak after laparoscopic cholecystectomy. *HPB (Oxford)*, 3, 165-8.

Vakil, N., Morris, A. I., Marcon, N., Segalin, A., Peracchia, A., Bethge, N., Zuccaro, G., Bosco, J. J. & Jones, W.F. (2001). A prospective, randomized, controlled trial of covered expandable metal stents in the palliation of malignant esophageal obstruction at the gastroesophageal junction. *Am J Gastroenterol*, 96, 1791-6.

van der Gaag, N. A., Rauws, E. A., van Eijck, C. H., Bruno, M. J., van der Harst, E., Kubben, F. J., Gerritsen, J. J., Greve, J. W., Gerhards, M. F., de Hingh, I. H., Klinkenbijl, J. H., Nio, C. Y., de Castro, S. M., Busch, O. R., van Gulik, T. M., Bossuyt, P. M. & Gouma, D. J. (2010). Preoperative biliary drainage for cancer of the head of the pancreas. *N Engl J Med*, 362, 129-37.

van Heel, N. C., Haringsma, J., Spaander, M. C., Bruno, M. J. & Kuipers, E. J. (2010) Short-term esophageal stenting in the management of benign perforations. *Am J Gastroenterol*, 105, 1515-20.

Van Steenbergen, W., Pelemans, W. & Fevery, J. (1992). Endoscopic biliary endoprosthesis in elderly patients with large bile duct stones: long-term follow-up. *J Am Geriatr Soc*, 40, 57-60.

Verschuur, E. M., Repici, A., Kuipers, E. J., Steyerberg, E. W. & Siersema, P. D. (2008). New design esophageal stents for the palliation of dysphagia from esophageal or gastric cardia cancer: a randomized trial. *Am J Gastroenterol*, 103, 304-12.

Vitale, G. C., Tran, T. C., Davis, B. R., Vitale, M., Vitale, D. & Larson, G. (2008). Endoscopic management of postcholecystectomy bile duct strictures. *J Am Coll Surg*, 206, 918-23.

Wadhwa, R. P., Kozarek, R. A., France, R. E., Brandabur, J. J., Gluck, M., Low, D. E., Traverso, L. W. & Moonka, R. (2003). Use of self-expandable metallic stents in benign GI diseases. *Gastrointest Endosc*, 58, 207-12.

Weber, A., Schneider, J., Neu, B., Meining, A., Born, P., Schmid, R. M. & Prinz, C. (2007). Endoscopic stent therapy for patients with chronic pancreatitis: results from a prospective follow-up study. *Pancreas*, 34, 287-94.

Weber, A., Mittermeyer, T., Wagenpfeil, S., Schmid, R. M. & Prinz, C. (2009). Self-expanding metal stents versus polyethylene stents for palliative treatment in patients with advanced pancreatic cancer. *Pancreas*, 38, e7-e12.

Wilcox, C. M. & Varadarajulu, S. (2006). Endoscopic therapy for chronic pancreatitis: an evidence-based review. *Curr Gastroenterol Rep*, 8, 104-10.

Williams, E.D. & Draganov, P.V. (2009). Endoscopic management of biliary strictures after liver transplantation. *World J Gastroenterol*, 15, 3725-33.

Williams, E. J., Green, J., Beckingham, I., Parks, R., Martin, D. & Lombard, M. for the British Society of Gastroenterology. (2008). Guidelines on the management of common bile duct stones. *Gut*, 57, 1004-21.

Wright, G., Lewis, H., Hogan, B., Burroughs, A., Patch, D. & O'Beirne, J. (2010). A self-expanding metal stent for complicated variceal hemorrhage: experience at a single center. *Gastrointest Endosc*, 71, 71-8.

Xinopoulos, D., Dimitroulopoulos, D., Theodosopoulos, T., Tsamakidis, K., Bitsakou, G., Plataniotis, G., Gontikakis, M., Kontis, M., Paraskevas, I., Vassilobpoulos, P. & Paraskevas, E. (2004). Stenting or stoma creation for patients with inoperable malignant colonic obstructions? Results of a study and cost-effectiveness analysis. *Surg Endosc*, 18, 421-6.

Zehetner, J., Shamiyeh, A., Wayand, W. & Hubmann, R. (2008). Results of a new method to stop acute bleeding from esophageal varices: implantation of a self-expanding stent. *Surg Endosc*, 22, 2149-52.

9

Usefulness of Bacteriological Monitoring of Endoscope Reprocessing

Julia Kovaleva and Astrid Buss
University Medical Center Groningen, Laboratory for Infectious Diseases Groningen, The Netherlands

1. Introduction

Flexible endoscopy is a widely used diagnostic and therapeutic procedure. In The Netherlands, a 26% increase in the number of endoscopies from 325.000 in 1999 to almost 410.000 in 2004 was found. The total number of endoscopic retrograde cholangiopancreatographies (ERCP) was estimated at 14.596 in 2004 (Terhaar sive Droste et al., 2006).
Contaminated endoscopes have been linked to more outbreaks of healthcare-associated infections than any other medical device. During the period 1974–2004, 70 outbreaks following endoscopy procedures were reported in the USA in 64 scientific articles (Seoane-Vazquez et al., 2006). A total of 10637 patients were exposed to contamination agents during 28 outbreaks. Inadequate decontamination procedures were the leading cause of contamination; equipment malfunction became the second cause of contamination during the period 1990–2004. More than 91% of the infections identified could be prevented if quality control systems are improved. However, the true transmission during endoscopy may go unrecognized because of inadequate surveillance or no surveillance at all, low frequency and absence of clinical symptoms (Srinivasan, 2003).
Endoscopes become heavily contaminated with blood, secretions and microorganisms during use, and because each endoscope may be used for different patients in a single day, it is essential to clean and disinfect them effectively between every endoscopic procedure in patients. Accurate reprocessing of flexible endoscopes must involve cleaning, followed by high level disinfection with further rinsing and drying before storage. Most contemporary flexible endoscopes cannot be heat-sterilized and are designed with multiple channels and ports which are exposed to body fluids and are difficult to clean and disinfect (Nelson et al., 2001). Growth of biofilms inside endoscope channels can result in failure of the endoscope reprocessing and is an important factor in the pathogenesis of endoscopy-related infections (Buss et al., 2008; Kovaleva et al., 2009). Such events should be prevented by well instructed personnel, well functioning washing, disinfection and drying equipment and observance of general hygiene guidelines in the endoscopy center.
Bacterial transmission from endoscopes to patients tends to be incidentally identified when an unusual species or a microorganism with an uncommon resistance profile is involved. The microorganisms most frequently associated with iatrogenic transmission during endoscopy are gram-negative bacteria (*Pseudomonas aeruginosa, Serratia marcescens* and *Salmonella* species), mycobacteria and yeasts (Buss et al., 2008; Kovaleva et al., 2009; Spach et

al., 1993). These microorganisms can be transferred from previous patients or contaminated cleaning sources (reprocessing equipment, water supply lines) by contaminated endoscopes or accessories (Srinivasan, 2003).
Endoscopy-related outbreaks are associated with high costs including the costs of the epidemiological investigation of the outbreak, the diagnosis and treatment of the affected patients, and the use of resources cost associated with endoscope unit inactivity (Seoane-Vazquez et al., 2006).
Microbiological surveillance of endoscope reprocessing is appropriate to trace contamination of endoscopes and to prevent contamination and infection in patients after endoscopic procedures. Routine microbiological monitoring of endoscope reprocessing has been recommended by several organizations (Beilenhoff et al., 2008; Systchenko et al., 2000).
The repeated detection of an infection with the same microorganism in patients after endoscopic procedures in the University Medical Center Groningen (UMCG), The Netherlands, led to the implementation of the surveillance system for evaluation of the efficacy of the endoscope reprocessing (Buss et al., 2008; Kovaleva et al., 2009).

2. Endoscopy-related infections

Flexible endoscopes belong to semi-critical devices which come in contact with mucus membranes or non intact skin during endoscopic procedures. Endoscopes for therapeutic procedures (bronchoscopy, ERCP) are used in sterile body cavities. They are frequently designed with small lumina and multiple channels which are difficult to clean and disinfect. Such endoscopes should be sterilized or receive an intensive disinfection procedure (Alvarado & Reichelderfer, 2000).
Infections related to endoscopes can be divided into two types: endogenous and exogenous. Endoscopic procedures most often result in endogenous infections (i.e., infections resulting from the patient's own microbial flora) and *Escherichia coli, Klebsiella, Enterobacter* species and enterococci are generally isolated (Spach et al., 1993). Endogenous infections are associated with endoscopy but can not be prevented by well controlled disinfection procedures. The exogenous microorganisms most frequently associated with transmission during bronchoscopy are *P. aeruginosa* and *Mycobacterium tuberculosis*, atypical *Mycobacterium* species, and *P. aeruginosa* the most common in gastrointestinal endoscopy (Nelson & Muscarella, 2006). These microorganisms can be transmitted from previous patients or contaminated reprocessing equipment by contaminated endoscopes or its accessory equipment. Exogenous infection should be prevented by strict endoscope disinfection procedures (Srinivasan, 2003).

2.1 Endoscopy-related infection associated with gastrointestinal endoscopy

Bacteraemia occurs in any situation where there is damage of the mucosal membrane (for example, during teeth cleaning). The presence of bacteraemia after an endoscopic procedure does not indicate that serious clinical infection is present. Microscopic tissue trauma occurring during endoscope insertion can result in the passage of microflora into the bloodstream. The microorganisms isolated from the blood cultures belong to the oropharyngeal commensal microflora and are general of low pathogenicity (O'Connor et al., 1983).
The important risk factors of endoscopy-related infections in gastrointestinal endoscopy are the number of microorganisms present inside the endoscope or its accessories or the growth

of a biofilm, invasive endoscopic procedures resulting in tissue damage, compromised immune status of the patient and the presence of infective foci (abscess, cholangitis) during an endoscopic procedure (Gastroenterological Society of Australia, 2006).

The role of antibiotic prophylaxis in gastrointestinal endoscopy is controversial. Prophylactic antibiotic administration is not recommended for any gastrointestinal endoscopic procedure (Hirota et al., 2003). Only patients with bile duct obstruction, immunosuppression or previous endocarditis may need the prophylaxis during ERCP or other therapeutic gastrointestinal endoscopic procedure (Cotton et al., 2008). Recent studies examining antibiotic prophylaxis prior to ERCP concluded that it may reduce the incidence of bacteraemia, but did not reduce the incidence of clinical sepsis or cholangitis. Optimum benefit of antibiotics is obtained if therapeutic levels are present in the tissues at the time of endoscopic procedure. Antibiotic prophylaxis should be started intravenously at least one to two hours before the procedure (Cotton et al., 2008; Harris et al., 1999; Gastroenterological Society of Australia, 2006).

Despite the large number of annually performed procedures, iatrogenic infections due to flexible gastrointestinal endoscopy are apparently rare. ERCP is the only endoscopic procedure which has been associated with a significant rate of procedure-induced infection (Christensen et al., 2004). The common pathogenic microorganisms encountered in the biliary tree are *P. aeruginosa, E. coli, Klebsiella, Bacteroides* species and enterococci.

A complication of ERCP can be defined as any event occurring during the 30-day period after the procedure that changed the health status of a patient negatively. Post-ERCP complications can be divided into mild (required up to 3 days in hospital), moderate (required 4 to 10 days of hospitalization) and severe complications (required more than 10 days of hospitalization, surgical intervention and/or resulted in the death of the patient) (Cotton et al., 1991).

Cholangitis and bacteraemia following ERCP can occur due to exogenous source (contaminated endoscope or accessories) or endogenous bacterial flora. Bloodstream infection is one of the most serious complications of this procedure, with the actual incidence varied from 0% to 27% in different populations and with the 8% - 20% mortality rate (Anderson et al., 2008; Kullman et al., 1992). Cholangitis, the most frequent infective complication of ERCP, most commonly results from inadequate drainage of infected and obstructive biliary duct system (Low et al., 1980). Post-ERCP cholangitis is defined by a typical clinical picture (temperature >38°C, upper abdominal colicky pain, cholestasis/jaundice) without evidence of other concomitant infections with/without positive gall cultures obtained during the biliary drainage (Masci et al., 2001).

2.1.1 Role of Pseudomonas aeruginosa in endoscopy-related infections

P. aeruginosa, a gram-negative opportunistic pathogen, is the most commonly reported organism responsible for transmission of infection during gastrointestinal endoscopy. It is known by its preference for a moist environment (wet endoscope channels after reprocessing, hospital water supply) (Nelson & Muscarella, 2006). *Pseudomonas* is well known to be able to form biofilms, and these biofilms are extremely difficult to remove from plumbing, automatic endoscope reprocessors and endoscope channels (Pajkos et al., 2004).

Pseudomonas contamination of endoscopes was first reported in the mid-70s (Bilbao et al., 1976) and is adequately documented as a serious clinical cause of ERCP-associated infection by 1980 (Low et al., 1980). Outbreaks of *P. aeruginosa* sepsis and cholangitis following ERCP continue to be reported. Frequently, the infection has not been recognized because of inadequate surveillance, low frequency and absence of clinical symptoms. It comes to light only as a result of infection control procedures.

According to the recent reports, *P. aeruginosa* transmission during gastrointestinal endoscopy has been attributed to (1) inadequate high-level disinfection of the endoscope channels after endoscope reprocessing prior to storage (Allen et al., 1987; Fraser et al., 2004), (2) colonization of the water supply to the endoscope (Bass et al., 1990) and (3) defective disinfecting machines, failure in design or defects in endoscope channels and accessories (Alvarado et al., 1991; Nelson & Muscarella, 2006). Serotype 10 of *P. aeruginosa* was predominating in the published reports of *Pseudomonas* transmission (Allen et al., 1987; Alvarado et al., 1991). This serotype persisted in the outbreaks despite the intensive disinfection procedures. This phenomenon was linked to biofilm formation but no explanation was found as to why this serotype was isolated.

Inadequate drying of the endoscope channels prior to storage was responsible for the outbreaks of *Pseudomonas* bacteraemia after ERCP (Allen et al., 1987; Classen et al., 1988). *P. aeruginosa* remaining in the endoscope moist channels after reprocessing can colonize and multiply to high numbers during storage. This situation can result in an increased risk of transmission to the first patient of the day during an ERCP procedure.

2.1.2 Example of an outbreak of Pseudomonas sepsis after ERCP

We have recently been confronted with an outbreak of multidrug-resistant *P. aeruginosa* sepsis affecting six patients after ERCP. Our registration system enabled us to retrieve one of three endoscopes daily in use as the possible source of infection. Epidemiologic investigation including microbiological sampling of the implicated endoscope, the washer disinfectors and the tubes connecting the washer disinfectors and the endoscopes was performed. The results of recent surveillance cultures from diagnostic and therapeutic endoscopes were reviewed. Environmental investigations to determine potential reservoirs or sources of contamination included wash tables, sinks, drying cabinets, hand soap and detergent soap for endoscopes. The medical records of all patients who underwent ERCP with this endoscope from introduction in service until it was removed from service were reviewed.

All of the cultures from the washer disinfectors, the connecting tubes, other endoscopes, and from the environmental surfaces in the endoscopy center were negative for *P. aeruginosa*. Epidemiologic investigation found that the implicated ERCP endoscope had contamination with *P. aeruginosa* in microbiological surveillances before the outbreak, despite intensive high level disinfection procedures. The endoscope was removed from service and underwent sterilization with ethylene oxide. Following gas sterilization, the implicated endoscope was found to have *P. aeruginosa*-negative cultures and was re-introduced into service. However, 4 months later, it was again contaminated with *P. aeruginosa*. The endoscope was sent to the manufacturer for repair. Structures suggesting the presence of biofilm were found on the inner surface of the undamaged endoscope channels. The endoscope channels were changed.

The available *P. aeruginosa* strains were subjected to molecular typing by repetitive DNA sequence-based polymerase chain reaction (rep-PCR) using the DiversiLab System for DNA fingerprinting (BioMérieux, France). The isolates from the six patients and from the endoscope channels, obtained before gas sterilization, showed matching patterns (similarity above 95%) (Kovaleva et al., 2009).

2.2 Endoscopy-related infection associated with bronchoscopy

During the period 1974-2004, bronchoscopy procedures accounted for 47.5% of the endoscopy-related infections in the USA and 21.1% of the infections in other countries (Seoane-Vazquez et al., 2007). Several studies have found bronchoscopy procedures to be relatively more prone to infection transmission than gastrointestinal endoscopic procedures (Seoane-Vazquez et al., 2007; Spach et al., 1993).

The microorganisms most frequently associated with transmission during bronchoscopy are gram-negative bacilli, particularly *P. aeruginosa* or *Enterobacteriaceae* or infection with *M. tuberculosis* or other mycobacteria (Cêtre et al., 2005; Nelson & Muscarella, 2006). While isolation of various *Enterobacteriaceae* from the lungs is not rare, severe nosocomial pneumonia is not frequently diagnosed in patients during infection outbreaks. It is possible that the incidence of pneumonia related to bronchoscopy is underestimated (Shimonom et al., 2008). The pathogens of nosocomial pneumonia are related to the timing of onset. Microorganisms responsible for early-onset nosocomial pneumonia are generally endogenous. In late-onset nosocomial pneumonia, the causative microorganisms include potentially multidrug-resistant nosocomial organisms such as *P. aeruginosa*.

Three large outbreaks of *P. aeruginosa* infections following flexible bronchoscopy associated with a loose port of the biopsy channel of the bronchoscope were reported in the literature (Cêtre et al., 2005; Kirschke et al., 2003; Srinivasan et al., 2003). Another two *Pseudomonas* outbreaks were associated with a damaged internal channel caused by defective biopsy forceps (Corne et al., 2005). A contaminated bronchoscope washer disinfector was the source of the several *Pseudomonas* outbreaks (Schelenz & French, 2000; Shimonom et al., 2008).

Numerous reports of mycobacterial transmission by flexible bronchoscopy have been reported. Mycobacterial infections during bronchoscopy have been related to contaminated suction valves (Wheeler et al., 1989), cracked biopsy channels (Pappas et al., 1982), contaminated topical anaesthetic solutions (Leers et al., 1980) and contaminated disinfecting machines (Bryce et al., 1993; Fraser et al., 1992).

The last two years we were confronted with repeated contaminations of flexible bronchoscopes with fastidiously growing *Methylobacterium. Methylobacterium* was also isolated from the broncho-alveolair lavages of the patients after bronchoscopy with the contaminated bronchoscopes. We consider *Methylobacterium* as a contaminant being the cause of pseudo-infections because no patient manifested true infection with this bacterium. *Methylobacterium* is a fastidious, slowly growing gram-negative rod that forms pink colonies on agar plates and is a common contaminant in water (Sanders et al., 2000). Nevertheless it has been described as opportunistic human pathogen and has been shown to be able to cause colonization and infections in immunocompromised patients (Kaye et al., 1992; Liu et al., 1997). Two publications of *Methylobacterium* contamination related to endoscopic procedures were found in the literature. One patient developed *Methylobacterium* bacteraemia following ERCP with the contaminated endoscope (Imbert et al., 2005). A pseudo-outbreak of *Methylobacterium mesophilicum* and *Mycobacterium chelonae* was described in patients who underwent bronchoscopy. *M. mesophilicum* was isolated from broncho-alveolar lavages obtained from ventilated patients. *Methylobacterium* grew from the bronchoscopes and automated washers which were revealed as the source of the contamination. The presence of biofilm was demonstrated on tubing from the manifold block to the top of the reservoir (Kressel & Kid, 2001).

3. Microbiological surveillance of endoscope reprocessing

Endoscopes, especially the instruments with highly refined technical properties, can be cleaned and disinfected but not sterilized after use. This implies the risk of settlement of biofilm producing species, which can not be removed with current cleaning and disinfection procedures. A currently applied surveillance protocol for endoscopes demonstrates recurrent colonization of these instruments. Occasionally this leads to series of infections in patients, who become severely ill with pathogenic species being part of the biofilm which has settled in the interior of the endoscope.

In The Netherlands the current guidelines advise no routine microbiological surveillance of endoscopes, only under special circumstances like a defect of the endoscope or in the disinfection process and also in case of an outbreak (Dutch Infection Prevention Working Party, 2004). In our opinion is a good working disinfection process no guarantee on "clean" endoscopes, because damage of the endoscope itself occurs during use, e.g. due to through scratches in the working channel by the biopsy forceps, and forms a niche for rising microbiological biofilm. Outbreaks can easily be overlooked and are often only recognized if special microorganisms are involved, like outbreaks caused by a multi-resistant *E. coli* in 2002 and by a multi-resistant *P. aeruginosa* in 2008 in patients after ERCP in the UMCG (Kovaleva et al., 2009). Recently in France hospitals duodenoscopes-related nosocomial infections due to *Klebsiella pneumoniae* producing extended-spectrum beta-lactamase (ESBL) occurred (Aumeran et al., 2010) and also of even more multidrug-resistant *K. pneumoniae* carbapenemase (KPC)-producing *K. pneumoniae* type 2 (Carbonne et al., 2010).

3.1 Endoscope reprocessing

Accurate reprocessing of flexible endoscopes must involve cleaning, followed by high level disinfection with further rinsing and drying before storage. If the programme does not include an adequate drying phase, like after manual disinfection, the instrument must be disinfected again if it has not been in use for longer than 4 hours (Dutch Infection Prevention Working Party, 2004). Because almost all outbreaks are related to breaches in reprocessing techniques, it is crucial that endoscope cleaning and disinfection are performed carefully. However, process control of the endoscope reprocessing does not guarantee prevention of settlement of biofilm and consequent shedding of bacteria during endoscopy. Disinfection and drying procedures may fail in the endoscope with a manufacturing defect or damaged internal channels when the decontamination process cannot reach all internal parts of the instrument, and biofilm formation will occur within the endoscope channels (Kovaleva et al., 2009; Srinivasan, 2003).

At the UMCG endoscope reprocessing is performed according to the recommendations of the Dutch national guideline (Dutch Infection Prevention Working Party, 2004) and to the manufacture's recommendations. After manual pre-cleaning and cleaning with detergent (Neodisher Mediclean, Dr. Weigert, Hamburg, Germany) and rinsing with water, endoscopes are disinfected 10 minutes at the temperature of 25 °C in one of the automatic washer disinfectors (WD 440, Wassenburg Medical Devices B.V., The Netherlands) with 1 % Neodisher Septo PAC (Dr. Weigert, Hamburg, Germany). This disinfectant contains a blend of peracetic acid (1 %), acetic acid (< 20%) and hydrogen peroxide (15-30%). After disinfection endoscopes are dried for 2 hours at 50 °C using sterile compressed air and hereafter are stored in drying cabinets with continuous flow of dry compressed air at room temperature. If a flexible endoscope is used for different patients in a single day, the disinfection and drying procedures will be performed between patients.

3.2 Surveillance algorithm

In the UMCG the surveillance system for evaluation of the efficacy of the endoscope reprocessing was implemented. According to our surveillance protocol, therapeutic gastro- and duodenoscopes are microbiologically tested monthly and diagnostic endoscopes once every 3 months (Buss et al., 2008; Kovaleva et al., 2009). A decision algorithm was designed for interpretation of the relevance of positive culture results (Figure 1).

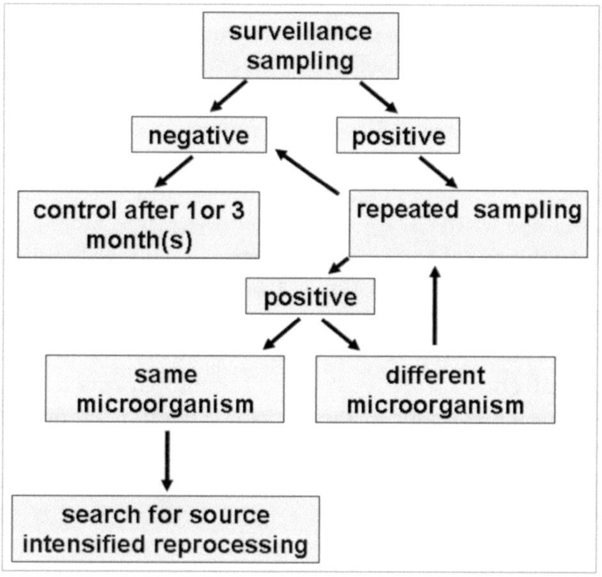

Fig. 1. Decision algorithm for endoscope surveillance.

If, in terms of the decision algorithm, a contamination problem occurs or clinical data suggest transmission, additional samples are taken from the washer disinfectors and also from the tubes connecting the washer disinfectors and the endoscopes and other endoscope accessories. Culturing of special microorganism (e.g. mycobacteria) might be indicated. After a single contamination with a relevant microorganisms (e.g., *Enterobacteriaceae, Candida* species, gram-negative nonfermenters, *Staphylococcus aureus*), the endoscope is taken out of service in patients and the results of repeat sampling are awaited. Such endoscopes undergo an intensive high level disinfection procedure. Endoscopes with positive cultures for the same clinically relevant microbial species in two consecutive tests after high level disinfection procedures stay out of use and undergo an additional reprocessing step using sterilization with ethylene oxide followed by microbiological testing before use.

A contaminated endoscope should be inspected for potential defects. Unfortunately, it is not possible to adequately check all internal endoscope channels. Cracking, splitting, channel wall holes can all be the source of bacterial contamination within the endoscope which can be difficult to impossible to detect by routine inspection and testing.

In the literature there are no standards about frequency of the testing intervals of surveillance cultures. The Gastroenterological Society of Australia guideline (2006) recommends the microbiologic monitoring of ERCP endoscopes and bronchoscopes every 4 weeks and all other gastrointestinal endoscopes every 4 months. According to the European Society of Gastrointestinal Endoscopy guideline, routine microbiological testing of endoscopes is advised to perform at intervals no longer than 3 months (Beilenhoff et al., 2007).
Every microbiological surveillance system has one important limitation. If there is a clinical demand for reuse of an endoscope in the mean time, surveillance culture results will likely not be obtained until after the endoscope is used on the next patient because cultures take a minimum of 24 to 48 hours to incubate (Beilenhoff et al., 2007).

3.3 Sampling technique

Sampling of patient-ready endoscopes can be performed with two different techniques. For anterograde sampling, the last rinse water from the endoscope is collected inside the washer disinfector at the distal end of the endoscope. At the endoscopy center in the UMCG, we use a retrograde technique to obtain surveillance specimens for culture from the biopsy/suction and the water/air endoscope channels (Buss et al., 2008; Kovaleva et al., 2009).
For retrograde sampling, the biopsy/suction channel and the water/air channel of the endoscope are each flushed with 20 ml sterile demineralised water manually outside the washer disinfector from the distal to the proximal end. To allow the water to enter the small distal openings of the channels, we connect the syringe with an adapter taken from a gastrointestinal dilator (Savary-Gilliard Dilators; Cook Medical, Bloomington, IN, USA). For sampling under sterile conditions this work has to be done by two persons. The water is collected at the proximal ends of the channels. The biopsy/suction channel is flushed a second time after collecting the water at the suction port and the endoscope is then turned upside-down in order to collect the fluid at the biopsy port. Sampling options can differ depending on the design of the endoscope and the washer disinfector. Samples should be processed shortly after collecting. All samples from endoscopes are sent for culturing. In case of positive results all isolated strains are stored.
If sampling of washer disinfectors is indicated samples from all water channels, the water inlet and the water reservoir and from the tubes connecting the washer disinfectors and the endoscopes should be taken. To enhance the sensitivity of culturing, the washer disinfector can be taken out of use at the end of a normal working day and samples should be taken several days later or at least after one overnight storage period. Following this procedure an auto-disinfection cycle can be run and one to several days later a second sampling can be performed.
The endoscopes have to be sampled in a retrograde manner, because anterograde sampling is not sensitive enough, as shown by our own data (Buss et al., 2008) and those of another study (Srinivasan et al., 2003). Srinivasan et al. (2003) and Cêtre et al. (2005) sampled the biopsy suction channel retrogradely using the suction button of bronchoscopes to suck back the sample fluid, used for flushing, to the proximal channel opening. In our approach the water and air channels of gastrointestinal endoscopes were sampled retrogradely. Alternatively, flushing through combined with brushing may be used (Rejchrt et al., 2004). During the endoscopy-related outbreak caused by ESBL-positive *K. pneumoniae* in France the epidemic strain was finally isolated from one duodenoscope by flushing and brushing the channels (Aumeran et al., 2010). We know no comparison of the sensitivities of these variants with that of our way of retrograde sampling. The mechanisms underlying the

higher sensitivity of retrograde sampling need to be further investigated. Probably, changing the direction of the water flow leads to easier removal of organic material and biofilm that have grown with the anterograde flow of the disinfection procedure. Niches inside the endoscopes that are not reached by the anterograde sampling flow may become more accessible.

3.4 Laboratory protocol

One hundred mL of each sample are inoculated on agar plates for aerobic culturing as follows: blood agar (BA; 5% blood sheep agar; Oxoid Ltd., Cambridge, UK), chocolate blood agar (CHOC; Oxoid), Sabouraud dextrose agar with 0.02 g/L aztreonam and 0.02 g/L vancomycin (SABav; Oxoid), and tryptone glucose extract agar (TGE; Oxoid). The cultures are incubated for 4 days at 35 °C (BA, CHOC, SABav) or 7 days at room temperature (TGE). In addition, 1 mL of each sample are added to an aerobic blood culture bottle and incubated for 4 days in the BacT/ALERT system (bioMérieux SA, Marcy l'Etoile, France). Alternatively to the use of a broth medium, samples can be filtrated to concentrate the microorganisms and the filters cultured.

Bacterial isolates and yeasts are identified according to standard determination schemes. If indicated, culturing of mycobacteria can be done following standard sampling procedures. We do not culture for anaerobic microorganisms nor do we carry out virus detection.

3.5 Culture results and interpretation

In 2008 208 retrograde samples from endoscopes were taken. With retrograde sampling, 20% (42/208) of all endoscope cultures were found to be contaminated with a microorganism; 5.3% (11/208) of the tests resulted in withdrawal of the contaminated endoscopes, followed by repeated intensified disinfection procedures and gas sterilization. Previous surveillance data from September 2002 until January 2005 demonstrate the much higher sensitivity of retrograde versus anterograde taken samples. The percentage of positive cultures of anterograde versus retrograde samples were 7.9% respectively 31% for all microorganisms and for yeasts alone 2.8% respectively 25% (Buss et al., 2008).

Various groups of bacteria were found in the surveillance cultures. The following microorganisms were frequently found: aerobic gram-positive cocci, *Enterobacteriaceae*, gram-negative nonfermenters (*Pseudomonas*, *Acinetobacter* species). Repeated endoscope contamination with *Stenotrophomonas maltophilia* and *Methylobacterium* is regularly demonstrated, after which intervention conform the protocol is implemented. Frequently more than one species was found in one culture; in many cases this was a mix of *Candida* species with gram-negative rods or nonfermenters.

In the course of time we found an increasing number of endoscopes positive for non-albicans *Candida* species, in particular *Candida parapsilosis* (77% of all further identified non-albicans *Candida* species). The persistent culturing of *C. parapsilosis* was generally an indicator of a disinfection problem and may be caused by a low disinfection temperature.

3.6 Economic burden of endoscope reprocessing and endoscopy-related infection

The literature related to the costs associated with endoscope reprocessing and the economic consequences of endoscope contamination is very limited. The economic evaluation of exogenous endoscopy-related outbreaks should include the analysis of outcomes (the number of prevented exogenous endoscopy-related infections) and the estimation of the health care, non-health care and indirect costs (Seoane-Vazquez et al., 2006). The health care costs include the costs of the epidemiological investigation of the outbreak, the diagnosis and treatment of the affected patients, and the use of resources cost associated with endoscope unit inactivity. A study of post-arthroscopy infections estimated the cost approximately at $9,155 per case (Babcock et al., 2003).

The economic evaluation of the microbiological surveillance should include a calculation of the costs for the microbiological tests, costs in time for nursing staff to collect the samples, costs of endoscope recall and extra disinfection procedures or service of the endoscopes. Recent articles pointed to the high cost of periodic monitoring of endoscopes, washer disinfectors and the environment. A recently published study analysed the cost of 4-weekly surveillance microbiological tests of bronchoscopes, duodenoscopes and automated washer disinfectors during a 5-year period. The overall cost of performed tests and cost in time for nursing staff to collect the samples was estimated at $AUD 100.400 (Gillespie et al., 2008). The costs of an outbreak with a number of clinical complications as described in our cases are usually a multiple of this amount. Microbiological surveillance of endoscope reprocessing and intervention protocol can save the high costs associated with incidental cases and outbreaks of endoscopy-related infections.

In the economic analyses performed in 2008 in the UMCG, the costs of the surveillance of the endoscope reprocessing (cost of tests and cost in time for staff) were estimated at € 25.967. Not calculated were the costs for reprocessing and/or revision of endoscopes by the manufacturer. It was estimated that the costs of the recent *Pseudomonas* outbreak, i.e. the direct health-care costs for the diagnosis, treatment and hospitalization of the six affecting patients, approximated € 157.729.

3.7 Summary and future prospects

The UMCG has 9 years of experience with the microbiological monitoring of flexible endoscopes, biofilm detection and intervention. Positive results of microbiological surveillance have been leading to withdrawal, additional disinfection and incidental gas sterilization of the contaminated endoscopes. The risk of contamination and infection were reduced for large groups of patients, and the expected costs of the post-endoscopic infectious complications were saved (Buss et al, 2008; Kovaleva et al., 2009). However, our surveillance and intervention did not prevent six serious infections by the genotypic similar strain of *P. aeruginosa*, due to the window period in between the surveillance procedures (1 month).

Our protocol is able to detect a structural problem in the endoscope disinfection process. Retrograde sampling is crucial for this purpose, because it has much higher sensitivity than anterograde sampling (Buss et al., 2008; Srinivasan et al., 2003). Endoscopes with damaged working channels often are the source of the contamination problems.

Our monitoring and decision algorithm is a product of a learning-by-doing process when we were confronted with contamination problems. If we had not done retrograde sampling we would not have recognized the structural disinfection problems of individual endoscopes. Ideally, an easily performed daily microbiological surveillance method will be developed in the future, which can replace culturing and give faster results. This technique might be based on adenosine triphosphate measuring or polymerase chain reaction detection (Obee et al., 2005; Sciortino et al., 2004).

Some investigators have begun exploring sterile-sheathed endoscopes with new technology to reduce the risk for infectious complications. The EndoSheath is an endoscope system in which all parts of the endoscope that come into contact with the patient are fully disposable (Colt et al., 2000; Srinivasan, 2003). The endoscope does not come in contact with the patient and does not require disinfection. The disposable sheath, which is in contact with the patient, includes the air/water, suction, and working channels. The main purposes of the sheath are to prevent the transmission of pathogens, and to reduce the need for high-level sterilization.

4. Impact of biofilms on endoscope reprocessing

4.1 Definition and properties of biofilm

Microorganisms in nature do not generally grow in nutrient-rich suspensions as in the laboratory, but prefer to grow in surface-associated communities, called biofilms (Bar-Or, 1990). The phenomenon of biofilm formation by microorganisms on inert surfaces has been extensively studied and there appears to be a direct relationship between the ability of the organism to form a biofilm and its pathogenicity (Shin et al., 2002).

A biofilm is an assemblage of microbial cells that is irreversibly attached to a surface and enclosed in an exopolysaccharide matrix (Donlan, 2002). Biofilms consist of a substratum to which the microorganism adheres, a conditioning film, the matrix and the liquid phase (Costerton et al., 1995). A typical biofilm will contain around 85% polysaccharide matrix and only 15% bacterial mass. Biofilms may form on different surfaces, including living or dead tissues, indwelling medical devices, water supply systems, or endoscope channels (Donlan, 2002; Pajkos et al., 2004).

Bacteria growing within biofilms have a number of characteristics that distinguish them from planktonic populations. Ability to form biofilms allows microorganisms to survive under conditions of drying, chemical and antibiotic exposure. Cells growing within biofilms are protected from host immune system and are frequently 1000 times more resistant to antibiotics than the non-attached planktonic cells. The increased resistance to antimicrobial agents can be explained by poor penetration of an antibiotic into a biofilm, slow growth rate and formation of resistant phenotypes of microorganisms within biofilms (Costerton et al., 1995; Patel, 2005).

Under adverse conditions, biofilms are capable to release their bacterial population into a planktonic state. This ability can be explained by intercellular communication within a biofilm (Davies et al., 2008). Signalling systems include quorum sensing (the release of signal chemicals in response to increasing population density), biosignal blockers, pheromones and butyrylhomoserine lactone. These signalling systems are important in regulation of a number of physiological processes, including antibiotic synthesis, plasmid transfer and the expression of virulence factors (van Delden & Iglewski, 1998).

With the increasing use of invasive medical procedures, infections involving biofilms form an important risk factor for infectious complications. It has been reported that bacterial biofilm causes about 65% of bacterial infections in the clinic (Chicurel, 2000). These infections often develop in immunocompromised patients and can be caused by a variety of different microorganisms. Biofilm infections show poor manifestation and recurring symptoms after antibiotic therapy (Costerton et al., 1995). Bacteria within biofilms are able to evade the host immune system. Antibodies are not effective against microorganisms within biofilms, and immune complex can damage the surrounding tissues (Cochrane et al., 1985).

4.2 Removal of biofilms

During endoscopy, the environment provides optimal conditions for the growth of biofilms. Modern endoscopes contain multiple channels and ports which allow for the collection of organic material. The presence of biofilms on the inner surface of endoscope channels has been reported in many publications (Buss et al., 2008; Kovaleva et al., 2009; Pajkos et al., 2004). Even if valid endoscope reprocessing protocols are applied, microbial accumulation can lead to the development of a mature biofilm inside narrow endoscope channels in time (Pajkos et al., 2004). Biofilm formation on the inner surface of the endoscope channels, especially, when these become scratched or damaged, can result in failure of the decontamination process. It can create a vicious circle of growth, disinfection, partial killing or inhibition and regrowth, resulting in outbreaks of endoscopy-related infections in patients who underwent an endoscopy with the biofilm-containing endoscope (Buss et al., 2008; Kovaleva et al., 2009).

Scanning electron microscopy is able to reveal incomplete removal of debris from the interior part of a dismantled endoscope after reprocessing. Figure 2 shows a bacterial biofilm inside an endoscope channel. This endoscope was contaminated not only the inside but also the outside of the channels.

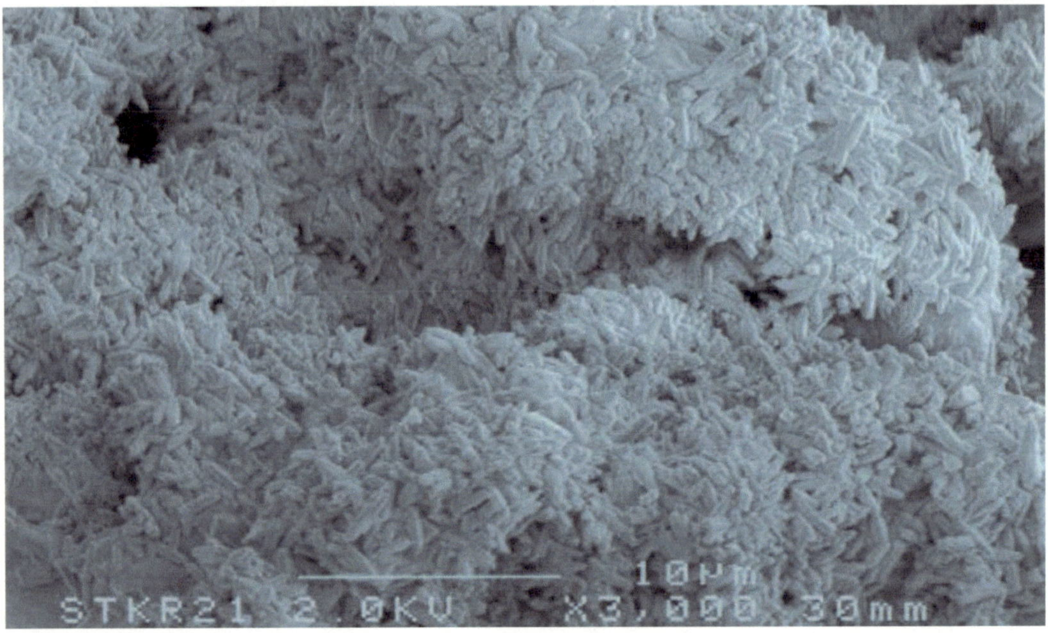

Fig. 2. Scanning electron microscopy picture of bacterial biofilm in an endoscope channel.

Oxidising agents are the most effective chemicals currently available for killing and removing biofilms. Peracetic acid is an oxidising agent usually used for high-level disinfection of flexible endoscopes. It is effective against bacteria, fungi, spores and viruses, minimally toxic and not corrosive at the concentration recommended for disinfection. The biocidal effect of peracetic acid on sessile microorganisms is well known (Henoun Loukili et al., 2004). However, the effect of this disinfectant on biological deposits, particularly its ability to fix or to remove biofilms from materials, is not completely studied.

To have potential action on biofilms, relatively high concentrations of the disinfecting agent are necessary. Current peracetic acid disinfectants are not used in high concentrations for endoscope reprocessing because of corrosive properties (Gastroenterological Society of Australia, 2006). According to Marion-Ferey et al. (2003), peracetic acid had a limited efficacy in biofilm removal from the silicone tubing in haemodialysis systems. Other studies demonstrated the ability of peracetic acid disinfectants to fix the *E. coli* biofilm and blood on to artificial materials (Henoun Loukili et al., 2004; Kampf et al., 2004)

Glutaraldehyde is also an effective agent in endoscope disinfection. It requires a much greater time to kill the biofilm and is less effective in causing shedding of the biofilm from the surface. However, glutaraldehyde is irritating to the skin, can cause allergic contact dermatitis, and may result in irritation of the eyes and nasal mucosa (Alvarado & Reichelderfer, 2000). Recently, resistance to glutaraldehyde against some *M. chelonae* strains has been described in the literature (van Klingeren & Pullen, 1993). Kovacs et al. (1998) reported a strain of *P. aeruginosa* responsible for three separate clinical episodes of ERCP-associated cholangitis and concluded that the organism developed adaptive chemical resistance to glutaraldehyde.

The use of anti-biofilm oxidising agents and disinfectants with antimicrobial coating inside washer disinfectors could reduce biofilm build-up inside endoscopes and endoscope washers and decrease the risk of transmitting infections (Marion et al., 2006; Rutala & Weber, 2001).

Sterilization can be helpful to destroy microorganisms within biofilms. However, flexible endoscopes cannot be heat-sterilized because of vulnerable elements. Low temperature hydrogen peroxide plasma and ethylene oxide gas sterilization can be used during endoscope reprocessing. Recent studies indicate problems with gas and plasma sterilization of long, narrow lumina in the presence of organic soil and salts (Gastroenterological Society of Australia, 2006).

4.3 Role of drying in biofilm removal

Accurate drying and storage are important factors in the maintenance of bacteria-free endoscopes. The potential for microbial growth inside endoscope channels after disinfection mainly depends on the conditions within the endoscope channels during drying and storage. Wet channels after reprocessing facilitate growth of such microorganisms as *Pseudomonas* and *Acinetobacter* species during storage (Alfa & Sitter, 1991). The drying procedure of the endoscopes after cleaning at 50 °C, followed by drying with a constant flow of compressed ambient air is applied in the UMCG.

According to the literature, endoscopes stay bacteria-free after prolonged storage if an adequate drying procedure was applied. When stored in the drying cabinet with a laminar air flow, no growth of bacteria and *Candida* species was found in endoscopes channels 5 days after reprocessing (Rejchrt et al., 2004). Allen et al. (1987) pointed the high efficiency of a drying procedure with suctioning 70% alcohol through endoscope channels, followed by compressed air in prevention of the further contaminations during the *P. aeruginosa* infection outbreak.

We recently demonstrated that routine cleaning procedures can not always remove biofilm reliably from endoscope channels if the accurate drying procedure is not applied. We

studied the ability for biofilm formation and the effects of the peracetic acid-based disinfectant, currently in use for endoscope reprocessing in the UMCG, with, and without additional drying on *Candida albicans, C. parapsilosis, P. aeruginosa* and *S. maltophilia* biofilms (Kovaleva et al., 2010).
The biofilms were prepared in sterile tissue culture polystyrene 96-well microtiter plates. After 72 h incubation, single- and dual-species biofilms were treated for 10 min with the disinfectant at concentrations conform the minimal bactericidal concentration of the strains tested and at 1% concentration, recommended for disinfection of flexible endoscopes by the company. In order to mimic the biofilm formation and to establish a possible regrowth of biofilms inside the endoscope channels after reprocessing, we developed an in vitro biofilm model which underwent the different steps of the disinfection and drying procedures applied for reprocessing of flexible endoscopes (Figure 3). The viability of the biofilm was quantified by using the tetrazolium salt (MTT) reduction assay and by counting colony-forming yeasts and bacteria of the 10-fold serial biofilm dilutions on agar plates.

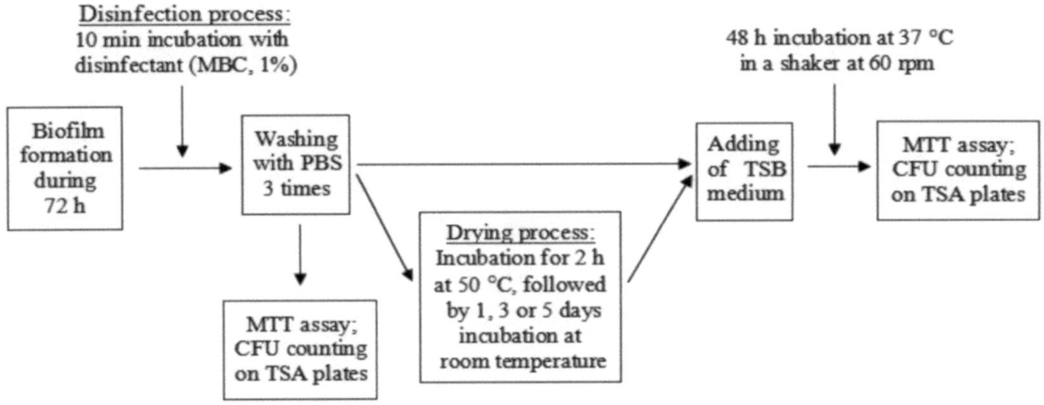

Fig. 3. In vitro biofilm model mimicking the different steps of the disinfection procedure without and with the drying process in a flexible endoscope. CFU, colony-forming units; MTT, tetrazolium salt reduction assay; MBC, minimal bactericidal concentration; TSA, trypticase soy agar; PBS, phosphate buffered saline.

A low MTT formazan signal was demonstrated in all biofilms directly after 10 min treatment with the minimal bactericidal concentration and 1% disinfectant (Figure 4a). A total inhibition of microbial growth in all biofilms on agar plates occurred after treatment with 1% disinfectant. Minimal bactericidal concentration caused a marked inhibition of microbial growth of all biofilms but not a 100% bactericidal and fungicidal efficacy. Regrowth of all biofilms occurred following 48 h incubation with trypticase soy broth directly after treatment with the minimal bactericidal concentration and 1% disinfectant if the drying procedure was skipped. No biofilm regrowth occurred in wells after a drying procedure for 1, 3 and 5 days in all biofilms (Figure 4b).

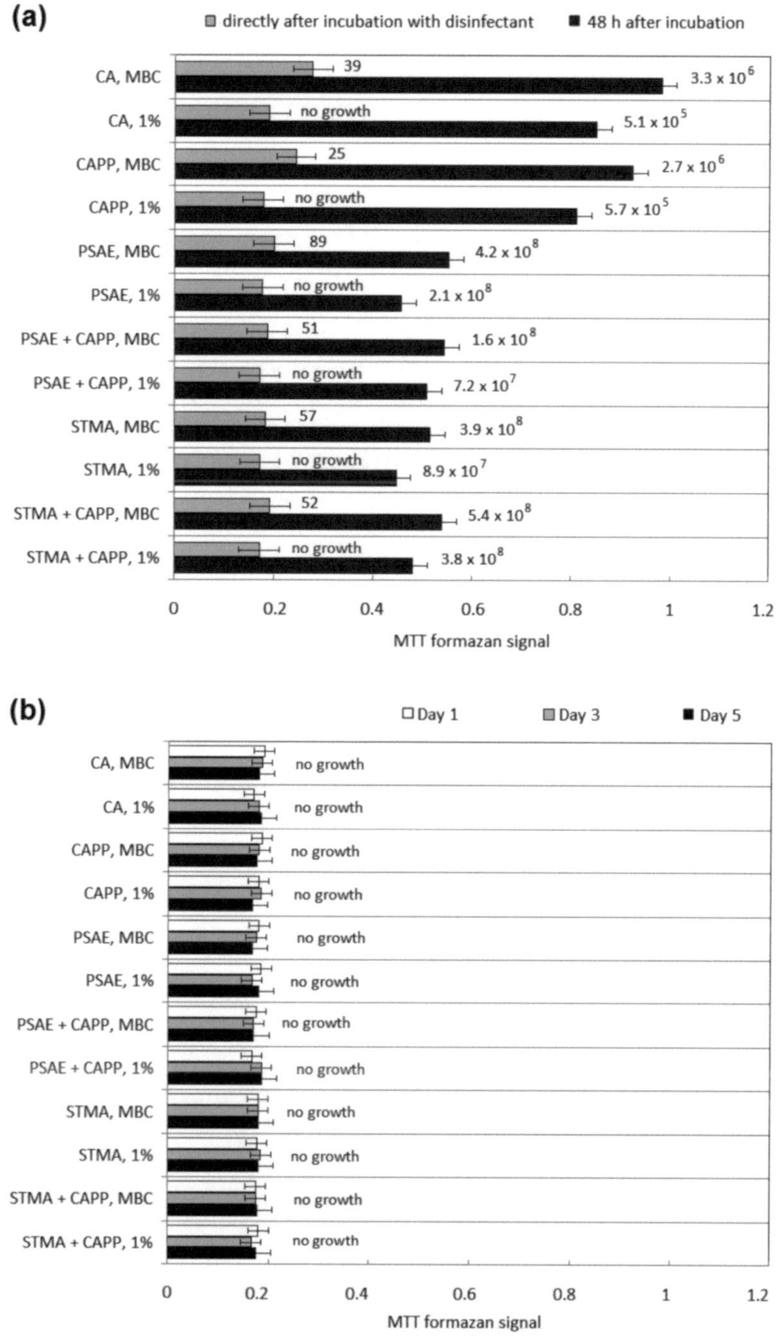

Fig. 4. Regrowth of the single- and dual-species *C. albicans* (CA), *C. parapsilosis* (CAPP), *P. aeruginosa* (PSAE) and *S. maltophilia* (STMA) biofilms expressed in vitality by measuring the MTT signal and expressed in viability in CFU per well after the disinfection procedure with MBC and 1% disinfectant (a) without additional drying and (b) with additional drying for 1, 3 and 5 days.

This study demonstrated the high efficacy of the drying procedure after the disinfection step against yeasts and bacteria in all single- and dual-species biofilms. Failure of decontamination endoscopes can be explained by an invalid drying procedure.

5. Conclusion

Contaminated endoscopes have been linked to many outbreaks of device-related nosocomial infections. The true incidence of endoscopy-related infections is unknown because of inadequate surveillance or no surveillance at all. Endoscopy-related infections can cause serious harm and can give rise to concerns over these procedures by physicians and patients in.

Flexible endoscopes can be cleaned and disinfected but not sterilized after use. This implies the risk of settlement of biofilm producing species. Routine cleaning and disinfection procedures do not remove biofilm reliably from endoscope channels if the accurate drying procedure is not applied. This may explain the failure of decontamination during endoscope reprocessing.

Process control of the washing and disinfection procedure is requested and implemented but does not guarantee prevention of settlement of biofilm and consequent shedding of bacteria during endoscopy. Implementation of a microbiological surveillance of endoscope reprocessing is appropriate to detect early colonization and biofilm formation in the endoscope and to prevent contamination and infection in patients after endoscopic procedures. However, the returns of prevention of endoscopy-related infections should be reasonably in balance with the costs of the technical and laboratory procedures resulting from surveillance and the costs of reprocessing or servicing of the contaminated endoscope.

6. Acknowledgment

The authors wish to thank Prof. Dr. John Degener and Prof. Dr. Henny van der Mei for their advice and support. We thank the staff of the Departments of Medical Microbiology and Endoscopy of the UMCG for technical assistance and collaboration.

7. References

Allen, J.; Allen, M.; Olson, M.; Gerding, D.; Shanholtzer, C.; Meier, P.; Vennes, J. & Silvis, S. Pseudomonas Infection of the Biliary System Resulting from Use of a Contaminated Endoscope. *Gastroenterology*, Vol.92, No.3, (March 1987), pp. 759-763, ISSN 0016-5085

Alfa, M. & Sitter, D. In-hospital Evaluation of Contamination of Duodenoscopes: a Quantitative Assessment of the Effect of Drying. *Journal of Hospital Infection*, Vol.19, No.2, (October 1991), pp. 89-98, ISSN 0195-6701

Alvarado, C. & Reichelderfer, M. APIC Guidelines for Infection Prevention and Control in Flexible Endoscopy. *American Journal of Infection Control*, Vol.28, No.2, (April 2000), pp. 138-155, ISSN 0196-6553

Alvarado, C.; Stolz, S. & Maki, D. Nosocomial Infections from Contaminated Endoscopes: a Flawed Automated Endoscope Washer. An Investigation Using Molecular Epidemiology. *The American Journal of Medicine*, Vol. 91, No.3B, (September 1991), pp. 272-280, ISSN 0002-9343

Anderson, D.; Shimpi, R.; McDonald, J.; Branch, M.; Kanafani, Z.; Harger, J.; Ely, T.; Sexton, D. & Kaye, K. Infectious Complications Following Endoscopic Retrograde Cholangiopancreatography: an Automated Surveillance System for Detecting Postprocedure Bacteraemia. *American Journal of Infection Control*, Vol.36, No.8, (October 2008), pp. 592-594, ISSN 0196-6553

Aumeran, C.; Poincloux, L.; Souweine, B.; Robin, F.; Laurichesse, H.; Baud, O.; Bommelaer, G. & Traoré, O. Multidrug-resistant Klebsiella Pneumoniae Outbreak after Endoscopic Retrograde Cholangiopancreatography. *Endoscopy*, Vol.42, No. 11, (November 2010), pp. 895-899, ISSN 0013−726X

Babcock, H.; Carroll, C.; Matava, M.; L'ecuyer, P. & Fraser, V. Surgical site infections after arthroscopy: outbreak investigation and case control study. *Arthroscopy: The Journal of Arthroscopic and Related Surgery*, Vol.19, No.2, (February 2003), pp. 172-181, ISSN 0749-8063

Bar-Or, Y. The Effects of Adhesion on Survival and Growth of Microorganisms. *Experientia*, Vol.46, No.8, (1990), pp. 823-826, ISSN 0014-4754

Bass, D.; Oliver, S. & Bornman, P. Pseudomonas Septicaemia after Endoscopic Retrograde Cholangiopancreatography - an Unresolved Problem. *South African Medical Journal*, Vol.77, No. 10, (May 1990), pp. 509-511, ISSN 0256-9574

Beilenhoff, U.; Neumann, C.; Rey, J.; Biering, H.; Blum, R.; Schmidt, V. & ESGE Guidelines Committee. ESGE-ESGENA Guideline for Quality Assurance in Reprocessing: Microbiological Surveillance Testing in Endoscopy. *Endoscopy*, Vol.39, No.2, (February 2007), pp. 175-181, ISSN 0013−726X

Bilbao, M.; Dotter, C.; Lee, T. & Katon, R. Complications of Endoscopic Retrograde Cholangiopancreatography (ERCP). *Gastroenterology*, Vol. 70, No.3, (March 1976), pp. 314-320, ISSN 0016-5085

Bryce, E.; Walker, M.; Bevan, C. & Smith J. Contamination of Bronchoscopes with Mycobacterium Tuberculosis. *Canadian Journal of Infection Control*, Vol.8, No.2, (Summer 1993), pp. 35-36, ISSN 1183-5702

Buss, A.; Been, M.; Borgers, R.; Stokroos, I.; Melchers, W.; Peters, F.; Limburg, A. & Degener, J. Endoscope Disinfection and its Pitfalls – Requirement for Retrograde Surveillance Cultures. *Endoscopy*, Vol.40, No.4, (February 2008), pp. 327-332, ISSN 0013−726X

Carbonne, A.; Thiolet, J.; Fournier, S.; Fortineau, N.; Kassis-Chikhani, N.; Boytchev, I.; Aggoune, M.; Séguier, J.; Sénéchal, H.; Tavolacci, M.; Coignard, B.; Astagneau, P. & Jarlier, V. Control of a Multi-hospital Outbreak of KPC-producing Klebsiella Pneumoniae Type 2 in France, September to October 2009. *Eurosurveillance*, Vol.48, No.15, (December 2010), pii: 19734, ISSN 1560-7917

Cêtre, J.-C.; Nicolle, M.-C.; Salord, H.; Pérol, M.; Tigaud, S.; David, G.; Bourjault, M. & Vanhems, P. Outbreaks of Contaminated Broncho-alveolar Lavage Related to Intrinsically Defective Bronchoscopes. *Journal of Hospital Infection*, Vol.61, No.1, (September 2005), pp. 39-45, ISSN 0195-6701

Chicurel, M. Bacterial Biofilms and Infections. Slimebusters. *Nature*, Vol.408, No.6810, (November 2000), pp. 284-286. ISSN 0028-0838

Christensen, M.; Matzen, P.; Schulze, S. & Rosenberg, J. Complications of ERCP: a Prospective Study. *Gastrointestinal Endoscopy*, Vol.60, No.5, (November 2004), pp. 721-731, ISSN 0016−5107

Classen, D.; Jacobson, J.; Burke, J.; Jacobson, J. & Evans, R. Serious Pseudomonas Infections Associated with Endoscopic Retrograde Cholangiopancreatography. *The American Journal of Medicine*, Vol.84, No.3, (March 1988), pp. 590-596, ISSN 0002-9343

Cochrane, D.; Brown, M.; Anwar, H.; Weller, P.; Lam, K. & Costerton, J. Antibody Response to Pseudomonas Aeruginosa Surface Protein Antigens in a Rat Model of Chronic Lung Infection. *Journal of Medical Microbiology*, Vol.27, No.4, (December 1988), pp. 255-261.

Colt, H.; Beamis, J.; Harrell, J. & Mathur, P. Novel Flexible Bronchoscope and Single-use Disposable-sheath Endoscope System. A Preliminary Technology Evaluation. *Chest*, Vol.118, No.1, (July 2000), pp. 183-187, ISSN 0012-3692

Corne, P.; Godreuil, S.; Jean-Pierre, H.; Jonquet, O.; Campos, J.; Jumas-Bilak, E.; Parer, S & Marchandin, H. Unusual Implication of Biopsy Forceps in Outbreaks of Pseudomonas Aeruginosa Infections and Pseudo-infections Related to Bronchoscopy. *Journal of Hospital Infection*, Vol.61, No.1, (September 2005), pp. 20-26, ISSN 0195-6701

Costerton, J.; Lewandowski, Z.; Caldwell, D.; Korber, D & Lappin-Scott, H. Microbial Biofilms. *Annual Reviews in Microbiology*, Vol.49, (October 1995), pp. 711–745, ISSN 0066-4227

Costerton, J.; Stewart, P. & Greenberg, E. Bacterial Biofilms: a Common Cause of Persistent Infections. *Science*, Vol.284, No.5418, (May 1999), pp. 1318-1322, ISSN 0036-8075

Cotton, P.; Connor, P.; Rawls, E. & Romagnuolo, J. Infection after ERCP and Antibiotic Prophylaxis: a Sequential Quality-Improvement Approach over 11 Years. *Gastrointestinal Endoscopy*, Vol.67, No.3, (March 2008), pp. 471-475, ISSN 0016−5107

Cotton, P.; Lehman, G.; Vennes, J.; Geenen, J.; Russell, R.; Meyers, W.; Liguory, C. & Nickl, N. Endoscopic Sphincterotomy Complications and their Management: an Attempt at Consensus. *Gastrointestinal Endoscopy*, Vol.37, No.3, (May-June 1991), pp. 383-393, ISSN 0016−5107

Davies, D.; Parsek, M.; Pearson, J.; Iglewski, B.; Costerton, J. & Greenberg, E. The Involvementof Cell-to-cell Signals in the Development of a Bacterial Biofilm. *Science*, Vol. 280, No.5361, (April 1998), pp. 295-298, ISSN 0036-8075

Dutch Infection Prevention Working Party (WIP). Guideline for Cleaning and Disinfection of Endoscopes. (April, 2004). Revision: April, 2009. Available at: http://www.wip.nl/UK/; follow links to Documentation - guideline downloads - Hospitals - Cleaning, disinfection and sterilization

Fraser, T.; Reiner, S.; Malczynski, M.; Yarnold, P.; Warren, J. & Noskin, G. Multidrug-resistant Pseudomonas Aeruginosa Cholangitis after Endoscopic Retrograde Cholangiopancreatography: Failure of Routine Endoscope Cultures to Prevent an Outbreak. *Infection Control and Hospital Epidemiology*, Vol. 25, No. 10, (October 2004), pp. 856-859, ISSN 0899-823X

Fraser, V.; Jones, M.; Murray, P.; Medoff, G.; Zhang, Y & Wallace, R. Contamination of Flexible Fiberoptic Bronchoscopes with Mycobacterium Chelonae Linked to an Automated Bronchoscope Disinfection Machine. *The American Review of Respiratory Diseases*, Vol.145, No.4, (April 1992), pp. 853-855, ISSN 0003-0805

Gastroenterological Society of Australia. (March, 2006). Infection control in endoscopy. Digestive Health Foundation, Available from: http://www.gesa.org.au/pdf/booklets/I_Control_2nd_Edition.pdf

Gillespie, E.; Kotsanas, D. & Stuart, R. Microbiological monitoring of endoscopes: 5-year review. *Journal of Gastroenterology and Hepatology*, Vol.23, No.7, (July 2008), pp. 1069-1074, ISSN 0815-9319

Harris, A.; Chan, C.; Torres-Viera, C.; Hammett, R. & Carr-Locke, D. Meta-analysis of Antibiotic Prophylaxis in Endoscopic Retrograde Cholangiopancreatography. *Endoscopy*, Vol.31, No.9, (November 1999), pp. 718-724, ISSN 0013−726X

Henoun Loukili, N.; Becker, H.; Harno, J.; Bientz, M. & Meunier O. Effect of Peracetic Acid and Aldehyde Disinfectants on Biofilm. *Journal of Hospital Infection*, Vol.58, No.2, (October 2004), pp. 151-154, ISSN 0195-6701

Hirota, W.; Petersen, K.; Baron, T.; Goldstein, J.; Jacobson, B.; Leighton, J.; Mallery, J.; Waring, J.; Fanelli, R.; Wheeler-Harbough, J. & Faigel, D. Guidelines for Antibiotic Prophylaxis for GI Endoscopy. *Gastrointestinal Endoscopy*, Vol.58, No.4, (October 2003), pp. 475-482, ISSN 0016−5107

Imberta, G.; Secciab, Y. & La Scola, B. Methylobacterium sp. Bacteraemia due to a Contaminated Endoscope. *Journal of Hospital Infection*, Vol.61, No.3, (November 2005), pp. 268-270, ISSN 0195-6701

Kampf, G.; Blo, R. & Martiny, H. Surface Fixation of Dried Blood by Glutaraldehyde and Peracetic Acid. *Journal of Hospital Infection*, Vol.57, No.2, (June 2004), pp. 139-143, ISSN 0195-6701

Kaye, K.; Macone, A. & Powel H. Catheter Infection Caused by Methylobacterium in Immunocompromised Hosts: Report of Three Cases and Review of the Literature. *Clinical Infectious Diseases*, Vol.14, No.5, (May 1992), pp. 1010-1014, ISSN 1058-4838

Kirschke, D.; Jones, T.; Craig, A.; Chu, P.; Mayernick, G.; Patel, J. & Schaffner, W. Pseudomonas Aeruginosa and Serratia Marcescens Contamination Associated with a Manufacturing Defect in Bronchoscopes. *New English Journal of Medicine*, Vol. 248, No.3, (January 2003), pp. 214-220, ISSN 0028-4793

Kovacs, B.; Aprecio, R.; Kettering, J. & Chen, E. Efficacy of Various Disinfectants in Killing a Resistant Strain of Pseudomonas Aeruginosa by Comparing Zones of Inhibition: Implications for Endoscopic Equipment Reprocessing. *The American Journal of Gastroenterology*, Vol.93, No.11, (November 1998), pp. 2057-2059, ISSN 0002-9270

Kovaleva, J.; Meessen, N.; Peters, F.; Been, M.; Arends, J.; Borgers, R. & Degener, J. Is Bacteriologic Surveillance in Endoscope Reprocessing Stringent Enough? *Endoscopy*, Vol.41, No.10, (October 2009), pp. 913-916, ISSN 0013−726X

Kovaleva, J.; Degener, J. & Van der Mei, H. Mimicking Disinfection and Drying of Biofilms in Contaminated Endoscopes. *Journal of Hospital Infection*, Vol.76, No.4, (December 2010), pp. 345-350, ISSN 0195-6701

Kressel, A. & Kidd, F. Pseudo-outbreak of Mycobacterium Chelonae and Methylobacterium Caused by Contamination of an Automated Endoscopy Washer. *Infection Control and Hospital Epidemiology*, Vol. 22, No.7, (July 2001), pp. 414-418, ISSN 0899-823X

Kullman, E.; Borch, K.; Lindstrom, E.; Ansehn, S.; Ihse, I. & Anderberg, B. Bacteremia Following Diagnostic and Therapeutic ERCP. *Gastrointestinal Endoscopy*, Vol.38, No.4, (July - Augustus 1992), pp. 444-449, ISSN 0016-5107

Leers, W. Disinfecting Endoscopes: How not to Transmit Mycobacterium Tuberculosis by Bronchoscopy. *Canadian Medical Association Journal*, Vol.123, No.4, (Augustus 1980), pp. 275-283, ISSN 1488-2329

Liu, J.; Wu, J.; Chen, H.; Huang, A.; Ko, W. & Chuang, Y. Methylobacterium Mesophilicum Synovitis in an Alcoholic. *Clinical Infectious Diseases*, Vol.24, No.5, (May 1997), pp. 1008-1009, ISSN 1058-4838

Low, D.; Mieflikier, A.; Kennedy, J. & Stiver, H. Infectious Complications of Endoscopic Retrograde Cholangiopancreatography. A Prospective Assessment. *Annals of Internal Medicine*, Vol.140, No.8, (Augustus 1980), pp. 1076-1077, ISSN 0003-4819

Marion, K.; Freney, J.; Bergeron, E.; Bergeron, J.; Renaud, F. & Costerton, J. Using an Efficient Biofilm Detaching Agent: an Essential Step for the Improvement of Endoscope Reprocessing Protocols. *Journal of Hospital Infection*, Vol.64, No.2, (October 2006), pp. 136-142, ISSN 0195-6701

Marion-Ferey, K.; Pasmore, M.; Stoodley, P.; Wilsony, S.; Husson, G. & Costerton, J. Biofilm Removal from Silicone Tubing: an Assessment of the Efficacy of Dialysis Machine Decontamination Procedures Using an in Vitro Model. *Journal of Hospital Infection*, Vol.53, No.1, (January 2003), pp. 64-71, ISSN 0195-6701

Masci, E.; Toti, G.; Mariani, A.; Curioni, S.; Lomazzi, A.; Dinelli, M.; Minoli, G.; Crosta, C.; Comin U.; Fertitta, A.; Prada, A.; Rubis Passoni, G. & Testoni, P. Complications of Diagnostic and Therapeutic ERCP: a Prospective Multicenter Study. *The American Journal of Gastroenterology*, Vol.96, No.2, (February 2001), pp. 417-423, ISSN 0002-9270

Nelson, D.; Barkun, A.; Block, K.; Burdick, J.; Ginsberg, G.; Greenwald, D.; Kelsey, P.; Nakao, N.; Slivka, A.; Smith, P. & Vakil, N. Technology Status Evaluation Report. Transmission of Infection by Gastrointestinal Endoscopy. *Gastrointestinal Endoscopy*, Vol.54, No.6, (December 2001), pp. 824-828, ISSN 0016−5107

Nelson, D. & Muscarella, L. Current Issues in Endoscope Reprocessing and Infection Control during Gastrointestinal Endoscopy. *World Journal of Gastroenterology*, Vol.12, No.25, (July 2006), pp. 3953-3964, ISSN 1007-9327

Obee, P.; Griffith, C.; Cooper, R.; Cooke, R.; Bennion, N. & Lewis, M. Real-time Monitoring in Managing the Decontamination of Flexible Gastrointestinal Endoscopes. *American Journal of Infection Control*, Vol.33, No.4, (May 2005), pp. 202-206, ISSN 0196-6553

O'Connor, H.; Hamilton, I.; Lincoln, C.; Maxwell, S. & Axon, A. Bacteremia with Upper Gastrointestinal Endoscopy - a Reappraisal. *Endoscopy*, Vol.15, No.1, (January 1983), pp. 21-23

Pajkos, A.; Vickery, K. & Cossart, Y. Is Biofilm Accumulation on Endoscope Tubing a Contributor to the Failure of Cleaning and Decontamination? *Journal of Hospital Infection*, Vol.58, No.3, (November 2004), pp. 224-229, ISSN 0195-6701

Pappas, S.; Schaaff, D.; DiCostanzo, M.; King, F. & Sharp, J. Contamination of Flexible Fiberoptic Bronchoscopes. *The American Review of Respiratory Diseases*, Vol.127, No.3, (March 1982), pp. 391-392, ISSN 0003-0805

Patel R. Biofilms and Antimicrobial Resistance. *Clinical Orthopaedics and Related Research*, No.437, (Augustus 2005), pp. 41–47, ISSN 0009-921X

Rejchrt, S.; Čermák, P.; Pavlatová, L.; Míčková, E. & Bureš J. Bacteriologic Testing of Endoscopes after High-level Disinfection. *Gastrointestinal Endoscopy*, Vol.60, No.1, (July 2004), pp. 76-78, ISSN 0016−5107

Rutala, W. & Weber, D. New Disinfection and Sterilization Methods. *Emerging Infectious Diseases*, Vol.7, No.2, (March – April 2001), pp. 348-353, ISSN 1080-6059

Sanders, J.; Martin, J.; Hooke, M. & Hooke, J. Methylobacterium Mesophilicum Infection: Case Report and Literature Review of an Unusual Opportunistic Pathogen. *Clinical Infectious Diseases*, Vol.30, No.6, (June 2000), pp. 936-938, ISSN 1058-4838

Schelenz, S. & French, G. An Outbreak of Multidrug-resistant Pseudomonas Aeruginosa Infection Associated with Contamination of Bronchoscopes and an Endoscope Washer-disinfector. *Journal of Hospital Infection*, Vol.46, No.1, (September 2000), pp. 23-30, ISSN 0195-6701

Sciortino, C.; Xia, E. & Mozee, A. Assessment of a Novel Approach to Evaluate the Outcome of Endoscope Reprocessing. *Infection Control and Hospital Epidemiology*, Vol. 25, No.4, (April 2004), pp. 284-290, ISSN 0899-823X

Shimonom, N.; Takuma, T.; Tsuchimochi N.; Shiose, A.; Kanamoto, M.; Uchida, Y.; Morita, S.; Matsumoto, H & Hayashi, J. An outbreak of Pseudomonas Aeruginosa Infections Following Thoracic Surgeries Occurring via the Contamination of Bronchoscopes and an Automatic Endoscope Reprocessor. *Journal of Infection and Chemotherapy*, Vol.14, No.6, (December 2008), pp. 418–423, ISSN 1341-321X

Shin, J.; Kee, S.; Shin, M.; Kim, S.; Shin, D.; Lee, S.; Suh, S. & Ryang, D. Biofilm Production by Isolates of Candida Species Recovered from Nonneutropenic Patients: Comparison of Bloodstream Isolates with Isolates from other Sources. *Journal of Clinical Microbiology*, Vol.40, No.4, (April 2002), pp. 1244-1248, ISSN 0095-1137

Seoane-Vazquez, E.; Rodriguez-Monguio, R.; Visaria, J. & Carlson, A. Exogenous Endoscopy-related Infections, Pseudo-infections, and Toxic Reactions: Clinical and Economic Burden. *Current Medical Research and Opinion*, Vol.22, No.10, (October, 2006), pp. 2007-2021, ISSN 1473-4877

Seoane-Vazquez, E.; Rodriguez-Monguio, R.; Visaria, J. & Carlson, A. Endoscopy-related Infections and Toxic Reactions: an International Comparison. *Endoscopy*, Vol.39, No.8, (Augustus 2007), pp. 742-778, ISSN 0013−726X

Spach, D.; Silverstein, F. & Stamm, W. Transmission of Infection by Gastrointestinal Endoscopy and Bronchoscopy. *Annals of Internal Medicine*, Vol.118, No.2, (January, 1993), pp. 117-128, ISSN 1539-3704

Srinivasan, A. Epidemiology and Prevention of Infections Related to Endoscopy. *Current Infectious Disease Reports*, Vol.5, No.6, (December, 2003), pp. 467-472, ISSN 1534-3146

Srinivasan, A.; Wolfenden, L.; Song, X.; Mackie, K.; Hartsell, T.; Jones, H.; Diette, G.; Orens, J.; Yung, R.; Ross, T.; Merz, W.; Scheel, P.; Haponik, E. & Perl, T. An Outbreak of Pseudomonas Aeruginosa Infections Associated with Flexible Bronchoscopes. *New English Journal of Medicine*, Vol.348, No.3, (January 2003), pp. 221-227, ISSN 0028-4793

Systchenko, R.; Marchetti, B.; Canard, J.; Palazzo, L.; Ponchon, T.; Rey, J.; Sautereau, D. & French Society of Digestive Endoscopy. Guidelines of the French Society of Digestive Endoscopy: Recommendations for Setting up Cleaning and Disinfection Procedures in Gastrointestinal Endoscopy. *Endoscopy*, Vol.32, No.10, (October 2000), pp. 807-818, ISSN 0013−726X

Terhaar sive Droste, J.; Craanen, M.; Kolkman, J. & Mulder, C. Dutch Endoscopic Capacity in the Era of Colorectal Cancer Screening. *The Netherlands Journal of Medicine*, Vol.64, No.10, (November 2006), pp. 371-373, ISSN 0300-2977

Van Delden, C. & Iglewski, B. Cell-to-cell Signalling and Pseudomonas Aeruginosa Infections. *Emerging Infectious Diseases*, Vol.4, No.4, (October - December 1998), pp. 551-560, ISSN 1080-6059

Van Klingeren, B. & Pullen, P. Glutaraldehyde Resistant Mycobacteria from Endoscope Washers. *Journal of Hospital Infection*, Vol.25, No.2, (October 1993), pp. 147-149, ISSN 0195-6701

Wheeler, P.; Lancaster, D. & Kaiser, A. Bronchopulmonary Cross-colonization and Infection Related to Mycobacterial Contamination of Suction Valves of Bronchoscopes. *The Journal of Infectious Diseases*, Vol.159, No.5, (May 1989), pp. 954-958, ISSN 0022-1899

10

Transgastrostomal Observation and Management Using an Ultrathin Endoscope After Percutaneous Endoscopic Gastrostomy

Shinji Nishiwaki[1], Hiroo Hatakeyama[1],
Masahide Iwashita[1] and Hiroshi Araki[2]
[1]*Department of Internal Medicine, Nishimino Kosei Hospital,*
[2]*Department of Gastroenterology, Graduate School of Medicine, Gifu University,*
Japan

1. Introduction

Recent developments have made ultrathin endoscopes available for routine esophagogastroduodenoscopy and also for unsedated transnasal observation (Shaker, 1994). Transnasal endoscopy is known to be less of a burden for patients (more tolerable) than transoral endoscopy and has benefits including fewer effects on respiratory and cardiovascular status and reduced recovery time after the procedure (Campo et al., 1998; Dumortier et al., 1999; Mori et al., 2008). Transnasal ultrathin endoscopy has also been applied for biliary drainage, insertion of a nasoenteral feeding tube or a long intestinal tube, and percutaneous endoscopic gastrostomy (PEG) (Fang et al., 2005; Itoi et al., 2008; Sato et al., 2008; Vitale et al., 2005). PEG has become the primary access for long term enteral feeding since its introduction in 1980 (Gauderer et al., 1980; Ponsky & Gauderer, 1981), being a very easy and rapid method compared with the previous surgical technique to place a gastrostomy tube.

The endoscopic approach from the gastrocutaneous tract was first described by Chaurasia , et al. for the insertion of a jejunal feeding tube through the PEG (PEG-J) tract (Chaurasia & Chang, 1995). Although they used a pediatric bronchoscope at that time, an ultrathin endoscope later took its place for this purpose (Adler et al., 2002). We have been employing an ultrathin endoscope through the gastrostomy tract for observation, diagnosis, and treatment of various digestive diseases from April 2003. We also investigated the usefulness of such transgastrostomal endoscopy (TGE) for management of patients who had undergone percutaneous endoscopic gastrostomy (PEG).

2. Procedure of transgastrostomal endoscopy (TGE)

Patients with a mature gastrocutaneous tract are candidates for this procedure. Patients before the maturation of the fistula (2 to 4 weeks after the PEG) have higher risk of fistula disruption. If it is necessary to perform TGE in an earlier phase or at the PEG, tight affixation of the stomach to the abdominal wall using a gastropexy device (Rogers, 1989) allows TGE to be performed.

2.1 Equipment

The endoscopes wc used were GIF-XP240, GIF-XP260 and GIF-XP260N (Olympus Optical Co., Ltd., Tokyo, Japan) (Fig. 1). The diameters of these endoscopes were 7.7, 6.5, and 5.2 mm, respectively. The diameter of the working channel of these endoscopes was 2.0 mm. GIF-XP240, GIF-XP260, and GIF-XP260N allow insertion through more than 24, 20 and 18 F fistula tracts, respectively.

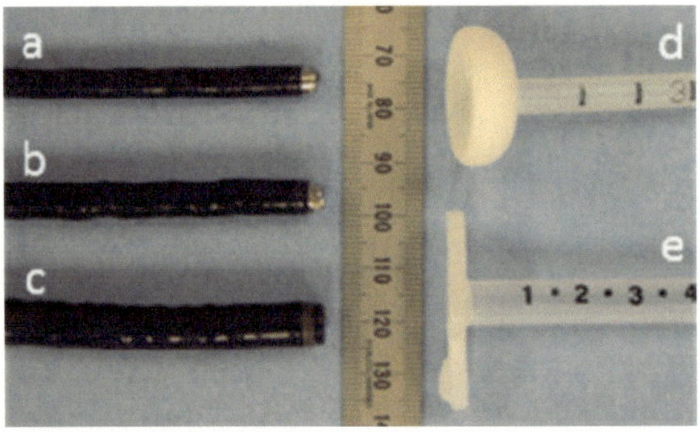

Fig. 1. Photograph of ultrathin endoscopes and gastrostomy tubes. a: GIF-XP260N, b: GIF-XP260, c: GIF-XP240 (Olympus Optical Co., Ltd., Tokyo, Japan), d: Ponsky NBR, 20F (Bard Access Systems, Inc., Salt Lake City, UT, USA), e: Securi-T, 24F (Boston Scientific, Natick, MA, USA)

2.2 Routine observation by TGE

The patient is usually infused with 500 ml of water instead of liquid feeds for several hours before the endoscopic examination to remove the gastric mucus. The patient is laid in the supine position and then the gastrostomy tube is removed. After applying lidocaine jelly around the stoma, an ultrathin endoscope is inserted through the fistural tract and proceeded into the gastric lumen (Fig. 2A). The endoscope is directed to the oral side and advanced to the esophagogastric junction (Fig. 2B). The junction can be observed in detail without disturbance, free from the shade of the endoscope. The endoscope is retrogradely inserted through the esophagus, and we can observe oral cavity as well as pharyngeal cavity if necessary. The endoscope is then withdrawn to the stomach and directed to the anal side. The endoscope is easily inserted up to the upper jejunum from the stoma (Fig. 2C). The endoscope is pulled back to the stomach and turned back to see around the stoma (Fig. 2D).

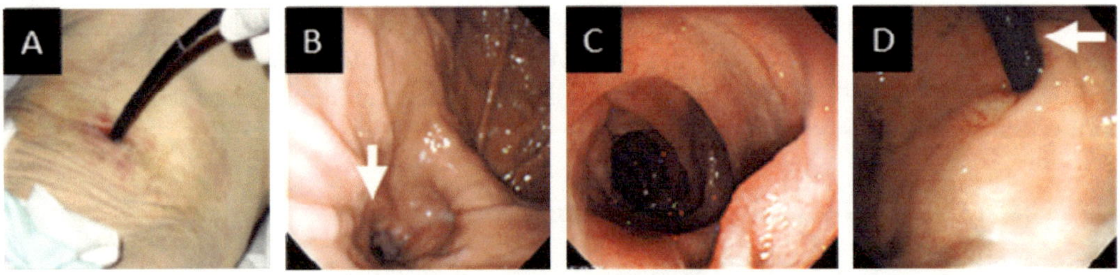

Fig. 2. A: Insertion of an ultrathin endoscope through the gastrostomy tract. B: Endoscopic view of esophagogastric junction (arrow) which is retrogradely observed from the stomach. C: Endoscopic view of upper jejunum. D: Endoscopic view of the stoma from the stomach. Arrow indicates the endoscope inserted through the stoma.

After the observation of the upper gastrointestinal tract, the endoscope is withdrawn from the stoma and a new gastrostomy tube is replaced via the skin incision.

3. Diagnostic application of TGE

Since most of patients who undergo PEG are of advanced age and also have comorbid diseases, they usually do not undergo esophagogastroduodenoscopy after PEG. As TGE is a less invasive procedure to perform even for critically ill patients, we have routinely conducted TGE at the periodical replacement of gastrostomy tubes. We have found variety of newly developed lesions in the upper gastrointestinal tracts and were able to treat them at an early stage without symptoms.

3.1 Cardiopulmonary tolerance during the procedure of TGE

TGE is a less invasive examination compared to transoral and transnasal endoscopy, because TGE does not pass through the pharynx. It requires neither local anesthesia of the pharynx or nasal tract nor conscious sedation before the procedure of TGE. We monitored blood pressure, heart rate, and percutaneous oxygen saturation concentration measurement of the arterial blood (SPO_2) during TGE procedures in 20 consecutive patients. The values were compared to those for patients with the same clinical background during the examination of transoral endoscopy in routine esophagogastroduodenoscopy. Table 1 shows the comparison of cardiopulmonary effects during the procedures of TGE and transoral endoscopy. None of the TGE examinations required sedation, while the transoral examinations required 1 to 4 mg of intravenous administration of midazolam. There were no significant differences in the fluctuation of blood pressure and heart rate between TGE and transoral endoscopy. TGE displayed no effects on SPO_2 during the procedure, while transoral endoscopy caused a decrease of SPO_2 in 46% of the patients.

	Transgastrostomal endoscopy (n=20)	Transoral endoscopy (n=13)	P value
Fluctuation of blood pressure (more than 20%)	5% (1/20)	23% (3/13)	$P = 0.157$
Fluctuation of heart rate (more than 20%)	15% (3/20)	15% (2/13)	$P > 0.5$
Decrease of SPO_2 (more than 3%)	0% (0/20)	46% (6/13)	$P < 0.01$

Table 1. The effects of TGE and transoral endoscopy on blood pressure, heart rate, and SPO_2.

3.2 Newly developed lesions in upper gastrointestinal tract after PEG

We have been conducting TGE for screening the upper gastrointestinal tract since April 2003. TGE was carried out 805 times in 245 PEG patients (Table 2) during routine replacement of gastrostomy tubes until November 2010. The demographic data are shown in Table 2. The mean age of the subjects was 80.8 years old, and the most frequent underlying disease was cerebrovascular disease. The endoscopic findings of TGE were compared to those at PEG placement. There were a variety of newly developed lesions after PEG.

Age (mean ± SD)	80.8 ± 8.9
Gender (male : female)	71 : 174
Underlying disease	
Cerebrovascular disease	143
Dementia	42
Neuromuscular disease	23
Pneumonia	20
Malignant tumor	6
Others	11

Table 2. Demographic data of patients who underwent TGE after PEG.

Reflux esophagitis was found in 35 patients (14.2%), which was the most frequent lesion after PEG. Among the 35 patients, reflux esophagitis was absent at the PEG tube placement in the 30 patients. There were 5 severe cases with symptoms of hematemesis and this had subsequently led to stricture of the lower esophagus in 3 patients (Fig. 3A). Although in these 3 patients, we were unable to insert a transoral endoscope into the stomach, we were able to conduct endoscopic observation of the stomach by TGE (Fig. 3B).

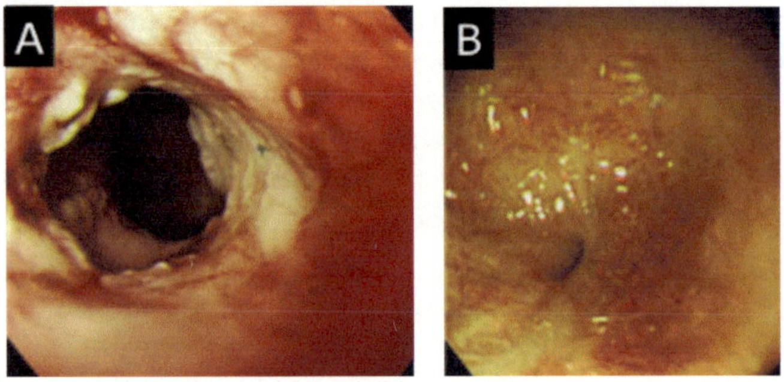

Fig. 3. Endoscopic view of severe reflux esophagitis after PEG. A: Circumferential ulcer was observed by emergency transoral esophagoscopy after the symptom of hematemesis. B: The stricture of the lower esophagus after administration of proton pump inhibitor was observed from the stomach by TGE.

The next most frequent lesion after PEG was polypoid lesion around the stoma. We classified polypoid lesions into 3 types according to their location e.g.; basal bumper type, peri-bumper type and opposite-bumper type. The basal-bumper type polyp was communicated with the fistural tract and the pathology was inflammatory granulation (Fig. 4A). The peri-bumper type polyp was located around the stoma and often observed in cases with decompression by a mushroom type gastrostomy tube (Fig. 4B). Pathological examination revealed hyperplasia of the gastric mucosa. The opposite-bumper type polyp was located on the contra lateral wall of the stoma, probably caused by the contact of the top of the bumper or tube (Fig. 4C). The pathology was hyperplasia. Most of the polypoid lesion was not significantly changed in the subsequent observation by TGE. One case with haemorrhage from the basal-bumper type granuloma was resected by polypectomy using TGE.

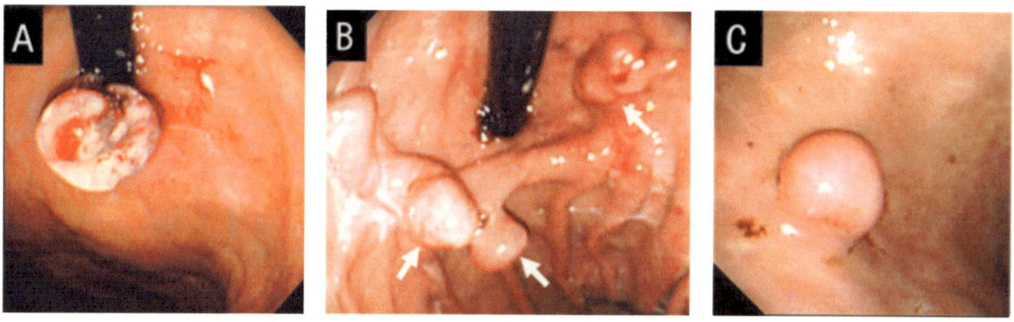

Fig. 4. Endoscopic views of polypoid lesions around the stoma. A: basal-bumper type, B: peri-bumper type, C: opposite-bumper type.

Gastric ulcer was observed in 6 patients. All of their lesions were accidentally found at TGE, because they did not complain of symptoms due to their comorbid diseases. Among the 6 patients, the lesions of 3 patients were supposed to have been caused by direct contact with the bumper. These ulcers were characterized by their location on the contralateral side of the bumper (Fig. 5A). The remaining 3 patients were sporadic cases (Fig. 5B). We have also experienced additional 2 cases of symptomatic gastric ulcer which were detected by transoral endoscopy. For their initial symptoms of hematemesis and tarry stool, emergent esophagogastroduodenoscopy was performed (Nishiwaki et al., 2010b). Hemostasis was obtained by endoscopic hemoclips and coagulation, respectively. TGE was not available for such therapy, because the working channel of the ultrathin endoscope was too narrow to insert the devices to achieve hemostasis.

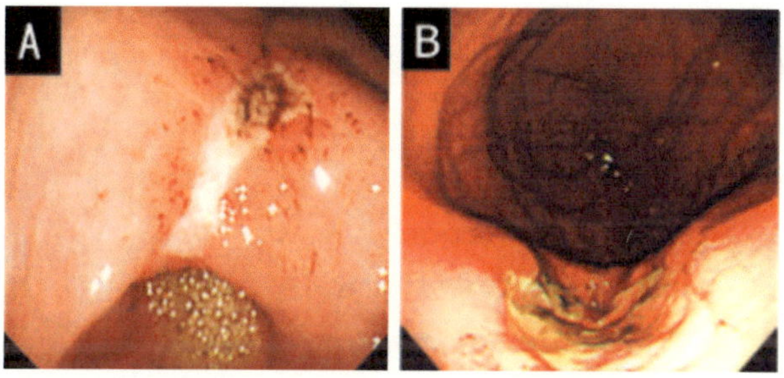

Fig. 5. A: Gastric ulcer was observed on the posterior wall of the lower body of the stomach, contralateral to the stoma. B: Peptic ulcer was observed on the lesser curvature of the upper body in the stomach.

Neoplastic lesions were also detected by TGE. We have experienced 3 cases of early gastric cancer and one case of carcinoid tumor that developed after PEG. One case was recurrence of early gastric cancer after endoscopic mucosal resection before the PEG. One case of early gastric cancer underwent coagulation therapy with argon plasma (Fig. 6A). The remaining two cancer (Fig. 6B) and one carcinoid tumor lesions were resected by endoscopic submucosal dissection assisted by TGE, the technique of which is described in section 4.2.1. The primary duodenal cancer was accidentally found by TGE at the first endoscopic examination 5 years after PEG.

Candida esophagitis was observed in 4 patients. All of the patients were administered proton pump inhibitor, which might have been involved in the development of the esophagitis.

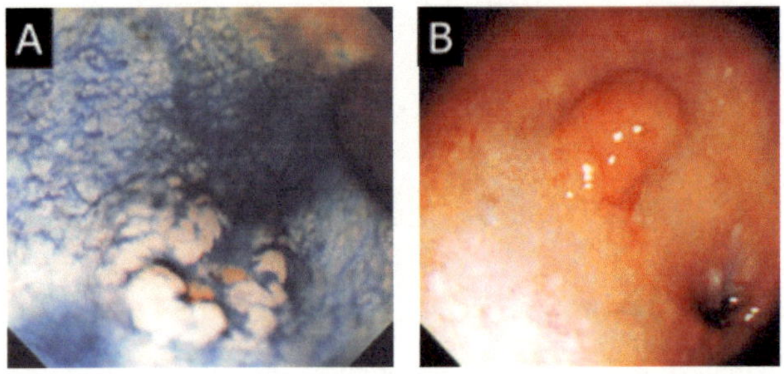

Fig. 6. A: Indigocarmine sprayed endoscopic view of early gastric cancer. Superficial depressed lesion (IIc) was observed on the greater curvature of the antrum. The biopsy specimen of the lesion was well-differentiated tubular adenocarcinoma. B: Superficial elevated lesion (IIa) was observed on the lesser curvature of the upper body of the stomach. Pathological finding of the biopsy specimen was well-differentiated tubular adenocarcinoma.

Table 3 summarizes newly developed lesions after PEG. TGE was useful for the early detection and follow up of these lesions.

Pathological conditions	Number of patients
Reflux esophagitis	30
Polypoid lesion around the stoma	28
Gastric ulcer	6
Neoplastic lesions	
Early gastric cancer	3
Gastric carcinoid tumor	1
Primary duodenal cancer	1
Candida esophagitis	4
Total	73

Table 3. Newly developed upper gastrointestinal lesions which were detected by TGE after PEG.

4. Therapeutic application of TGE

TGE also offers several advantages for endoscopic treatments compared with a transoral endoscope. TGE can easily access up to the upper jejunum with less patient discomfort. TGE covers treatments for lesions from the upper esophagus to upper jejunum. Table 4 shows the list of TGE we have conducted for therapeutic purposes. .

	No. of trial	No. of success
Establishement of direct jejunal feeding access		
Placement of jejunal feeding thorough the PEG (PEG-J)	27	27
Direct percutaneous endoscopic jejunostomy (DPEJ)	36	33
Resection of upper gastrointestinal tumors		
TGE assisted endoscopic submucosal dissection (ESD)	5	5
Endoscopic mucosal resection	1	1
Polypectomy	1	1
Palliative therapy for gastrointestinal obstruction		
Transgastrostomal gastroduodenal stenting	5	4
Placement of long intestinal decompression tube	2	2
Other usage for endoscopic treatments		
Recovery of disrupted gastrocutaneous tract	5	5
Transgastrostomic biliary drainage	1	1

Table 4. Reference chart of TGE for therapeutic purposes and their outcomes.

4.1 Establishment of direct jejunal feeding access

Since the introduction of endoscopic placement of a gastrostomy tube, PEG has been the primary choice for long-term enteral access. However, there are some situations which postpyloric or jejunal feeding is preferable to gastric feeding. The indications for jejunal feeding include a high risk of aspiration, previous gastric resection, gastric pull-up, gastric outlet obstruction, an obstructed or nonfunctioning gastrojejunostomy, and gastric dysmotility (Shike & Latkany, 1998). The access for jejunal feeding was initially established as two methods, i.e.; transnasal insertion of a feeding tube and surgical placement of a jejunostomy tube. Alternative accesses methods for jejunal feeding have been developed; placement of a jejunal feeding tube through the PEG (PEG-J) and direct percutaneous endoscopic jejunostomy (DPEJ). We utilized TGE for the establishment of the two access methods.

4.1.1 Placement of a jejunal feeding tube through the PEG (PEG-J)

PEG-J was first described in 1984 (Ponsky & Aszodi, 1984). This technique was usually conducted for patients with high risk of aspiration due to gastroesophageal reflux of food after PEG (Nishiwaki et al., 2006). The tube is usually placed under fluoroscopic guidance. However, it is sometimes difficult to pass the feeding tube through the pyloric ring and duodenum using only fluoroscopy. A technique to assist the tube passage into the duodenum by transoral endoscopy has been reported (Duckworth et al., 1994; Leichus L et al., 1997). A transgastric technique using a pediatric bronchoscope or an ultrathin endoscope was described first in 1995 (Adler et al., 2002; Chaurasia & Chang, 1995).

We treated 27 patients using this technique with the following procedures: 1. Remove the gastrostomy tube. 2. Insert an endoscope through the gastrostomy and proceed up to the jejunum (Fig. 7A). 3. Insert a guidewire through the working channel of the endoscope. 4. Remove the endoscope retaining the guidewire (Fig. 7B). 5. Place a jejunal feeding tube over the guidewire through the PEG under fluoroscopic guidance (Figs. 7 C & D).

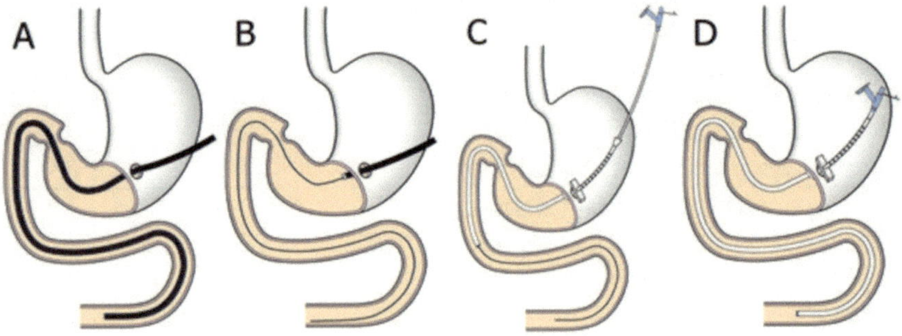

Fig. 7. Schematic procedure of PEG-J using TGE.

The jejunal feeding tubes (J-tube, Boston Scientific, Natick, MA, USA, or Jejunal Feeding Tube, Bard Access Systems, Inc., Salt Lake City, UT, USA) were successfully placed in all 27 patients. The duration of the procedure ranged from 4 to 20 minutes, which was remarkably quick compared with the procedure using only fluoroscopic guidance.

4.1.2 Direct percutaneous endoscopic jejunostomy (DPEJ)

Direct percutaneous placement of the jejunostomy tube was first described in 1987 (Shike et al., 1987). The first case series were for patients with previous gastric resection, and the technique was subsequently applied for patients with intact stomach. Becuase the length of the endoscope for the performance of DPEJ in the transoral route is 160 cm or longer, it requires the use of a long colonoscope or a small intestinal scope (Shike et al., 1991). However, the transgastrostomal approach facilitates access to the upper jejunum without difficulty. DPEJ using TGE was first described in 2002 (Baron, 2002). Although they successfully placed a jejunostomy tube through the mature gastrostomy tract, the gastrocutaneous tract was disrupted by passing through the bumper of the jejunostomy tube. We modified the procedure (Fig. 8) so that the jejunostomy tube does not pass the gastrostomy tract (Nishiwaki et al., 2009b).

After conscious sedation with intravenous administration of midazolam (1 to 2 mg) in most patients, an ultrathin endoscope was inserted through the gastrocutaneous tract immediately after the removal of the gastrostomy tube. The endoscope was inserted up to the jejunum and the site for placement was determined by transillumination to the abdominal wall and finger pressure against the jejunum (Fig. 8A). The abdominal skin surface of the placement area was cleansed with povidone-iodine, and local anesthesia was done administering 1% lidocaine. After test-puncturing with a 21-gauge needle, one or two point sutures were made using gastropexy devices (Create Medic Co., Ltd., Yokohama, Japan, or Easy Tie, Boston Scientific Japan K.K., Tokyo, Japan) to fix the jejunum against the abdominal wall. A 16- or 18-gauge Seldinger needle was inserted through the abdomen toward an open snare inserted through the TGE and a loop wire was passed through the outer sheath of the needle. The loop wire was grasped by the snare and pulled out through the gastrocutaneous tract with the endoscope (Fig. 8B). In most cases, the loop wire was then grasped in the stomach by biopsy forceps of an orally inserted endoscope (Fig. 8C) and pulled out via the mouth (Fig. 8D). In a few cases, the loop wire was directly brought out from the mouth by transgastrostomic endoscopy. Next, an jejunostomy tube was connected to the loop wire and the tube was placed in the jejunum by the pull-through technique (Fig. 8E). The systems to place the jejunostomy tube were One Step Button (Boston Scientific Co., Natick, MA, USA) or Bard Ponsky Pull PEG (Bard Access Systems, Inc., Salt Lake City, UT, USA)

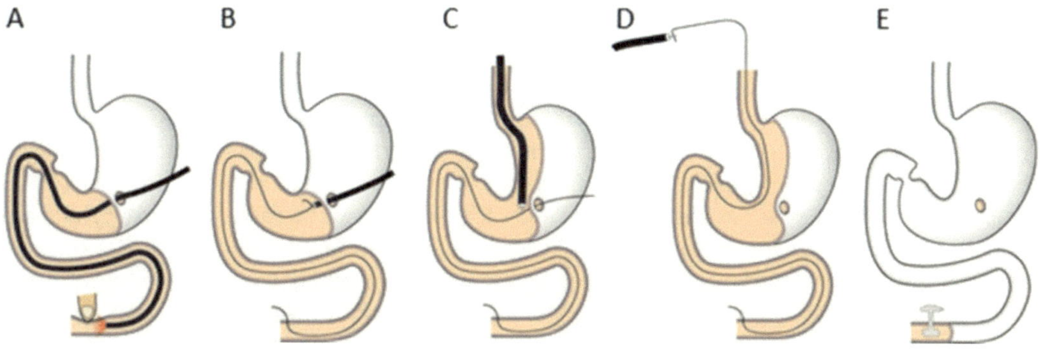

Fig. 8. Schematic procedure of DPEJ using TGE.

Thirty six DPEJ procedures were attempted in 35 patients, with 33 (92%) successful placements. One unsuccessful placement was due to jejunum migration away from the abdominal wall during the puncture; this patient was maintained by feeding via the PEG-J. The other two failures were due to the lack of transillumination. The average $\pm$ SD of duration of procedure, from insertion of the endoscope to the placement of the jejunostomy tube, was 29.6 $\pm$ 13.1 (15 to 70) min.

Procedure-related complications consisted of 1 case each of pneumonia, colocutaneous fistula, and pneumoperitoneum. Of these, pneumonia and colocutaneous fistula were considered major complications. In the former case, placement of the jejunostomy tube took 50 min, and pneumonia occurred before administration of nutrients. The patient died 4 days after DPEJ due to respiratory failure. In the latter case, the fact that the jejunostomy tube had been placed penetrating through the colon was revealed at the second replacement of the jejunostomy tube. The colocutaneous fistula was naturally closed after removal of the replaced tube and DPEJ was successfully completed 28 days after the removal. Pneumoperitoneum, a minor complication, was observed in a severely obese patient.

4.2 Resection of upper gastrointestinal tumors

Endoscopic techniques to remove gastrointestinal tumors have been established as snare polypectomy and endoscopic mucosal resection (EMR). EMR allows the removal of flat lesions by injection with saline into the submucosal layer, but it is difficult to remove larger tumors. Recent development of the technique of endoscopic submucosal dissection (ESD) facilitates the removal of widely-spread neoplastic lesions compared to the EMR. We utilized TGE for these resection techniques of the upper gastrointestinal tumors.

4.2.1 TGE assisted endoscopic submucosal dissection (ESD)

ESD is a new technique for the resection of early gastric cancer (Ono et al., 2001). This technique allows en bloc resection even for larger lesions and allows for precise histological analyses. However, this method has a high incidence of complications such as bleeding and perforation, and the technique requires skill and a longer time for resection compared to conventional EMR (Gotoda 2006). One of the technical problems of ESD is the difficulty of maintaining a clear view of the submucosal layer of the gastric wall during submucosal dissection. We developed the technique of ESD assisted by TGE to dissolve the problem (Nishiwaki et al., 2009a).

Five patients previously established with PEG underwent TGE-assisted ESD (Table 5). ESD was carried out by a single-channel videoendoscope, GIF H260 (Olympus Optical Co., Ltd, Tokyo), attached with a short hood. The high-frequency electrosurgical unit was the Erbotom ICC 200 in Cases 1-3, and the VIO 300D in Cases 4 and 5 (ERBE Elektromedizin GmbH, Tubingen, Germany). After circumferential markings around the lesion, submucosal injection was carried out using a mixture of hyaluronic acid and glycerol containing indigocarmine, according to the method described by Fujishiro, et al (Fujishiro et al., 2006). Circumferential mucosal cutting and submucosal dissection were carried out using a needle knife, a Flex knife, an insulation-tipped (IT) knife, or a combination of the three. TGE was inserted through the mature gastrocutaneous tract and grasped the edge of the resecting specimen to achieve appropriate counter-traction during submucosal dissection (Figs. 9A-C). Hemostatic forceps were used when active bleeding took place during the procedure or to prevent bleeding from large vessels before cutting in soft coagulation mode. TGE also worked for additional submucosal injection, washing with water, aspiration of gastric fluid.

Case I.D.	1	2	3	4	5
Age/Gender	83/M	82/F	72/M	79/F	82/F
Pathology	tub 1	tub 1	adenoma	tub 1	carcinoid tumor
Location	a.w. antrum	l.c. body	p.w. antrum	g.c. body	a.w. body
Dissection size (mm)	24 X 22	20 X 20	60 X 30	30 X 22	15 X 10
Operative duration (min)	21	18	105	55	80

tub 1: well differentiated tubular adenocarcinoma, a.w.: anterior wall, l.c.: lesser curvature, p.w.: posterior wall, g.c.: greater curvature

Table 5. Summary of the patients who underwent TGE-assisted ESD.

A laparoscopic port with a trocar is inserted into the gastric lumen percutaneously and assists in the ESD using an IT knife (Kondo et al., 2004). However these methods are thought to be limited for some tumor locations, as the assisting devices are not flexible. EMR assisted by a magnetic anchor has also been reported to create strong counter traction (Kobayashi et al., 2004). In our methods, an ultrathin endoscope is inserted through the gastrocutaneous tract after PEG, and assisted ESD is performed with an orally inserted videoendoscope. TGE can cover the whole stomach and esophagus and create appropriate counter traction for dissection of the lesion. Furthermore, TGE not only can provide traction control but can also support diverse procedures of ESD, such as marking, submucosal injection, washing out or aspiration of the intragastric contents. TGE facilitates ESD by this type of assistance, and the operation duration of TGE-assisted ESD has been found to be relatively short compared to the single-scope ESD in our hospital.

One of the problems of this method is light interference between the two endoscopes (Fig. 9D). When the two endoscopes faced each other, the position of the TGE had to be changed to eliminate the light interference. The other problem of this method is that it might be difficult to perform TGE before maturation of the gastrocutaneous tract. In the present case series, gastric tumors were found after PEG in three cases, but two tumors were found at the placement of PEG catheter. In general, it takes 3-4 weeks to complete the stoma. ESD was conducted in the two cases 3-4 weeks after PEG, after waiting for maturation of the gastrocutaneous tract. Pneumoperitoneum occurred after ESD in Case 3, although it recovered spontaneously. The use of gastropexy devices enabled us to fix the abdominal and gastric walls more tightly, such that pneumoperitoneum might be prevented even with prolonged endoscopic treatment. Narrowing of the ultrathin endoscope would be helpful for this method. Therefore, simultaneous PEG and TGE-assisted ESD using a gastropexy device and an ultrathin endoscope might be possible for large, difficult lesions.

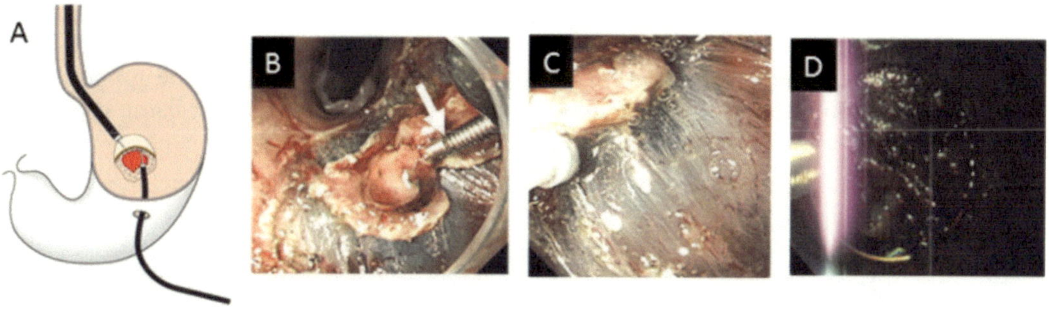

Fig. 9. TGE-assisted ESD. A. Schematic illustration of ESD assisted by TGE. B. Endoscopic view from transoral endoscope in Case 4. A grasping forceps was inserted through the TGE and grasped the edge of the gastric tumor (arrow). C. Endoscopic view from transoral endoscope in Case 4. Counter traction of the exfoliating lesion by TGE facilitated the submucosal dissection by a Flex knife. D. Endoscopic view from transoral endoscope in Case 1. Light from the TGE impeded the procedure of ESD when the endoscope faces each other. The position of TGE should be changed so as not to disturb the procedure.

4.2.2 Endoscopic mucosal resection (EMR) and polypectomy

The performance of ESD by TGE alone is quite difficult because the working channel of the ultrathin endoscope is too narrow to insert the devices for ESD. However, TGE itself can be used for polypectomy and EMR by using an appropriate injection needle and snare for the ultrathin endoscope. We carried out resection of two benign polyps by TGE. One case was a hyperplastic polyp on the prepylorus, and the other was inflammatory granuloma on the gastric stoma (Fig. 4A). Both polyps showed a tendency to develop during the periodical observation by TGE. Transgastric resections were successfully conducted without conscious sedation.

4.3 Palliative therapy for gastrointestinal obstruction using TGE

One of the indications of PEG is decompression of gastrointestinal content in cases of obstruction of gastrointestinal tract. On the other hand, some cases develop gastrointestinal obstruction after PEG. TGE also facilitates the palliative therapy in such cases.

4.3.1 Transgastrostomal stenting on gastroduodenal outlet obstruction

Endoscopic deployment of stents for malignant gastroduodenal outlet obstruction has been reported as a less invasive palliative therapy compared to a surgical bypass operation (Yim et al., 2001). It is more difficult to place the stent across the postpyloric lesion compared to the esophagus, because the delivery system often forms a loop in the stomach before passing through the obstruction. When the gastrostomy site is adjacent to the obstructed lesion, a transgastric approach for stenting is easier than a transoral approach. Transgastrostomic stenting for malignant duodenal obstruction was first described in 1993 (Keymling et al., 1993).

The schematic procedure of transgastrostomal stenting is shown in Fig. 10. An ultrathin endoscope is inserted through the mature gastrocutaneous tract followed by removal of the gastrostomy tube. A guidewire is advanced through the stenosis (Fig. 10A). The endoscope is once removed from the gastrostomy keeping the position of the guidewire. A balloon catheter is inserted over the guidewire and the stenosis is dilated with the balloon catheter (Fig. 10B). The ultrathin endoscope is inserted after the removal of the balloon catheter and advanced to the upper jejunum (Fig. 10C). A guidewire is inserted deeply in the jejunum through the endoscope and the endoscope is removed again, retaining the guidewire. A stent is finally deployed over the guidewire across the obstructed lesion using a delivery device (Figs. 10D & E).

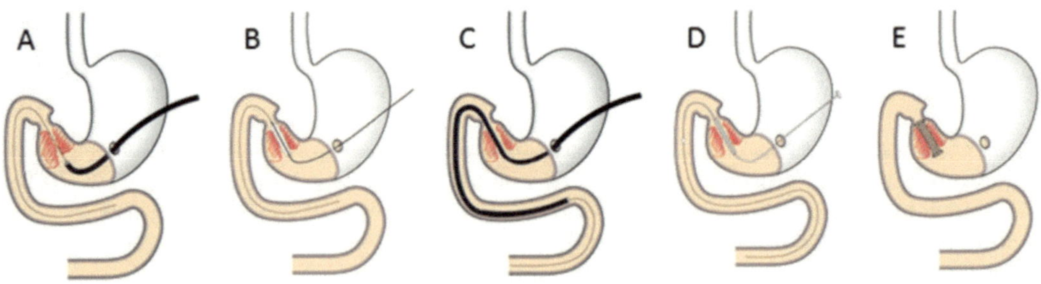

Fig. 10. Schematic procedure of the placement of an expandable metallic stent on the pyloric stenosis.

We tried this procedure for 5 patients in whom we had failed to place a stent by the transoral approach (Table 6). In 4 out of 5 patients, a non-covered expandable metallic stent was successfully deployed (Ultraflex, Boston Scientific Co., Natick, MA, USA). The one case (#5) of failure was changed to the placement of a jejunal feeding tube through the obstruction. The duodenal obstruction of this case was too severe to pass the delivery device but a 12F jejunal feeding tube was successfully inserted through the obstruction. All of the patients could successfully feed again after the procedure.

Case I.D.	1	2	3	4	5
Age/Gender	88/F	82/F	84/M	75/M	72/F
Tumors	Stomach	CBD	Stomach	CBD	Gall bladder
Obstruction	Pylorus	Duodenum	Pylorus	Duodenum	Duodenum
Operative duration (min)	20	27	15	45	
Outcome	Success	Success	Success	Success	Failure

CBD: common bile duct

Table 6. Summary of the cases with transgastrostomal stenting.

4.3.2 Placement of long intestinal decompression tube

Placement of a long intestinal decompression tube was carried out for malignant lower intestinal obstructions. A series of radiographs of the procedure in the case with ascending colon cancer is shown in Fig. 11. The procedure was the same as for the placement of a PEG-J tube as described in 4.1.1. The benefit of this procedure is that it is more comfortable for the patient, especially in the prolonged period of decompression, compared to transnasal placement.

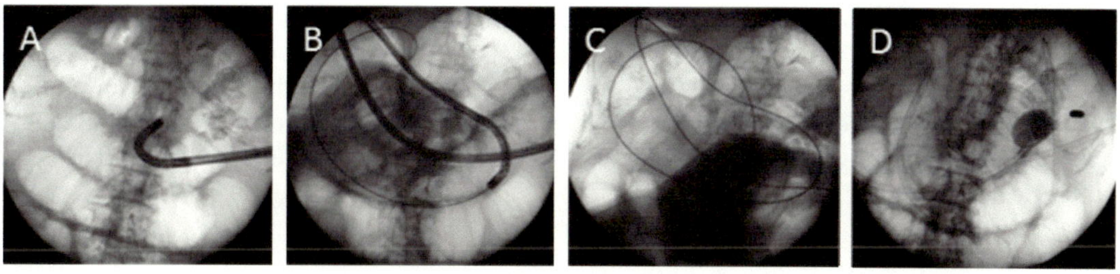

Fig. 11. Radiographs of the placement of a long intestinal decompression tube. A. An ultrathin endoscope was inserted into the stomach after removal of the gastrostomy tube. B. The endoscope was advanced to the upper jejunum. C. A guidewire was passed through the endoscope. D. A long intestinal decompression tube (CLINY Ileus Tube, Create Medic Co. Ltd., Yokohama, Japan) was placed over the guidewire.

4.4 Other usage for endoscopic treatments

We utilized TGE to treat other pathological conditions. The applications for pancreaticobiliary and esophageal diseases have been reported. Alternative possibilities for the usage of TGE are discussed in this section.

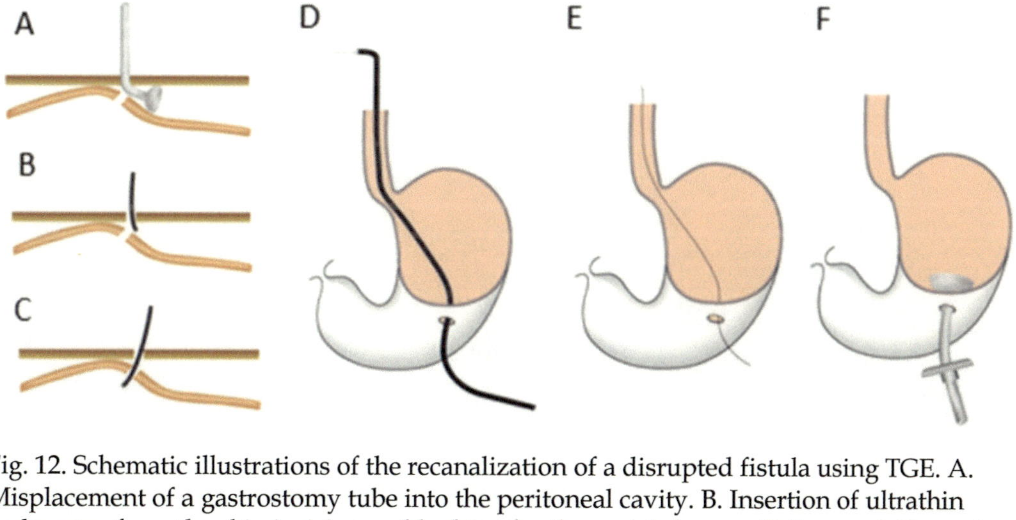

Fig. 12. Schematic illustrations of the recanalization of a disrupted fistula using TGE. A. Misplacement of a gastrostomy tube into the peritoneal cavity. B. Insertion of ultrathin endoscopy from the skin incision and looking for the gastric lumen. C. Successful insertion into the stomach. D. Passing the endoscope through the esophagus to the oral cavity. E. Insertion of a loop wire from the stoma out of mouth. F. A new gastrostomy tube is replaced by the pull-thorough technique.

4.4.1 Recovery of disrupted gastrocutaneous tract

Fistula disruption usually occurs upon early dislodgement of the gastrostomy tube or upon replacement of the tube. It might cause the serious complication of peritonitis due to leaking of gastric contents or feeding materials into the peritoneal cavity (Fang, 2007; McQuaid & Little, 1992; Romero et al., 1996). In order to place a new gastrostomy tube, a PEG procedure is often performed adjacent to the disrupted fistula (Galat et al., 1990). We employed TGE for recanalization of the disrupted fistula at the tube replacement (Nishiwaki et al., 2009 c). Schematic illustrations of the procedure are shown in Fig. 12.

We tried this technique for 5 patients with fistula disruption and in all of the patients, the disrupted fistula tract was successfully recovered. Before the introduction of this procedure, we inserted a guidewire to search for the gastric lumen from the skin incision under fluoroscopic guidance. However, in 2 out of 5 trials, we failed to reestablish a gastrocutaneous tract. The endoscopic view of TGE is helpful to locate the intragastric route from the skin incision.

4.4.2 Transgastrostomic biliary drainage

Endoscopic retrograde cholangiopancreatography from the gastrostomy have been reported (Baron & Vickers, 1998; Mori et al., 2007). Since all ultrathin endoscopes are forward-viewing, it is more difficult to insert a canula into a pancreatic or bile duct. Moreover, endoscopic treatment has limitations because of the limited availability of therapeutic devices. However, there is a benefit of direct access into the bile duct after sphincterotomy and the ability to conduct direct endoscopic observation of the bile tract (Larghi & Waxman, 2006).

We only experienced one case with transgastrostomal biliary drainage for obstructive jaundice in a patient with primary sclerosing cholangitis (Fig. 13). Placement of a transgastrostomal drain tube is more comfortable than that of a transnasal drain tube.

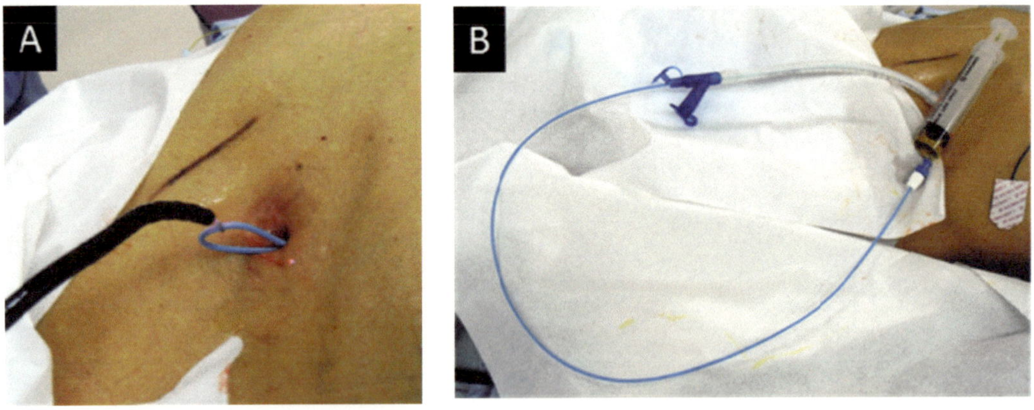

Fig. 13. Establishment of transgastrostomal biliary drainage. A. Endoscopically placed retrograde biliary drainage tube (FLEXIMA Single-Use Biliary Stent System, 6F, Boston Scientific, Maple Grove, MN, USA) was retrieved from the gastric stoma by TGE. B. The tube was passed through a 12F Jejunal Feeding Tube (Bard Access Systems, Inc., Salt Lake City, UT, USA). This procedure allowed the patient to continue to feed through the gastric decompression port of the tube.

4.4.3 Transstomal endoscopy other than gastrostomy

Transstomal endoscopy is also available via other routes than the gastrostomy tract. We experienced two cases of endoscopic placement of a jejunal extension tube through direct endoscopic jejunostomy. The first case had undergone DPEJ and showed repeated aspiration due to jejunoesophageal reflux of the feeding materials. We inserted the top of a feeding tube to 40 cm anal direction from the jejunostomy site using a transjejunostomal endoscope (Fig. 14). Another case was jejunal obstruction caused by inflammatory granuloma of the jejunostomy site (Nishiwaki et al., 2007). We could successfully place a feeding tube on the anal side of the obstruction by transjejunostomal endoscope. Although a similar procedure has previously reported under fluoroscopic guidance (Luttman et al., 2005), it might be easier to place a feeding tube using the transjejunostomal endoscope.

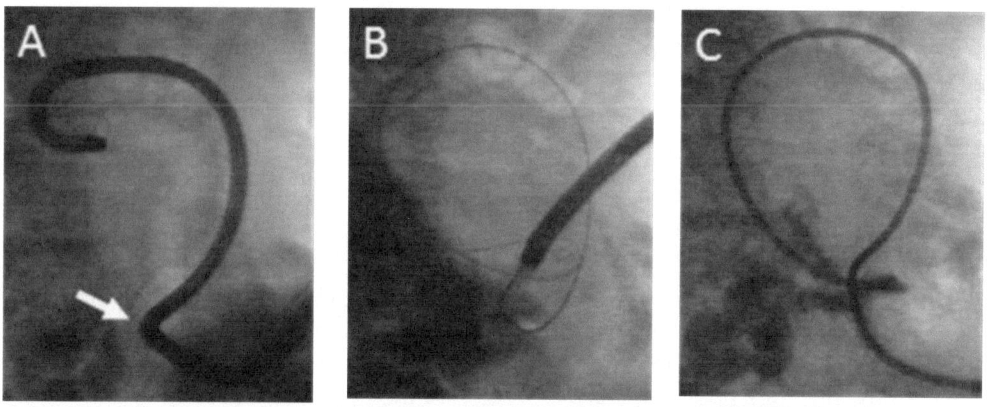

Fig. 14. Placement of an extension feeding tube through the DPEJ. A. An ultrathin endoscope was inserted through the jejunostomy site (arrow) and advanced to the anal side. B. A guidewire was placed through the endoscope. C. J-tube (Boston Scientific, Natick, MA, USA) was placed over the guidewire.

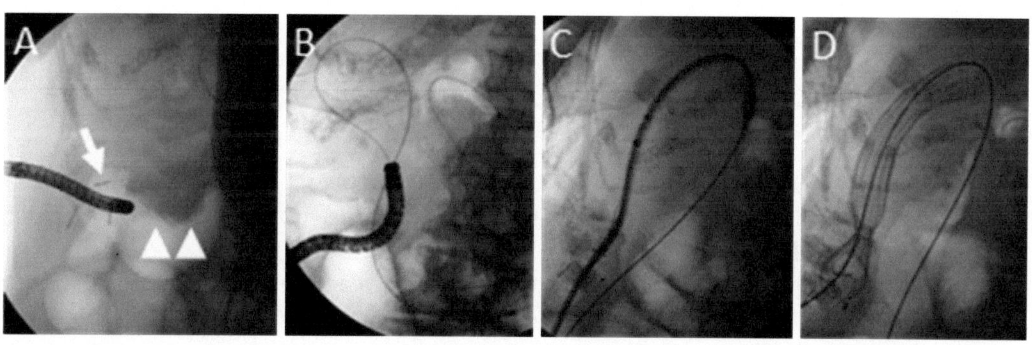

Fig. 15. Placement of an expandable metallic stent (Ultraflex, Boston Scientific, Natric MA, USA) across the obstructed ascending cancer. A. Insertion of an ultrathin endoscope through the cecostomy (arrow). Arrow heads indicate the location of the tumor. B. A guidewire was passed through the obstruction and inserted deeply along the anal side of the bowel under the guidance of fluoroscopy. C. Delivery system of the Ultraflex was

inserted through the obstruction over the guidewire. D. Ultraflex was deployed across the tumor.

We additionally experienced one case of transcecostomal endoscopy for stent placement across the ascending colon cancer (Nishiwaki et al., 2010b). The patient was too critically ill to undergo surgical treatment, and we were also unable to place a colonic stent by colonoscopy. After establishment of ultrasonography-guided percutaneous cecostomy, transcecostomal endoscopy facilitated the passing of a guidewire thorough the obstruction. The procedure of the stent deployment is shown in Fig. 15.

4.4.4 Other applications

TGE was reported to be useful for the dilatation of radiation-induced complete esophageal obstruction (Maple et al., 2006). The rendezvous technique for the dilatation of esophageal stricture was conducted by cooperative use of transoral endoscope and TGE. The use of TGE made the procedure more safe and effective.

Recent developments in super ultrathin endoscopes allow for insertion through the gastrostomy tube. The endoscope is then utilized for verification of a replaced gastrostomy tube into the stomach.

5. Conclusions

TGE offers a less invasive way to observe the upper gastrointestinal tract and allows for the detection of early stage gastrointestinal lesions. TGE also facilitates endoscopic treatments which might be more difficult by transoral endoscope. However, the narrow working channel of the ultrathin endoscope is a limitation of therapeutic TGE. Further improvements to the endoscope and applicable devices will be expected in the future.

6. Acknowledgements

We express our appreciation to Dr. Saito, Nishimino Kosei Hospital, for generous advice on these procedures. We also appreciate the members of the endoscopy unit of Nishimino Kosei Hospital (Dr. Maeda, Dr. Hayashi, Dr. Tagami, and Dr. Takada) for their assistance with the endoscopic procedures.

7. References

Adler D. G.; Gostout C. J. & Baron T. H. (2002) Percutaneous transgastric placement of jejunal feeding tubes with an ultrathin endoscope. *Gastrointest. Endosc.*, Vol.55, No.1, (Jan 2002), pp. 106-110, ISSN 0016-5107

Baron T. H. & Vickers S. M. (1998) Surgical gastrostomy placement as access for diagnostic and therapeutic ERCP. *Gastrointest. Endosc.*, Vol.48, No.6, (Dec 1998), pp. 640-641, ISSN 0016-5107

Baron T. H. (2002) Direct percutaneous endoscopic jejunostomy through a mature gastrostomy tract. *Gastrointest. Endosc.*, Vol.56, No.6, (Dec 2002), pp. 946-947, ISSN 0016-5107

Campo R.; Montserrat A. & Brullet E. (1998). Transnasal gastroscopy compared to conventional gastroscopy: a randomized study of feasibility, safety, and tolerance. *Endoscopy.* Vol.30, No.5, (Jun 1998), pp. 448-452, ISSN 0013-726X

Chaurasia O. P. & Chang K. J. (1995) A novel technique for percutaneous endoscopic gastrojejunostomy tube placement. *Gastrointest. Endosc.,* Vol.42, No.2, (Aug 1995), pp. 165-168, ISSN 0016-5107

Duckworth P. F. Jr.; Kirby D. F.; McHenry L.; DeLegge M. H. & Foxx-Orenstein A. (1994) Percutaneous endoscopic gastrojejunostomy made easy: a new over-the-wire technique. *Gastrointest. Endosc.,* Vol.40, No.3, (May-Jun 1994), pp. 350-353, ISSN 0016-5107

Dumortier J.; Ponchon T.; Scoazec J. Y.; Moulinier B.; Zarka F.; Paliard P. & Lambert R. (1999) Prospective evaluation of transnasal esophagogastroduodenoscopy: feasibility and study on performance and tolerance. *Gastrointest. Endosc.,* Vol.49, No.3, (Mar 1999), pp. 285-291, ISSN 0016-5107

Fang J. C.; Hilden K.; Holubkov R. & DiSario J. A. (2005) Transnasal endoscopy vs. fluoroscopy for the placement of nasoenteric feeding tubes in critically ill patients. *Gastrointest. Endosc.,* Vol.62, No.5, (Nov 2005), pp. 661-666, ISSN 0016-5107

Fang J. C. (2007) Minimizing endoscopic complications in enteral access. *Gastrointest. Endosc. Clin. N. Am.,* Vol.17, No.1, (Jan 2007), pp. 179-196, ISSN 1052-5157

Fujishiro M.; Yahagi N.; Nakamura M.; Kakushima N.; Kodashima S.; Ono S.; Kobayashi K.; Hashimoto T.; Yamamichi N.; Tateishi A.; Shimizu Y.; Oka M.; Ogura K.; Kawabe T.; Ichinose M. & Omata M. (2006) Successful outcomes of a novel endoscopic treatment for GI tumors: endoscopic submucosal dissection with a mixture of high-molecular-weight hyaluronic acid, glycerin, and sugar. *Gastrointest. Endosc.,* Vol.63, No.2, (Feb 2006), pp. 243-249, ISSN 0016-5107

Galat S. A.; Gerig K. D.; Porter J. A. & Slezak F. A. (1990) Management of premature removal of the percutaneous gastrostomy. *Am Surg.,* Vo.56, No.11 (Nov 1990) pp. 733-736, ISSN 0003-1348

Gauderer M. W.; Ponsky J. L. & Izant R.J. Jr. (1980) Gastrostomy without laparotomy: a percutaneous endoscopic technique. *J Pediatr Surg.,* Vol.15, No.6, (Dec 1980) pp. 872-875, ISSN 0022-3468

Gotoda T. (2006) Endoscopic resection of early gastric cancer: the Japanese perspective. *Curr Opin Gastroenterol.,* Vol.22, No.5, (Sep 2006) pp. 561-569, ISSN 0267-1379.

Itoi T.; Kawai T.; Itokawa F.; Sofuni A.; Kurihara T.; Tsuchiya T.; Ishii K.; Tsuji S.; Ikeuchi N.; Takeuchi M.; Sakai Y. & Moriyasu F. (2008) Initial experience of transnasal endoscopic biliary drainage without conscious sedation for the treatment of acute cholangitis (with video). *Gastrointest. Endosc.,* Vol.67, No.2, (Feb 2008), pp. 328-332, ISSN 0016-5107

Keymling M.; Wagner H. J.; Vakil N. & Knyrim K. (1993) Relief of malignant duodenal obstruction by percutaneous insertion of a metal stent. *Gastrointest. Endosc.,* Vol.39, No.3, (May-Jun 1993), pp. 439-441, ISSN 0016-5107

Kobayashi T.; Gotohda T.; Tamakawa K.; Ueda H. & Kakizoe T. (2004) Magnetic anchor for more effective endoscopic mucosal resection. *Jpn J Clin Oncol.,* Vol.34, No.3, (Mar 2004) pp. 118-123, ISSN 0368-2811

Kondo H.; Gotoda T.; Ono H.; Oda I.; Kozu T.; Fujishiro M.; Saito D. & Yoshida S. (2004) Percutaneous traction-assisted EMR by using an insulation-tipped electrosurgical knife for early stage gastric cancer. *Gastrointest. Endosc.*, Vol.59, No.2, (Feb 2004), pp. 284-288, ISSN 0016-5107

Larghi A. & Waxman I. (2006) Endoscopic direct cholangioscopy by using an ultra-slim upper endoscope: a feasibility study. *Gastrointest. Endosc.*, Vol.63, No.6, (May 2006), pp. 853-857, ISSN 0016-5107

Leichus L.; Patel R. & Johlin F. (1997) Percutaneous endoscopic gastrostomy/jejunostomy (PEG/PEJ) tube placement: a novel approach. *Gastrointest. Endosc.*, Vol.45, No.1, (Jan 1997), pp. 79-81, ISSN 0016-5107

Luttmann A.; Deppe H,; Wejda B. U.; Huchzermeyer H. & Dormann A. J. (2005) Placement of a jejunal enteral tube through a percutaneous endoscopic jejunostomy to prevent recurrent aspiration during intestinal feeding. *Gastrointest. Endosc.*, Vol.61, No.3, (Mar 2005), pp. 492-493, ISSN 0016-5107

Maple J. T.; Petersen B. T.; Baron T. H.; Kasperbauer J. L.; Wong Kee Song L. M. & Larson M. V. (2006) Endoscopic management of radiation-induced complete upper esophageal obstruction with an antegrade-retrograde rendezvous technique. *Gastrointest. Endosc.*, Vol.64, No5, (Nov 2006), pp. 822-828, ISSN 0016-5107

McQuaid K. R. & Little T. E. (1992) Two fatal complications related to gastrostomy "button" placement. *Gastrointest. Endosc.*, Vol.38, No.5, (Sep-Oct 1992), pp. 601-603, ISSN 0016-5107

Mori A.; Ohashi N.; Maruyama T.; Tatebe H.; Sakai K.; Inoue H.; Takegoshi S. & Okuno M. (2007) Endoscopic retrograde cholangiopancreatography through a gastric stoma using an ultrathin endoscope: a novel approach. *Endoscopy* Vol.39, Suppl.1, (Feb 2007), E. 323, ISSN 0013-726X

Mori A.; Ohashi N.; Maruyama T.; Tatebe H.; Sakai K.; Shibuya T.; Inoue H.; Takegoshi S. & Okuno M. (2008) Transnasal endoscopic retrograde cholangiopancreatography using an ultrathin endoscope: a prospective comparison with a routine oral procedure. *World J Gastroenterol.*, Vol.14, No.10, (Mar 2008), pp. 1514-1520, ISSN 1007-9327

Nishiwaki S.; Araki H.; Goto N.; Niwa Y.; Kubota M.; Iwashita M.; Onogi N.; Hatakeyama H.; Hayashi T.; Maeda T. & Saitoh K. (2006) Clinical analysis of gastroesophageal reflux after PEG. *Gastrointest. Endosc.*, Vol.64, No.6, (Dec 2006), pp. 890-896, ISSN 0016-5107

Nishiwaki S.; Shirakami Y.; Hayashi T. & Saitoh K. (2007) Jejunal inflammatory granuloma: a complication of direct percutaneous endoscopic jejunostomy. *Endoscopy* Vol.39, Suppl.1, (Feb 2007), E. 116, ISSN 0013-726X

Nishiwaki S.; Araki H.; Shirakami Y.; Niwa Y.; Iwashita M.; Hatakeyama H. & Saitoh K. (2009a) Transgastrostomic endoscopy-assisted endoscopic submucosal dissection. *Endoscopy* Vol.41, Suppl.2, (Feb 2009), E. 13, ISSN 0013-726X

Nishiwaki S.; Araki H.; Shirakami Y.; Kawaguchi J.; Asano T.; Iwashita M.; Tagami A.; Hatakeyama H.; Hayashi T.; Maeda T.; Naganawa S. & Saitoh K. (2009b) Direct percutaneous endoscopic jejunostomy using a transgastrostomic endoscope in patients with previous endoscopic gastrostomy. *Endoscopy* Vol.41, Suppl.2, (Mar 2009), E. 36-37, ISSN 0013-726X

Nishiwaki S.; Araki H.; Takada J.; Watanabe N.; Asano T.; Iwashita M.; Tagami A.; Hatakeyama H.; Hayashi T.; Maeda T. & Saitoh K. (2009c) Usefulness of an ultrathin endoscope in recanalization of a disrupted fistulous tract following percutaneous endoscopic gastrostomy or jejunostomy. *Endoscopy* Vol.41, Suppl.2, (Oct 2009), E. 273-274, ISSN 0013-726X

Nishiwaki S.; Hatakeyama H.; Takada J.; Watanabe N.; Iwashiwa M.; Araki H. & Saito K. (2010a) Transcecostomal colonic stent placement after US-guided percutaneous cecostomy. *Gastrointest. Endosc.*, Vol.71, No.6, (May 2010), pp. 1097-1099, ISSN 0016-5107

Nishiwaki S.; Araki H.; Takada J.; Watanabe N.; Asano T.; Iwashita M.; Tagami A.; Hatakeyama H.; Hayashi T.; Maeda T. & Saito K. (2010b) Clinical investigation of upper gastrointestinal hemorrhage after percutaneous endoscopic gastrostomy. *Dig Endosc.*, Vol.22, No.3, (Jul 2010), pp. 180-185, ISSN 0915-5635

Ono H.; Kondo H.; Gotoda T.; Shirao K.; Yamaguchi H.; Saito D.; Hosokawa K.; Shimoda T. & Yoshida S. (2001) Endoscopic mucosal resection for treatment of early gastric cancer. *Gut,* Vol.48, No.2, (Feb 2001), pp. 225-229, ISSN 0017-5749

Ponsky J. L. & Gauderer M. W. (1981) Percutaneous endoscopic gastrostomy: a nonoperative technique for feeding gastrostomy. *Gastrointest. Endosc.*, Vol.27, No.1, (Feb 1981), pp. 9-11, ISSN 0016-5107

Ponsky J. L. & Aszodi A. (1984) Percutaneous endoscopic jejunostomy. *Am J Gastroenterol.*, Vol.79, No.2, (Feb 1984), pp.113-116, ISSN 0002-9270

Rogers B. H.; Kaminski M. V. Jr & All J. (1989) Stabilizing sutures for percutaneous endoscopic gastrostomy. *Gastrointest. Endosc.*, Vol.35, No.3, (May-Jun 1989), pp. 241-243, ISSN 0016-5107

Romero R.; Martinez F. L, Robinson S. Y.; Sullivan K. M. & Hart M. H. (1996) Complicated PEG-to-skin level gastrostomy conversions: analysis of risk factors for tract disruption. *Gastrointest. Endosc.* Vol.44, No.3, (Sep 1996), pp. 230-234, ISSN 0016-5107

Sato R.; Watari J.; Tanabe H.; Fujiya M.; Ueno N.; Konno Y.; Ishikawa C.; Ito T.; Moriichi K.; Okamoto K.; Maemoto A.; Chisaka K.; Kitano Y.; Matsumoto K.; Ashida T.; Kono T. & Kohgo Y. (2008) Transnasal ultrathin endoscopy for placement of a long intestinal tube in patients with intestinal obstruction. *Gastrointest. Endosc.*, Vol.67, No.6, (May 2008), pp. 953-957, ISSN 0016-5107

Shaker R. (1994). Unsedated trans-nasal pharyngoesophagogastroduodenoscopy (T-EGD): technique. *Gastrointest. Endosc.*, Vol.40, No.3, (May-Jun 1994), pp. 346-348, ISSN 0016-5107

Shike M.; Schroy P.; Ritchie M. A., Lightdale C. J. & Morse R. (1987) Percutaneous endoscopic jejunostomy in cancer patients with previous gastric resection. *Gastrointest. Endosc.*, Vol.33, No.5, (Oct 1987), pp. 372-374, ISSN 0016-5107

Shike M.; Wallach C.; Likier H. Direct percutaneous endoscopic jejunostomies. *Gastrointest. Endosc.*, Vol.37, No.1, (Jan-Feb 1991), pp. 62-65, ISSN 0016-5107

Shike M.; Latkany L. Direct percutaneous endoscopic jejunostomy. (1998) *Gastrointest. Endosc Clin N Am.*, Vol.8, No.3, (July 1998), pp. 569-580, ISSN 1052-5157

Vitale M. A.; Villotti G.; D'Alba L.; De Cesare M. A.; Frontespezi S. & Iacopini G. (2005) Unsedated transnasal percutaneous endoscopic gastrostomy placement in selected patients. *Endoscopy*, Vol.37, No.1, (Jan 2005), pp. 48-51, ISSN 0013-726X

Yim H. B.; Jacobson B. C.; Saltzman J. R.; Johannes R. S.; Bounds B. C.; Lee J. H.; Shields S. J.; Ruymann F. W.; Van Dam J. & Carr-Locke D. L. (2001) Clinical outcome of the use of enteral stents for palliation of patients with malignant upper GI obstruction. *Gastrointest. Endosc.*, Vol.53, No.3, (Mar 2001), pp. 329-332, ISSN 0016-5107

11

Therapeutic Uses of Spiral Enteroscopy

Marco Balzarini, Marco Orsello and Mario Del Piano
SCDO di Gastroenterologia, Azienda Ospedaliero,
Universitaria Maggiore della Carità, Novara
Italy

1. Introduction

Not long ago, the small intestine was an unexplored frontier in gastrointestinal endoscopy. New developments in enteroscopes have opened up this region of the gastro-intestinal tract but it remains a difficult organ to access. Until recently, it was not possible to access most of the small bowel using endoscopic techniques without concomitant surgery.

Capsule endoscopy and balloon-assisted enteroscopy thus represent decisive breakthroughs in this field. Small bowel enteroscopy was considered a technically challenging procedure often requiring much time. In the past diagnostic and therapeutic options for small bowel conditions have traditionally been limited and frustrating for endoscopists.

With the development of balloon-assisted enteroscopy and most recently, spiral enteroscopy, endoscopic diagnosis and treatment of the entire small intestine are now feasible without operative intervention.

As indications expand and caseloads grow, it is important for gastroenterologists to know how these procedures are done and to be familiar with their potential complications.

2. Indication for deep enteroscopy

The indications for enteroscopy of the small intestine are rising so small bowel endoscopy is enjoying a significant renaissance.

Deep enteroscopy offers the potential advantages of biopsy, treatment of bleeding lesions, and other therapeutic maneuvers including stricture dilation, and stent placement.

Lesions located within the proximal two thirds of the small bowel transit time on capsule endoscopy are thought to be amenable to deep enteroscopy performed via the anterograde approach. Table 1 summarizes reported indications, relating to spiral enteroscopy [1 2 3 4 5 6 7].

The majority of the outcomes literature on deep enteroscopy pertains to double ballon enteroscopy (DBE), because publications on single ballon enteroscopy and spiral enteroscopy remain limited. A summary of the published DBE literature has demonstrated similar diagnostic yields to capsule endoscopy. In a summary of 16 published studies to date, the overall mean diagnostic yield was 67% with a treatment success rate of 64%.[8]. Double balloon enteroscopy has been reported to be diagnostic in a small percentage of patients with normal capsule examinations, particularly in the situation of ongoing acute obscure hemorrhage[9]

- Abnormal capsule endoscopy
- Abnormal radiologic imaging
- Anastamotic stricture
- Celiac disease
- Chronic abdominal pain
- Chronic diarrhea
- Fistula plug placement for enterocutaneous fistula
- Push enteroscopy (PE)
- Hepatojejunostomy stricture
- History of intestinal polyps (familial adenomatous polyposis, Gardner's syndrome)
- Iron deficiency anemia
- Obscure-occult gastrointestinal bleeding
- Obscure-overt gastrointestinal bleeding
- Small bowel fistula
- Small bowel obstruction
- Suspected small bowel Crohn's disease
- Therapeutic ERCP after Roux-en-Y gastric bypass

Table 1. Indication for spiral enteroscopy

Approximately 5% of patients presenting with acute or chronic gastrointestinal (GI) hemorrhage will have a responsible source located in the small intestine[10]. For patients residing in the United States or Europe, lesions most responsible for small bowel hemorrhage include arteriovenous malformations in 30%–40%[11], ulcerations, other vascular disorders including Dieulafoy lesions, and small bowel neoplasms in 1%–3% of patients.[12]. Small bowel follow-through radiographs have demonstrated a low yield (3%–20%) for pathologic findings in patients with obscure bleeding, and the findings are dependent upon the skill and time allotted by the radiologist for fluoroscopy[13].
Other indications for deep enteroscopy other gastrointestinal hemmorhage are similar to capsule endoscopy and include evaluation of patients with polyposis syndromes, refractory celiac sprue, and other ulcerative small bowel disorders. Similar to capsule endoscopy, the yield of DBE in patients with chronic abdominal pain is very low

3. Evolution of enteroscopy

Intraoperative enteroscopy was initially performed in the 1950s with a rigid sigmoidoscope passed through an operative laparotomy. By the 1970s fiberoptic endoscopes were used for intraoperative enteroscopy .[14] Intraoperative enteroscopy has a high diagnostic yield but has largely been replaced because of its high complication rate, need for a surgeon as well as an endoscopist, and postprocedural hospital stay.
Sonde enteroscopy was introduced in 1986 as an alternative to intraoperative enteroscopy, but it was eventually abandoned because it was labor intensive for the endoscopist and uncomfortable for the patient.

Push enteroscopy was the most widely used endoscopic procedure, but only about 60 to 120 cm of small bowel can be visualized [15]. Further advancement is generally limited by intragastric or small-bowel looping. Advanced skill or training is not typically required to perform this procedure. The procedure is performed under conscious sedation and takes between 15 and 45 minutes. The overall complication rate from PE is approximately 1%[16]. Care must be taken to avoid trauma to the thin-walled duodenum and jejunum during advancement of the relatively stiff enteroscope.
Device-assisted enteroscopy techniques, including double balloon endoscopy (DBE), single-balloonenteroscopy (SBE), and spiral enteroscopy (SE), have both diagnostic and therapeutic capabilities. Double-balloon enteroscopy (DBE) emerged as an option for small bowel imaging in the United States in 2004; single-balloon enteroscopy (SBE) and spiral enteroscopy were introduced into the US market in 2007

4. Device assisted enteroscopy

Device-assisted enteroscopy is the modality of choice for evaluating disorders of the mid-gut whenever tissue acquisition or therapeutic intent is cogent. This new term, *mid-gut,* refers to the small bowel between the ampulla and the ileocecal valve.[17].
Although capsule endoscopy can visualize the entire small intestine, a main disadvantage is the inability to obtain biopsy specimens, navigate altered anatomy, or perform therapeutic maneuvers via this procedure.

4.1 Ballon assisted enteroscopy

New techniques such as DBE and SBE use techniques designed to pleat the small bowel on the endoscope and overtube. They work on the principle of push-pull advancement through the small bowel by alternately inflating and deflating the balloons on the overtube and the enteroscope (in DBE) [18]

4.1.1 Double ballon enteroscopy

The concept of DBE was introduced in 1997[19] and was subsequently introduced into the United States in 2004 (Fujinon Inc, Saitama, Japan). The development of DBE was based on the concept that "stretching" of the small intestinal wall prevents further endoscopic advancement, and that the usage of a balloon would grip the intestinal wall and prevent subsequent loop formation[20].
The diagnostic enteroscope (EN450P5) has a 200-cm working length, an endoscope diameter of 8.5 mm, and an accessory channel of 2.2 mm. The therapeutic enteroscope (EN450T5) has a diameter of 9.4 mm and an accessory channel of 2.8 mm.

4.1.2 Single ballon enteroscopy

The SBE system (Olympus Corporation, Tokyo, Japan) was developed in 2006 and introduced subsequently into the commercial market in 2007.[21]
The rationale behind development of the SBE system was to reduce the learning curve for balloon-assisted enteroscopy, avoid the difficulty of attaching the enteroscope balloon to the distal tip of the scope encountered in DBE, and eliminate the requirement of inflating and deflating 2 balloons in multiple steps with the current DBE insertion technique.

4.2 Spiral enteroscopy

In addition to balloon assisted enteroscopy using double or single balloons, the novel technique of spiral enteroscopy (SE) has recently been reported.

This technique uses a flexible over-tube threaded with a pliable plastic spiral to grip the small bowel (Figure 1)

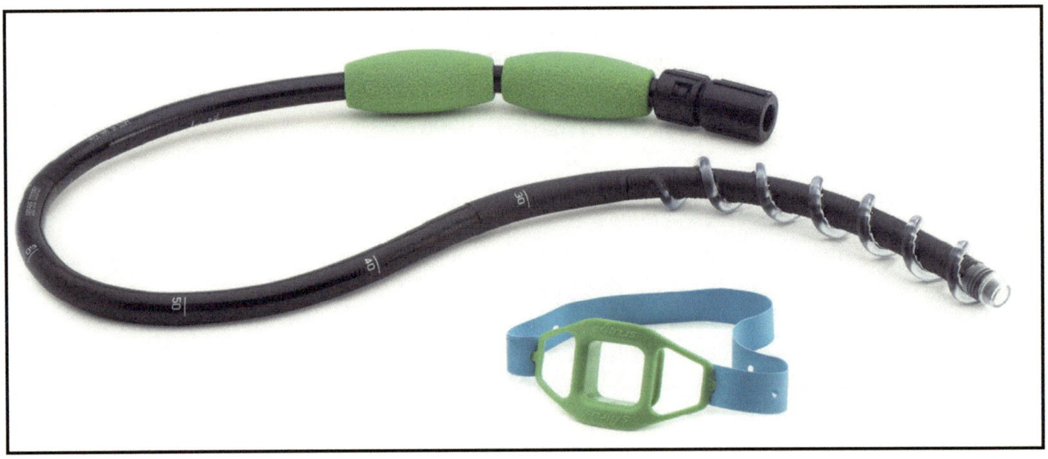

Fig. 1. Spiral overtube

Although the earlier prototypes were placed over a pediatric colonoscope, the newer devices are used with enteroscopes.

Rotational torque applied by the operator is converted into plication of the small bowel over the over-tube as the enteroscope advances.

Anterograde enteroscopic introduction with the spirus overtube helps to advance compatible enteroscopes beyond to Ligament of Treitz, the fixed portion of small bowel within the abdominal cavity. Rotation of the overtube beyond the Ligament of Treitz, allows a spiral to pleat the segment of the small bowel where disease is most commonly found (Figure 2).

The first case utilizing rotate to advance was performed in 2006 by Drs. Akerman and Cantero[22].

Spiral enteroscopy can also be performed in post-gastric surgery patients, and can be used in Roux-en-Y patients requiring endoscopic retrograde cholangiopancreatography.

The Endo-Ease Discovery SB system is an overtube with an outer spiral, which was cleared for enteroscopy by the FDA in 2008. The device is 118 cm long with a hollow spiral 5.5 mm high and 22 cm long with a locking device on the proximal end. The Discovery SB has an outer diameter of 16 mm and an internal diameter of 9.8 mm. The tube lightly connects to the existing enteroscopes by a "gentle lock" and rotates independently from the enteroscope. The lock can be disengaged and reengaged, allowing the option of advancing the enteroscope through the overtube when unlocked or performing spiral enteroscopy with the spiral overtube when locked.

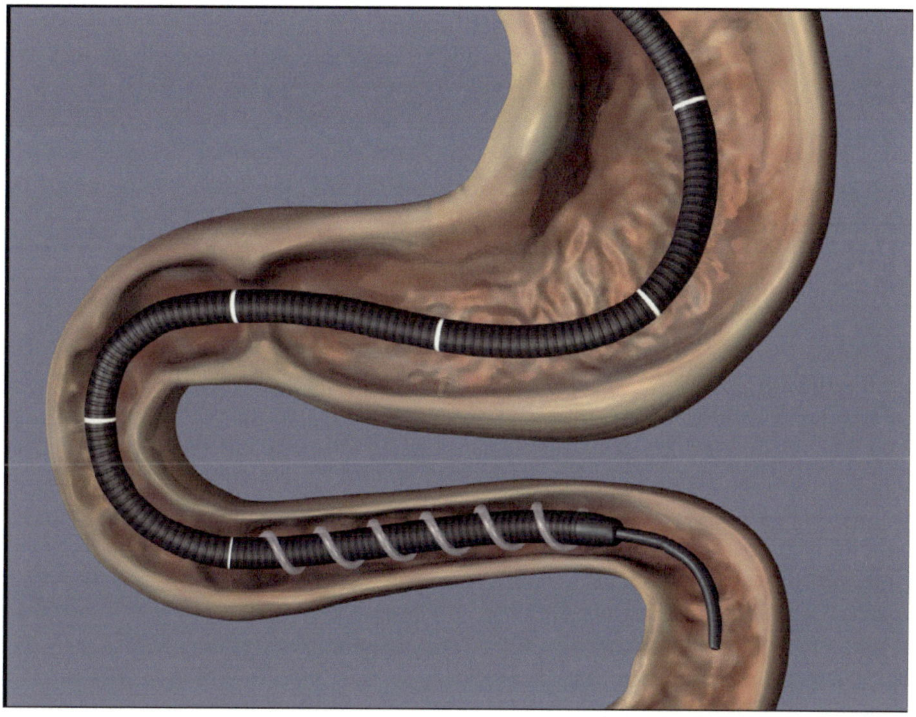

Fig. 2. Concept of "rotate to advance."

The Spirus overtube can be paired with existing enteroscopes measuring up to 9.4 mm . The product is a single use device sterilized.

An in vitro porcine model was created to demonstrate spiral advancement and pleating tecniques.

Spiral enteroscopy is possible also with retrograde approach. For this use exists a dedicated spiral tip overtube (Vista overtube, tube length 100 cm, tube outer diameter 1.85 cm, outer diameter includes spirals 3.33 cm). This overtube can be preloaded onto pediatric colonoscope or enteroscope. Initaial experience with this device are reported.[23]

While all three of these methods allow intubation of the deep small bowel, these techniques provide unique challenges involving patient sedation. Preliminary reports detailing the use of spiral enteroscopy have used anesthesiologist-guided monitored anesthesia care exclusively for sedation.[24] When standard sedation is used, spiral enteroscopy is technically feasible, clinically useful, and safe. Deep small bowel enteroscopy using the spiral overtube can be successfully and safely accomplished with gastroenterologist- guided, nurse-administered standard sedation also in a patient population with multiple comorbidities and a high prevalence of diagnostic findings requiring endoscopic therapy.

Although some of them only published in abstract form, some studies have compared SE with DBE and shown that SE required significantly shorter time than DBE to insert to similar depths[25] [26]. Initial studies of deep enteroscopy focused on presenting narrative experiences with the individual techniques. Comparative trials have been conducted to compare the utility of these various techniques in terms of their diagnostic yield, deep of maximal insertion allowed, efficacy, and complications[27]

In one prospective study on 35 patients DBE showed a clinically higher diagnostic yield than spiral enteroscopy but there was non difference in investigation performance, as assessed by time o insertion, duration of enteroscopy and amount of sedoanalgesia required.[28]

Khashab et al.[29] reported the first study comparing SE and SBE. Although SE yielded greater depth of maximal insertion than SBE, both techniques had similar diagnostic yields and procedure times. In addition, both techniques were safe and were particularly useful in evaluation and treatment of patients with obscure gasto-intestinal bleeding.

As seen above, the strengths of SE are rapid advancement in the small bowel and better control of the endoscope, which makes it easy to conduct endoscopic interventions.

4.2.1 Complications

Serious complications of deep small bowel enteroscopy occur infrequently. In published series, severe complications occur in deep small bowel enteroscopy in 0.3 to 4% of cases.

There are 2950 patients who have undergone spiral enteroscopy from August 2006 until May 2009. Cases have been performed in North America and Europe. Severe complications were defined as pancreatitis, nontransient intussusception, bleeding requiring transfusion or admission to the hospital, cardio-pulmonary arrest during a procedure and perforation. There were no reported complications of esophageal or gastric perforations, severe bleeding requiring transfusion, or cardio-pulmonary arrest during or resulting from the spiral enteroscopy procedures. There were 9 reported severe complications (0.3%) and no deaths reported as a result of the procedure. There were eight small bowel perforations (0.27%), all were recognized immediately. Four small bowel perforations occurred in the jejunum. Three duodenal perforations occurred while pushing to advance the scope through the duodenum. Two of four jejunal perforations occurred during therapeutic interventions. One perforation occurred in a Roux en Y patient. None of the perforations appeared to occur during rotation of the overtube to pleat the small bowel. Five perforations occurred when the experience of the physician was less than 10 cases.

Perforations may be minimized by advancing the enteroscope only when the lumen is clearly visualized and maintaining the scope tip 25-30 cm from the end of the Discovery SB overtube.

Also in a typical US patient population with multiple comorbidities and high prevalence of pathologic finding spiral enteroscopy is a technically feasible and safe way to perform diagnostic and therapeutic deep small bowel enteroscopy and in conclusion Spiral enteroscopy is a safe procedure with a low rate serious complications.

4.2.2 Procedure

Spiral enteroscopy applies the mechanical advantage of a screw to convert rotational force into linear force and pleat the small bowel on the enteroscope.

The patients is placed in the left lateral decubitus position for the procedure and received monitored anesthesia with propofol/midazolam hydrochloride/fentanyl or general anesthesia, according to the anesthesiologist's preference. Before performing the procedure, a proprietary lubricant is applied thoroughly to the overtube channel and than the DSB device is placed over the enteroscope. The distal end of the DSB is positioned 25 cm from the tip of the enteroscope and locked into place with the DSB proximal collar. When locked tightly onto the coupler at the proximal end of the overtube at the 140 cm mark, the scope is inserted into the esophagus. All subsequent movements of the scope must be done with gentle rotation of the overtube except when the overtube coupler has been unlocked. Engagement of the spiral in the duodenum may be difficult and it requires backing up of the scope and the overtube.

To rotate the tube, the hands are placed on the 2 soft handles located just below the lock. A special curved mouthpiece with a bigger aperture to accommodate the DSB and the enteroscope is used. Once past the ligament of Treitz the mobile small bowel can be plated on the overtube using spiral technique (Figure 3).

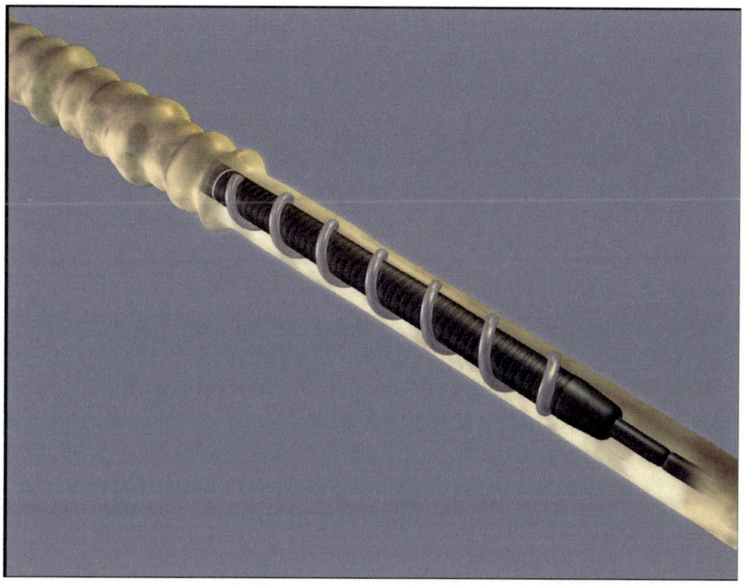

Fig. 3. Rotation pleats the small bowel.

Two operators are required, one for spiralling and a second for steering and insufflation to maximize insertion. Minimal insufflation is used. Spiral advancement is continued as long as the overtube rotates easily and the small bowel continues to be pleated onto the overtube. When advancement slow or rotations become difficult the overtube may be straightened and pulled back to remove loops. This achives a stray scope that is optimal for spiral advancement. When working optimally the spiral advancement has a rapid one to one advancement whith a minimal slippage of the overtube.

Fluoroscopic guidance can be helpful but not necessary to assist in advancing through the small bowel.

The overtube let maneuver the enteroscope if needed while it remains in place indeed the endoscope can be withdrawn completely from the overtube and reinserted without loss of position.

Withdrawal of the overtube and endoscope is accomplished by counter clockwise rotation of the overtube. The counter clockwise rotation unpleats the small bowel from the overtube By rotation of the DSB, advancement can be continued until the pleating of small bowel with rotation is no longer effective. The enteroscope is then unlocked from the DSB and pushed through the overtube for added depth of small bowel intubation. The DSB is then gradually withdrawn by anticlockwise rotation of the DSB, and the small-bowel mucosa examined.

Small-bowel pleating is accomplished without apparent twisting of the small bowel because the mesentery attachment to the small bowel resists the rotation of the small bowel.
In a setting when prompt endoscope extubation may have become necessary, rapid anticlockwise rotation would have achieved rapid withdrawal of the DSB.
The DSB has many features that make it a safe and easy device to use.
The shaft is uniformly more flexible at the distal end and transitions gradually to a less flexible proximal end, resulting in optimal integration of torque transmission and flexibility.
The locking device on the DSB allows spiral enteroscopy and standard push enteroscopy techniques to be used in conjunction to advance the enteroscope through the small bowel.
During withdrawal of the enteroscope, the DSB is rotated anticlockwise, which results in the pleated small bowel gradually coming off the device, allowing for controlled, careful examination of the small-bowel mucosa.
Spiral enteroscopy also has potential advantages over DBE and SBE, including speed of advancement through the small bowel, excellent controlled withdrawal especially useful for therapeutic maneuvers, and ability to completely withdraw the enteroscope and maintain position in the small bowel.
SE allows similar insertion depths to be reached as with DBE but the positioning with SE for collecting samples and for therapy is more stable than with DBE.
When using retrograde approach the endoscope is introduced in the usual fashion through the anus and advanced to where the colon lumen straightened out, usually in the descending or transverse colon. The overtube is disengaged and advanced over the endoscope using clockwise rotation; thus, the colonoscope served as a "guidewire" for the overtube. Since this maneuver usually resulted in simultaneous advancement of the tip of the colonoscope, it is important to always maintain good visibility of the lumen. When visualization of the lumen is not possible, overtube insertion is stopped, and water irrigation is performed to expose the lumen. Insufflation is kept to a minimum, and carbon dioxide can be used. If this failed, the scope can be gently pulled back while holding the overtube, and rarely spinning the overtube counter-clockwise, until the lumen is seen. The tip of the endoscope is usually advanced to the transverse colon or distal ascending colon in this fashion, where maximal overtube insertion usually occurred. The cecum is reached by disengaging the overtube and, while holding the handle at the anus, pushing the endoscope through the overtube. Once the ileum is intubated, the endoscope is exclusively advanced by pushing.
Table 2 shows a list of reported diagnostic/therapeutic interventions with spiral enteroscopy.
In particular management of patients with small-bowel obstruction distal to the third part of the duodenum can be challenging. These patients are often poor surgical candidates, and placement of a self-expanding metal stent can be technically demanding. Deploying a stent distal to an endoscope is technically challenging, requiring a stable position to effectively traverse the stricture and deploy a self-expanding metal stent. The configuration of the spirals of the overtube is such that the bowel is held in a very secure position, providing stability at the distal tip, which greatly assists self-expanding metal stent placement and other interventions[30]. The accessory channel of commercially available enteroscopes is not large enough to admit an enteral stent. This problem is overcome by using the DSB overtube as a vehicle for deploying SEMS and conceivably other therapies. However, this is a relatively new technique, and, as such, larger numbers of cases and further experience are required to determine whether there are any significant side effects.

- Biliary:
  - Balloon sphincteroplasty and sludge extraction
  - Cannulation/sphincterotomy
  - Pancreatic stent placement
  - Stent removal with stricture dilation
  - Stone extraction and biliary stent placement

- Lumenal:
  - Argon plasma coagulation
  - Biopsy
  - Bipolar cauterization
  - Enteral stent placement (for malignant obstruction)
  - Fistula plug placement
  - Foreign body retrieval (percutaneous endoscopic gastrostomy tube bumper)
  - India ink tattoo
  - Polypectomy

Table 2. Diagnostic/therapeutic interventions with spiral enteroscopy

4.2.3 Spiral enteroscopy in surgically altered gastrointestinal anatomy

Surgically altered gastrointestinal anatomy presents considerable impediments for accessing the pancreaticobiliary tree. Endoscopic methods for accessing the biliary and pancreatic ducts in patients with surgically altered anatomy can be difficult and patients with surgically altered upper gastro-intestestinal tract anatomy pose a challenge to endoscopic biliary interventions.

Endoscopic treatments are preferable because they are less invasive than either transhepatic or surgical options.

Performance of ERCP's in cases of Roux-en-Y anastamosis has presented particular challenges with success rates at reaching the biliary and pancreatic orifices using standard endoscopic techniques up to a maximum of 50%. One of the most common causes of difficulty is the inability of the endoscope to reach the papilla of Vater or the bilio-enteric anastomosis, due to the length of the passage or the angle of the anastomosis.

Cholelithiasis occurs in up to 38% of gastric bypass patients within 6 months of surgery. Cholecystectomy is not routinely performed in asymptomatic individuals with gallstones, leaving choledocolithiasis as a potential complication following gastric bypass.

Because of the length of the Roux limb and the acute angle of the jejunal-jejunal anastomis, ERCP is especially challenging and may not be feasible with standard equipment.

Wire guided passage of a duodenoscope has a demonstrated cannulation success rate of only 67%. Invasive techniques such as percutaneous gastrostomy tube placement and transhepatic access may carry additional risk and comorbidity.

Recently, balloon enteroscopy (BE) techniques such as double-balloon enteroscopy (DBE) or single-balloon enteroscopy (SBE) have made it easier to perform ERCP in these patients[31]

Although data on the use of SE are limited, the usefulness of SE for ERCP in patients with surgically altered anatomy is expected to be equal to or more than that of balloon enteroscopy.

Although only published in abstract form, some studies on SE-assisted ERCP have been reported.

Chandrasekharaet al.[32] reported a series of 5 patients undergoing ERCP with SE. Three patients had Roux-en-Y gastric bypass and 2 were status post-pancreaticoduodenectomy. All procedures were performed using the Olympus SIF-Q 180 enteroscope and DSB, and the success rate was 80%.

Shah[33] reported a series of 13 patients undergoing SE-assisted ERCP. Post-surgical anatomy included Roux-en-Y gastric bypass (n = 6), liver transplant (n = 6), and hepaticojejunostomy post liver resection (n = 1). Access to the papilla or anastomosis was achieved in 11/13 patients (85%) and ERCP was successfully performed in 9/13 (62%). Complications were seen in 2 patients, including mild pancreatitis and self-limiting hypopharyngeal trauma.

Sanjay et al.[34] reported that SE-assisted ERCP was performed in 3 patients including 2 patients for whom DBE-assisted ERCP had failed once. Successful selective cannulation and therapeutic intervention were achieved in all 3 cases. Mean total procedure time was 117 min.

In conclusion Spiral enteroscopy ERCP is a new technique that is a highly effective platform for reaching the pancreaticobiliary orifice in Roux-en-Y patients. Spiral enteroscopy ERCP also provides excellent stability for high success rates for completion of ERCP's.

Spirus enteroscopy reaches the biliary-enteric anastomosis or papilla in most patients with altered surgical anatomy and is associated with technical success in the majority of patients in whom access to the afferent limb is achieved. Modification of enteroscope-length ERCP accessories may improve success.

5. Clinical case

Our patient is a 26 yrs old woman, with Peutz-Jeghers syndrome and history of multiple abdominal surgeries: ileal resection for occlusion and for polyps removal in distal ileum.

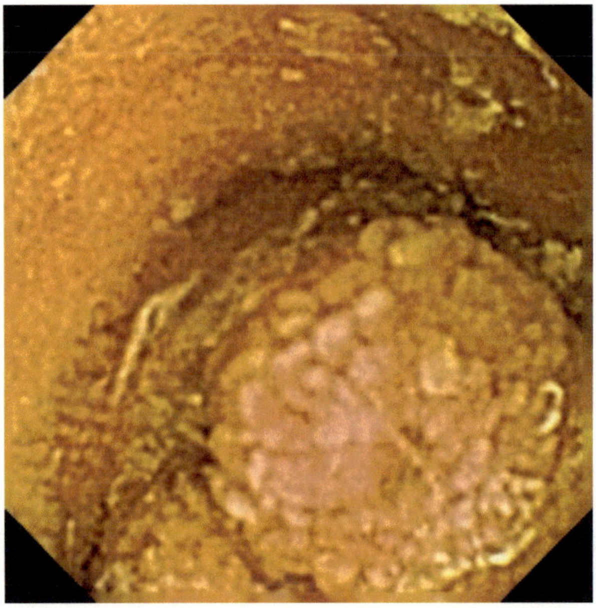

Fig. 4. Jejunal polyp at videocapsule endoscopy

In May 2010 she was submitted on video capsule (that revealed many penducolated and sessile polyps in the distal jejunum and not in the ileum, Figure 4) and enteroscopy with single balloon (retrograde and anterograde approach) with the detection of large polyps in II-III part of duodenum (not seen by video capsule) and small polyps in distal jejunum.
In July 2010 we performed spiral enteroscopy in general anesthesia in surgical room with surgeon in stand-by for the high risk of complication. More than 15 polipectomies were done (figure 5).

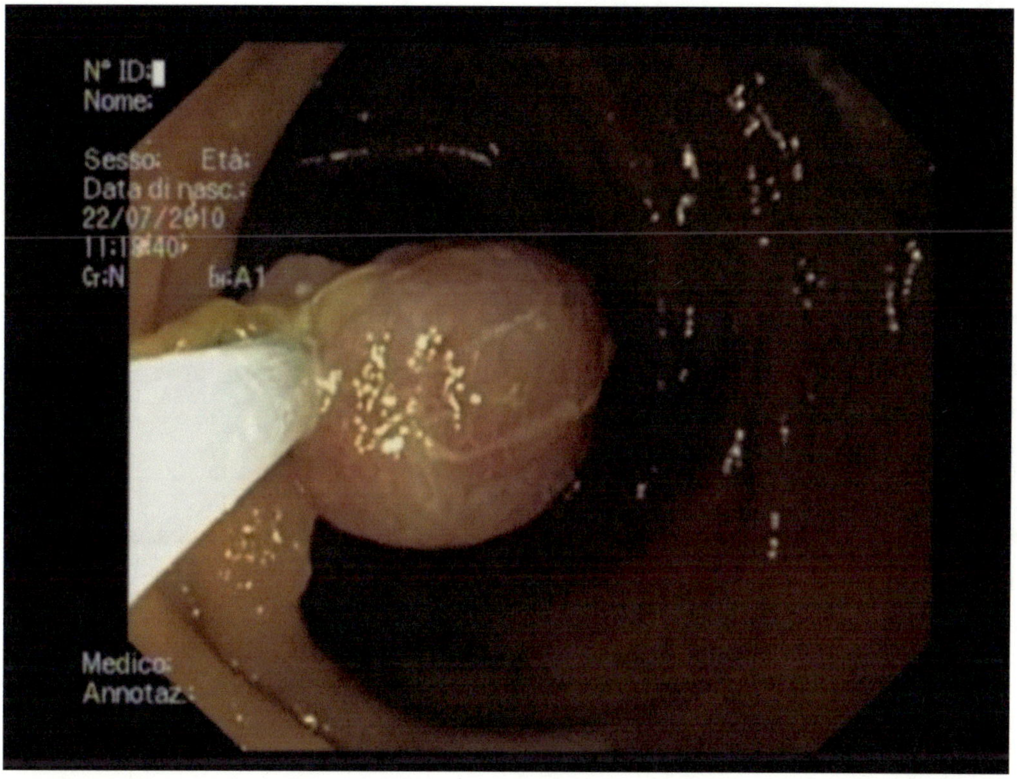

Fig. 5. Jejunal Polyp

We found small and large polyps , from 5 mms to 5 centimeters , penduncolated and sessile, the resection was en bloc or piece meal, with taking every specimen for histological evaluation (all was amartomas).
The time of endoscopy was 4 hours . 24 hours later, we recorded an elevation of transaminases (1.5 x) and total bilirubin (1.3 x) without abdominal symptom ; the patient was discharged 48 hour after the procedure, with normalization of blood tests.

5.1 Conclusion

Because of great number of large polyps, the spiral procedure seems to be better than other assisted enteroscopy : the over tube, that fix the endoscope with a coupler during spiral advancement and permit to disengage it for conventional manipulation, allows the scope to be removed and reintroduced after every polipectomy while holding the position deep in the small bowel (Figure 6).

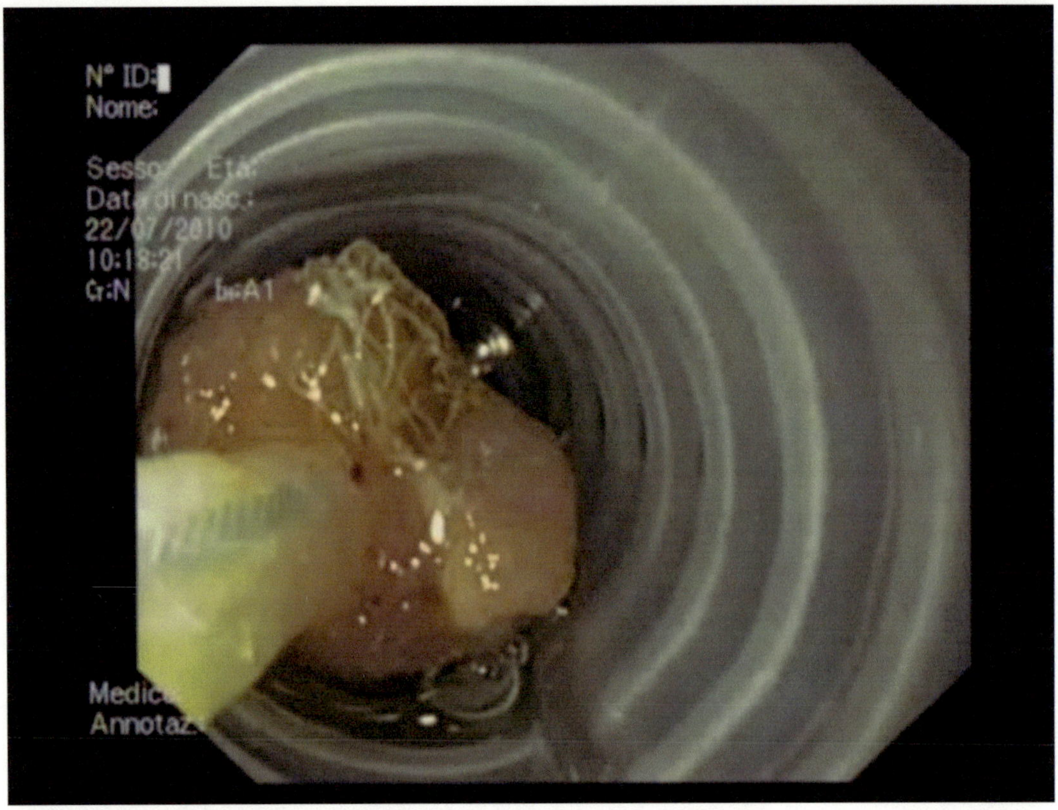

Fig. 6. Enteroscope through the overtube, polyp retrieved

Moreover, the disengagement and the rotation of the endoscope permits the best approach particularly to big polyps.
No major complications (perforation or bleeding) occurred during the procedure; the elevation of transaminases is related to transient edema in ampullary region due to trauma of the device.

6. References

[1] Akerman PA, Agrawal D, Cantero D, et al. Spiral enteroscopy with the new DSB overtube: a novel technique for deep peroral small-bowel intubation. *Endoscopy*. 2008 Dec;40(12):974-8.

[2] Morgan DR, Upchurch BR, Draganov PV, et al. Spiral enteroscopy: prospective multicenter US trial in patients with small bowel disorders. *Gastrointest Endosc*. 2009;69:AB127-8.

[3] Esmail S, Odstrcil EA, Mallat D, et al. A single center retrospective review of spiral enteroscopy. *Gastrointest Endosc*. 2009;69:AB197.

[4] Buscaglia JM, Dunbar KB, Okolo PI, 3rd, et al. The spiral enteroscopy training initiative: results of a prospective studyevaluating the Discovery SB overtube device during small bowel enteroscopy (with video). *Endoscopy*. 2009 Mar;41(3):194-9.

[5] Riccioni ME, Cianci R, Spada C et al. Use of spiral enteroscopy in a tertiary endoscopy center: initial experience. *Endoscopy*. 2009 Sep;41(9):820.

[6] Shin EJ. Enteral stent placement using spiral enteroscopy for malignant mid-jejunal obstruction. *The Dave Project* 2009.

[7] Raju GS, Gerson L, Das A, et al. American Gastroenterological Association (AGA) Institute technical review on obscure gastrointestinal bleeding. Gastroenterology 2007;133:1697- 1717.

[8] Ross A, Mehdizadeh S, Tokar J, et al. Double balloon enteroscopy detects small bowel mass lesions missed by capsule endoscopy. Dig Dis Sci 2008;53:2140–2143.

[9] Rockey DC. Occult gastrointestinal bleeding. N Engl J Med 1999; 341:38–46.

[10] Hartmann D, Schmidt H, Bolz G, et al. A prospective two-center study comparing wireless capsule endoscopy with intraoperative enteroscopy in patients with obscure GI bleeding. Gastrointest Endosc 2005;61:826–832.

[11] Rondonotti E, Pennazio M, Toth E, et al. Small-bowel neoplasms in patients undergoing video capsule endoscopy: a multicenter European study. Endoscopy 2008;40:488–495.

[12] Costamagna G, Shah SK, Riccioni ME, et al. A prospective trial comparing small bowel radiographs and video capsule endoscopy for suspected small bowel disease. Gastroenterology 2002;123: 999–1005.

[13] Huprich JE, Fletcher JG, Alexander JA, et al. Obscure gastrointestinal bleeding: evaluation with 64-section multiphase CT enterography— initial experience. Radiology 2008;246:562–571.

[14] Pennazio M. Small-bowel endoscopy [review]. Endoscopy 2004;36:32-41.

[15] DiSario JA, Petersen BT, Tierney WM, et al. Enteroscopes. *Gastrointest Endosc.* 2007 Nov;66(5):872-80.

[16] Ell C, May A. Mid-gastrointestinal bleeding: capsule endoscopy and push-and-pull enteroscopy give rise to a new medical term. Endoscopi 2006;38:73-5.

[17] Gerson LB. Double-balloon enteroscopy: the new gold standard for small-bowel imaging? Gastrointest Endosc 2005;62:71-5.

[18] Sugano KYH, Kita H. Double-balloon endoscopy: theory and practice. New YorK: Springer, 2006.

[19] Yamamoto H, Sekine Y, Sato Y, et al. Total enteroscopy with a nonsurgical steerable double-balloon method. Gastrointest Endosc 2001;53:216–220.

[20] Hartmann D, Eickhoff A, Tamm R, et al. Balloon-assisted enteroscopy using a single-balloon technique. Endoscopy 2007; 39(Suppl 1):E276.

[21] Akerman PA, Cantero D. Spiral enteroscopy and push enteroscopy. Gastrointest Endosc *Clin N Am.* 2009 Jul;19(3):357- 69.

[22] Luis F. Lara, Shailender Singh, Jayaprakash Sreenarasimhaiah. Initial experience with retrograde overtube-assisted enteroscopy using a spiral tip overtube. *Proc (Bayl Univ Med Cent)* 2010;23(2):130–133.

[23] Buscaglia JM, Dunbar KB, Okolo PI, et al. The spiral enteroscopy training initiative: results of a prospective study evaluating the discovery SB overtube device during small bowel enteroscopy. Endoscopy. 2009;41:194–199.

[24] Mantas A, Masand A, DeMarco D. A single center retrospectivecomparison of double balloon and spiral enteroscopy. *Am JGastroenterol.* 2009;104(Suppl 3):S508.

[25] Aldler A, Eckardt E, Veltzke-Schlieker W, Papnikolau I, Giannakoulopoulou E, Wiedemann B, Rosch T. Is Spirale Enteroscopy superior to double ballon enteroscopy in diagnosing the small intestine? First resul of a large prospective randomized comparative study. *Presented at DGBE-BV 2010 (German society for endoscopy and imaging)*

[26] May A, Farber M, Aschmoneit I, et al. Prospective multicenter trial comparing push-and-pull enteroscopy with the single- and double-balloon techniques in patients with small-bowel disorders. *Am J Gastroenterol2010*; 105:582-4.

[27] Frieling T, Heise J, Sassenrath W, Hulsdok A, Kreysel C. Prospective comparison between doble-balloon enteroscopy and spiral enteroscopy. *Endoscopy*. 2010;42: 885-8

[28] Khashab MA, Lennon AM, Dunbar KB, Singh VK, Chandrasekhara V, Giday S, et al. A comparative evaluation of singleballoon enteroscopy and spiral enteroscopy for patients with midgut disorders. *Gastrointest Endosc*. 2010;72:766–72.

[29] Anne Marie Lennon, MD, PhD, Vinay Chandrasekhara, MD, Eun Ji Shin, MD, Patrick I. Okolo,III, MD, MPH Spiral-enteroscopy–assisted enteral stent placement for palliation of malignant small-bowel obstruction (with video) *Gastrointestinal Endoscopy* Volume 71, No. 2 : 2010

[30] Aabakken L, Bretthauer M, Line PD. Double-balloon enteroscopy for endoscopic retrograde cholangiography in patients with a Roux-en-Y anastomosis. *Endoscopy*. 2007;39:1068–71.

[31] Chandrasekhara V, Lennon AM, Singh V, Liang D, Okolo P. ERCP using spiral enteroscopy in patients with altered gastrointestinal anatomy. *Am J Gastroenterol*. 2009;104(Suppl 3):S384

[32] Shah RJ. Spiral enteroscopy-assisted ERCP in patients with longlimb surgical biliary bypass. *Endoscopy*. 2009;41(Suppl 1):A25.

[33] Sanjay RH, Sharon D, Kevan I, Stephen JH, Jeffrey LT, Oleh H. Overtube-assisted ERCP in patients with surgically altered anatomy: a single center one-year experience. *Gastrointest Endosc*. 2009;69:AB193.

12

Endoscopic Resection of Large Colorectal Lesions

David Martínez Ares,
Pamela Estévez Boullosa and José Ignacio Rodríguez Prada
Gastroenterology Department,
Complejo Hospitalario Universitario de Vigo,
Spain

1. Introduction

The colorectal cancer (CRC) is one of the most common tumors in Western countries. It is the most common gastrointestinal tumor and it is estimated that between 5 and 6% of the population will suffer it along their lives. Colorectal cancer is a tumor in which it is possible to perform primary and secondary prevention. Primary prevention consists of all actions aimed to prevent the development of cancer or precancerous lesions, whereas secondary prevention is the detection and removal of these premalignant lesions, avoiding then the development of colorectal cancer (CRC).

CRC is a disease with a well-known natural history, fulfilling in most cases the adenoma-carcinoma sequence (Figure 1), and its natural history is long enough so it can be interrupted by various diagnostic and therapeutic strategies. In fact, in sporadic CRC, which represents most cases, the time since the appearance of a polyp in a colon without neoplastic disease, the posterior growing and degeneration of the lesion to finally become an invasive cancer, is usually not lower than 10-15 years. We therefore have a long time, enough to detect and remove these lesions, interrupting then the natural history of the disease and preventing the development of CRC; so endoscopic polypectomy is a therapeutic key point in the prevention of colorectal carcinoma.

Not all polyps degenerate into cancer and, consequently, not all colonic polyps should be removed. Although we already have endoscopic technology that allows us to accurately differentiate neoplastic from hyperplastic polyps, the standard practice is to remove all polyps. Definitely the result of histological examination of the polyp is which determines the way to approach in the future. The technique for the removal of polyps depends on several factors, such as size, location and morphology of the lesions. We can solve most pedunculated and sessile polyps with a simple polypectomy. Most colonic polyps are small and pedunculated, and its removal becomes relatively easy. When sessile polyps are located in the right colon due to the reduced thickness of the colonic wall in this location, injection of drugs into the submucosa before polypectomy decreases the risk of perforation. In large pedunculated polyps with thick pedicles, it can be helpful to use techniques to prevent bleeding after colonic polypectomy. Submucosal adrenaline injection at the base of the polyp or the placement of endoloop or hemostatic clips on the pedicle can prevent the development of bleeding complications. But this is not the aim of this work. Then we would try to describe in a practical way the different techniques for treatment of large sessile or flat lesions that can be found in the colon.

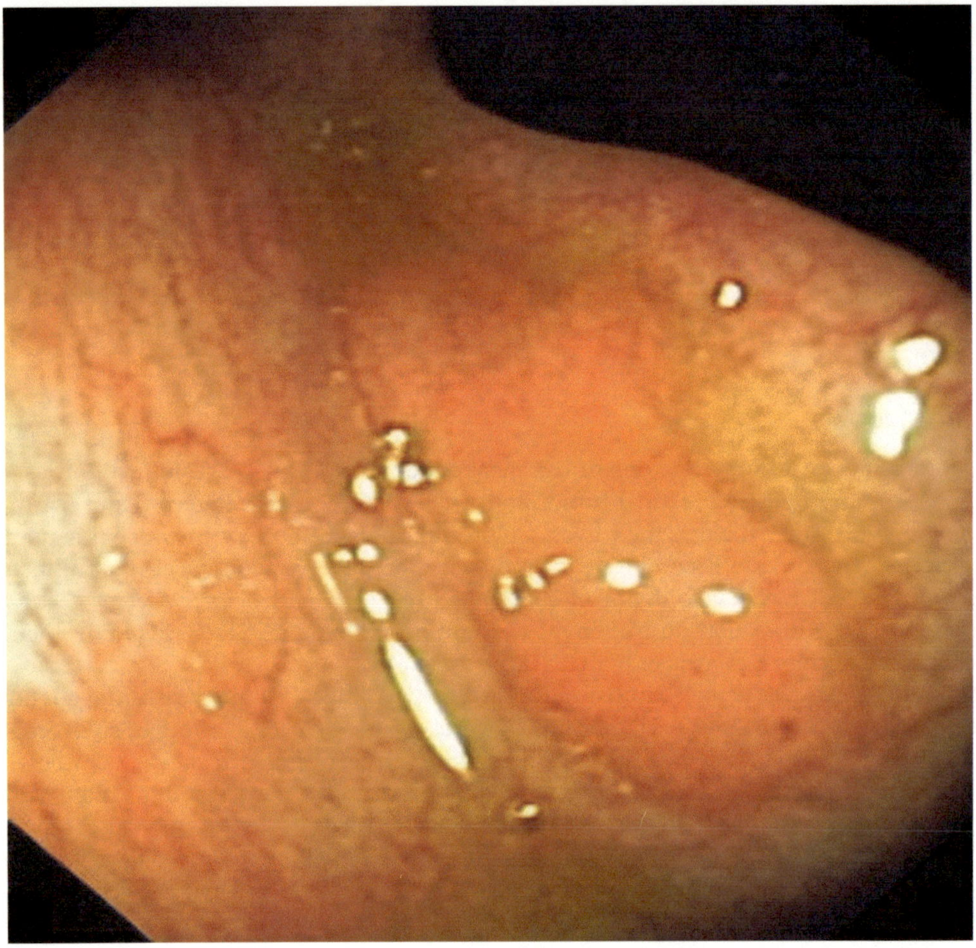

Fig. 1. The picture shows a conventional endoscopy where a flat lesion, slightly elevated and with indistinct edges can be observed.

We consider that sessile or flat lesions are large when they exceed 20 mm in diameter and giant polyps would be those whose size exceeds 30 mm. As well as polyps smaller than 2 cm can be removed en bloc in most cases, those larger than 2 cm are not always achieved, and lesions larger than 3 cm are almost never achieved. It is accepted that lesions of this size or greater should not be removed on a single piece using a polypectomy snare. The risk of perforation is extremely high in these cases so it is recommended to perform a piecemeal resection of these lesions. The performance of this technique to achieve success, understanding it as a complete resection of the lesion, the absence of recurrence of the lesion, and the absence of complications, requires the knowledge and practice of a number of endoscopic skills that we would describe below. In many centers, these large lesions are considered in most cases for surgical treatment. We should not forget that surgery, even in case of laparoscopic surgery, involves a large increase of health costs and it is not free of morbidity and mortality. We should also consider that many of the patients in whom these lesions are detected have an advanced age and high comorbidity, which increases the surgical risk. On the other hand, the use of CRC screening programs makes it more frequent to diagnose this type of lesions. Therefore, adopting therapeutic strategies with lower risk to patients, lower consumption of economic resources, greater respect to organ´s functionality and similar outcomes for patients seem to be more than reasonable. Naturally, we must correctly select the cases that can be solved endoscopically, avoiding then unnecessary risks and consumption of resources that will not prevent to refer patients to other interventions. Finally, treatment options that can be offered to an individual patient depend on the possibilities of each place. In very large series from reference hospitals where there are expert endoscopists show that up to two thirds of the benign lesions that are referred to surgery can be endoscopically resolved.

2. Endoscopic resection of large colorectal lesions

2.1 Endoscopic Mucosal Resection (EMR)

As it is well known this is a technique that is not exceedingly challenging from the endoscopic point of view, with little risk for complications but, rarely, it may allow removing en bloc lesions larger than 2 cm in diameter. However, as we will explain below, we believe that it does have an important role in colorectal neoplastic disease. It should not be, of course, a universal technique, but it would have its indications based on its benefits and its limitations.

2.1.1 Detection and characterization of the lesion

Nonpolypoid lesions are those consisting of dysplastic tissue that does not protrude or that protrudes a little into the intestinal lumen, reaching a maximum thickness of two times that of the surrounding mucosa. Flat lesions are often undetectable with conventional endoscopy, being essential to use endoscopic techniques such as chromoendoscopy (Figure 2), virtual chromoendoscopy or Narrow Band Imaging for the correct demarcation of the lesions. The nonpolypoid lesions of the colon can be flat and reach large dimensions but instead of growing into the intestinal lumen, they expand along the colonic wall, and they are called laterally spreading tumors (LST). These lesions have an invasive growth risk significantly lower than sessile lesions of the same size. Initially, what differentiates them it is its appearance, but there are great differences regarding their biological behavior, so in both cases, the therapeutic attitudes may be slightly different. This is, quite often, the presentation form of the lesions diagnosed in patients with long-standing ulcerative colitis and in the context of Lynch syndrome.

In order to plan the most appropriate therapeutic approach for a particular lesion we should correctly characterize it. According to most authors there are three aspects to consider in order of predicting the degree of invasion of the lesion. Some authors support performing whenever it is possible, an echoendoscopic study with high frequency miniprobes to evaluate the involvement of the colonic wall by the neoplasm. Other authors argue that endosonographic study is not essential since endoscopic appearance can greatly predict the degree of invasion of the lesion. First, the general appearance of the lesion must be defined, being strongly recommended the use of the Paris classification of superficial neoplastic lesions (2003). Most superficial endoscopic lesions are classified according to type 0. Polypoid lesions are subtype 0I (including two variants: pedunculated (0Ip) and sessile

(0Is)). Non-polypoid lesions are classified in subtype 0II (slightly elevated 0IIa, completely flat 0IIb and slightly depressed without ulcer 0IIc). Finally, subtype 0III represents non-polypoid lesions with a frank ulcer. The risk of malignant degeneration of the lesion depends on the existence of submucosa invasion, being the maximum risk in subtype III and the minimum risk in type I lesions. Thus, those benign lesions (flat adenomas and laterally spreading tumors) and adenocarcinoma IIa lesions with a diameter less than 20 mm and IIb and IIc lesions less than 10 mm. can be subsidiaries of endoscopic treatment. In lesions classified as subtype III (ulcerated) will never be indicated endoscopic treatment, so surgery would be unavoidable.

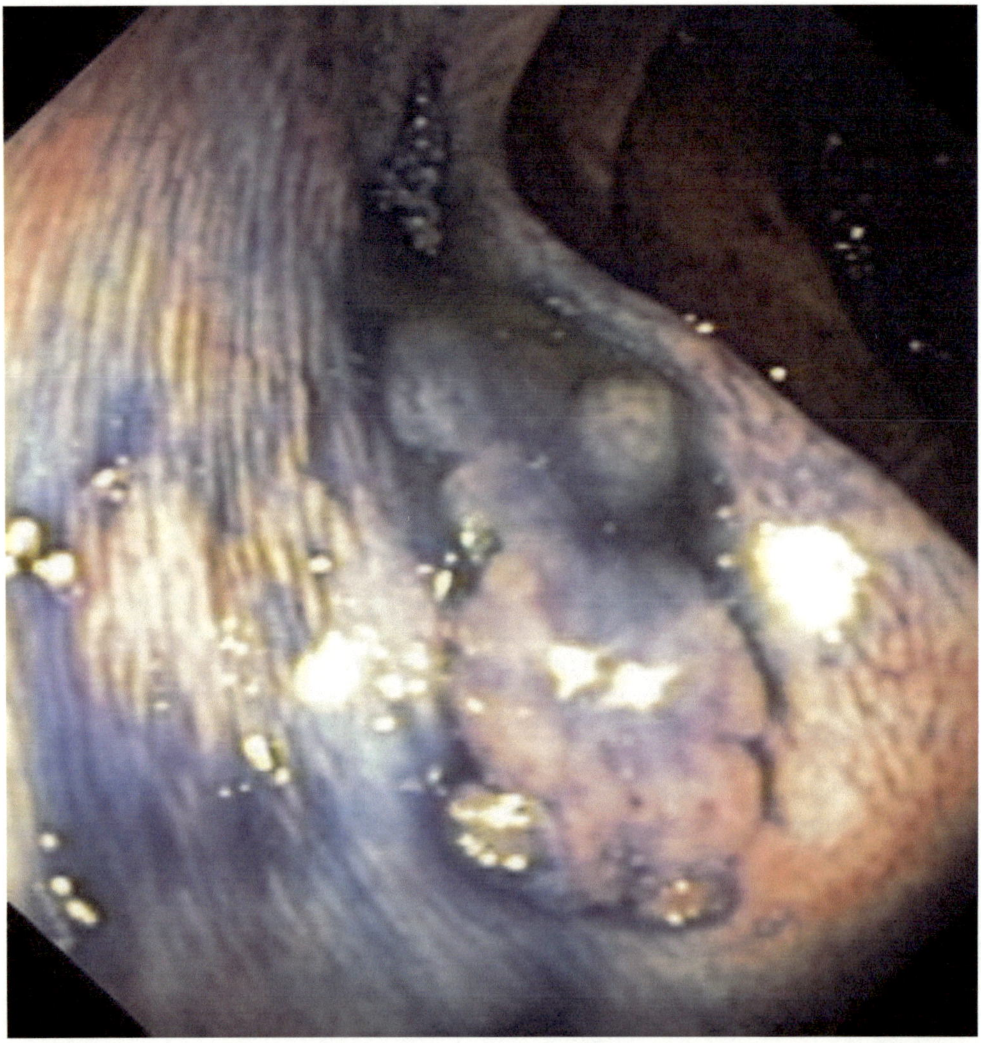

Fig. 2. Staining with indigo carmine 0.2% shows in greater detail the surface of the lesion with well defined edges.

Secondly, the appearance of the surface of the lesion has also a great transcendence, especially in LST. These LST are classified into two types according to their morphology, granular type (LST-G) (figure 3) and non-granular type (LST-NG) (Figure 4). LST-G lesions may reach large dimensions without presenting invasive growth, by contrast, this fact is much more likely in LST-NG. Therefore, endoscopic piecemeal mucosal resection (that is a lower complex technique and that is more available for any endoscopist) can be a therapeutic strategy for LST-G and en bloc resection with endoscopic submucosal dissection (ESD) should be applied to LST-NG, which is technically much more complex and with an increased risk of complications.

Finally, the study of crypts patterns according to Kudo´s classification using chromoendoscopy and magnification endoscopy has shown a great accuracy in predicting the invasive behavior. This classification states that: type I crypt pattern consists of regular round crypts, type II consists of stellar or papillary crypts, type IIIL consists of large roundish or tubular pits, type IIIS consists of small roundish or tubular pits, type IV consists of sulcus, branch, or gyrus-like crypts, and type V consists of irregular or severely distorted crypts. Types I and II are non-neoplastic (hyperplasic lesions) and excepting some circumstances they do not require treatment. Type IIIL, IIIS and IV are non-invasive lesions so endoscopic removal can be performed and type V represents invasive lesions so surgical resection is the best choice for treatment.

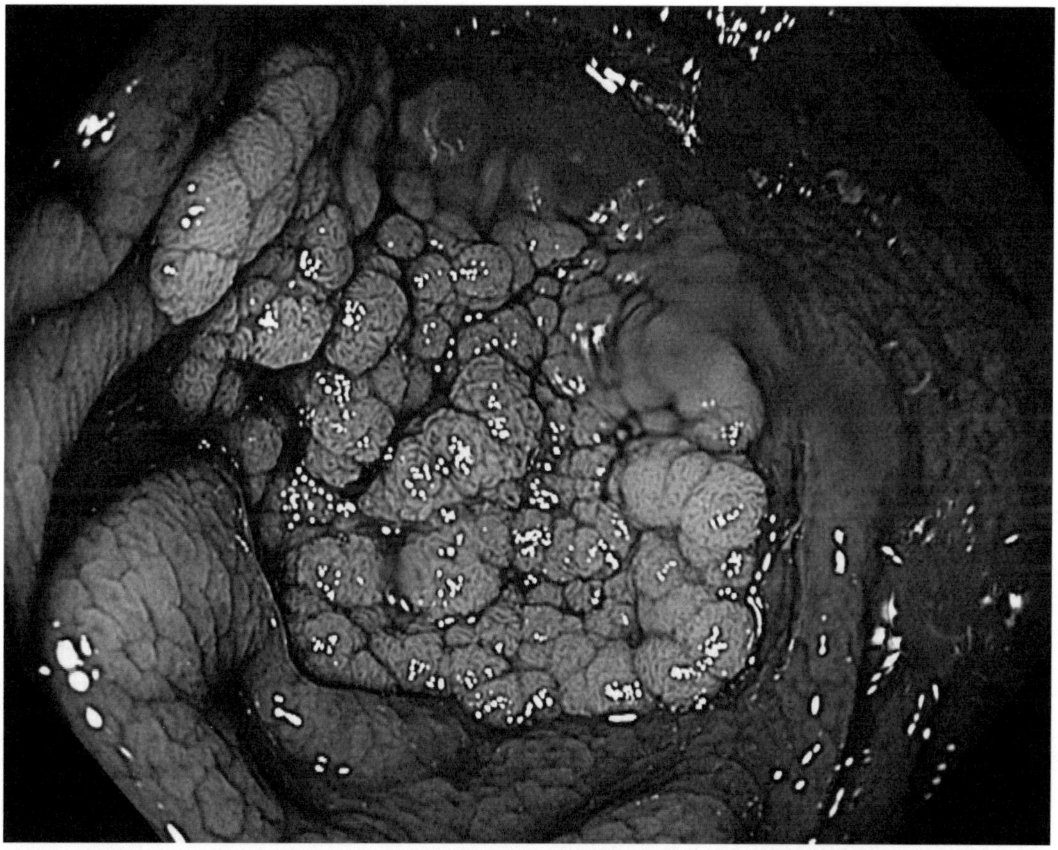

Fig. 3. Laterally spreading tumor with granular surface. It is classified as LST-G, and after its endoscopic resection a villous adenoma with low grade dysplasia was confirmed.

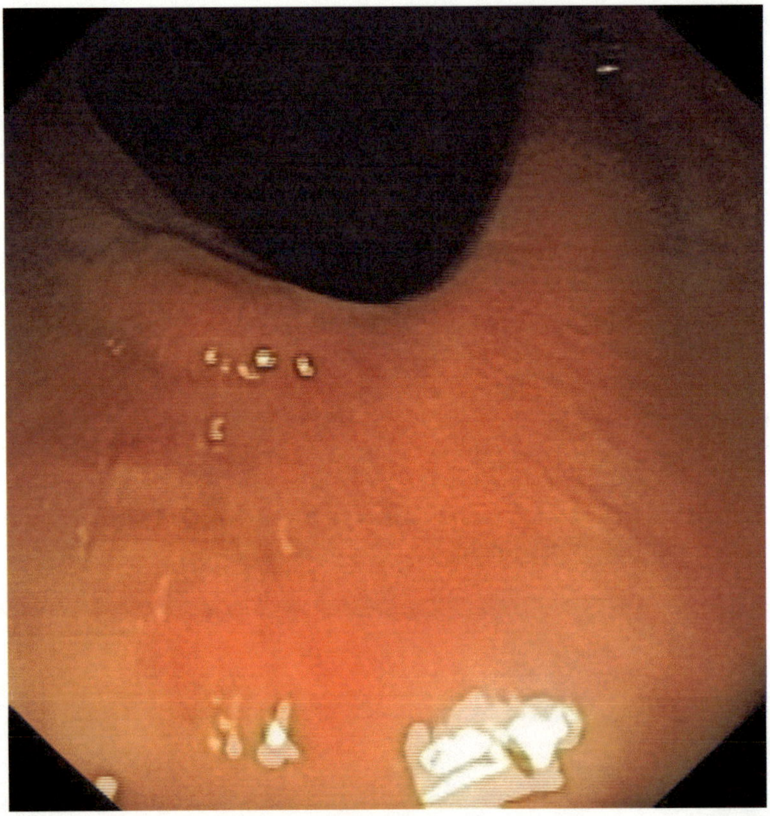

Fig. 4. Laterally spreading tumor with a smooth surface, not granular. Surgical resection was refused and the histological analysis revealed the presence of an invasive adenocarcinoma over a villous adenoma.

In conclusion, the characteristics of the lesion determine the correct treatment options: surgical or endoscopic resection. LST-NG lesions have twice the risk of presenting invasive growth, especially if pit pattern is suggestive of malignancy Kudo (V), lesions are greater than 20 mm of diameter and sclerotic changes are evident in the intestinal wall close to the lesion. In these cases it may be indicated surgical treatment, or in any case, a technique that allows "en bloc" resections of the lesion. In LST-G, the probability of invasive growth is increased if nodular areas larger than 10 mm or depressed areas are present or if the sign called "no lifting" after submucosal injection is present. So, LST-G have an infiltrative growth in less than 6% of cases, and if this takes place, more than 84% of the lesions present large nodular areas. In the absence of these data, piecemeal resection, technically easier, can be a good choice. There are some other endoscopic data that could be associated with an increased risk of invasive growth, although they do not achieve statistical significance in multivariate analysis, like for example colonic chicken skin mucosa, the presence of erythema over the lesion and the convergence of folds to the lesion.

2.1.2 Delimitation the edges of the lesion

The most experienced endoscopists suggest that it is essential to resect at least 1-2 mm of healthy edge to guarantee a complete resection of the lesion and to reduce the risk of recurrence. Some studies also suggest that ablation the edges of the lesion with argon plasma would reduce the risk of recurrence. However, other authors state that removing the entire lesion and including a small portion of healthy tissue in the surgical specimen would achieve the same result.

When an en bloc resection is achieved, this is less important. But when there is a large lesion that requires a piecemeal resection, the burn deforms tissue and it is more difficult to demark the lesion. Although the use of chromoendoscopy and NBI may be useful to detect the remaining tissue, it seems more useful to have a correct demarcation of the lesion before to start the resection. On the other hand, performing submucosal injection for lifting the lesion may distort its appearance by making the edges difficult to identify at the time of resection. Therefore, our standard practice is to define the edges of the lesion with a minimum burn that can be easily seen, which can be performed with argon plasma or with the tip of the polypectomy snare (Figure 5). These burns are easily recognizable; marking the entire periphery of the lesion. They are located at 1-2 mm from the edge of the lesion and they are separated from each other by 5-6 mm. At the end of resection of the lesion, if none of these burns is visible, we can be sure that we have performed a resection as extensive as originally planned.

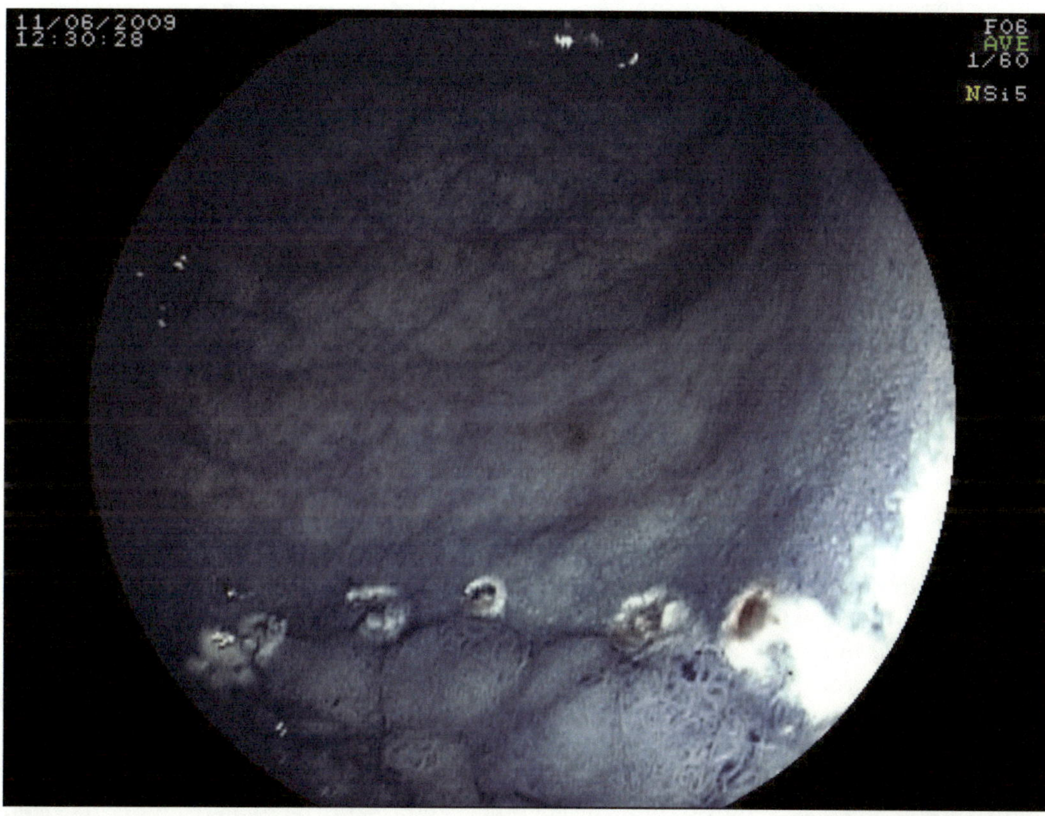

Fig. 5. After clearly limit the edges of the lesion using chromoendoscopy, in this case, computed virtual chromoendoscopy (CVC-FICE). The edges can be marked by burns performed with plasma argon or with snare tip from 3-5 mm at the edge of the lesion.

In our center, to correctly identify the edges of the lesion we usually use indigo carmine 0.2% (Figure 6). In recent years, since we have Computerized Virtual chromoendoscopy (CVC-FICE) (Figure 7) both techniques are used without distinction with identical results.

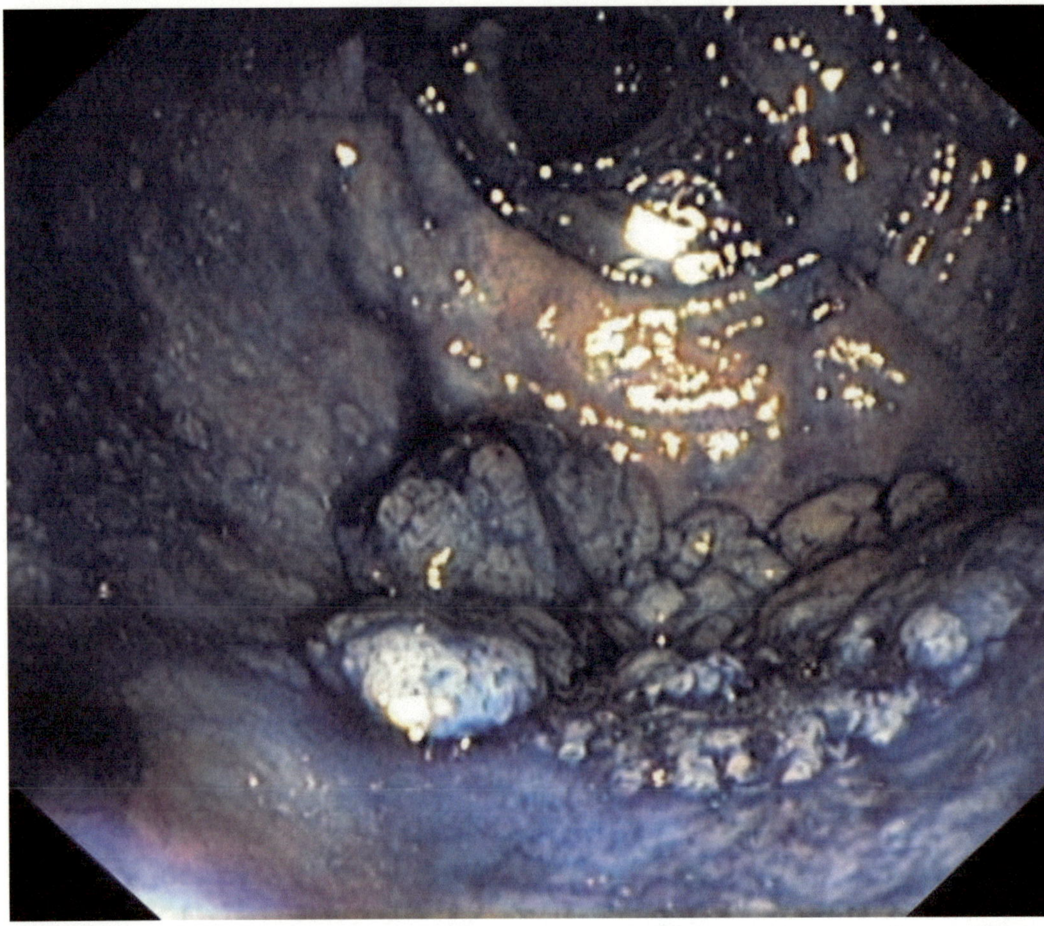

Fig. 6. Flat lesion, stained with 0.2% indigo carmine, which highlights the surface of the lesion and clearly defines the edges.

2.1.3 Submucosa injection

The injection of drugs into the submucosa aims to create a space between the mucosa and submucosa and muscular layer. Thus, resection of sessile or flat lesions is easier, and the risk of complications is reduced, especially perforation. The substance normally used is saline, with or without epinephrine. Since it is an isotonic substance, it spreads quickly, so the lifting disappears, that is why it is important to perform multiple injections, especially in large lesions. We have used other substances, such as glycerol, hyaluronic acid, hydroxypropylmethylcellulose or autologous blood anticoagulated with citrated substances. The lifting they generate is more lasting, allowing a small number of injections. Its major limitation is their high cost so they are no available in most centers. Hypertonic solutions of dextrose 50% with epinephrine have also been used, with better results than normal saline solution, allowing to remove lesions with lower volume of solution injected, fewer number of injections and less time consuming to complete resection. These differences are only significant in case of large lesions. However, it is found a higher frequency of postpolypectomy syndrome that can suggest a possible damage of the colonic wall, probably due to vascular disturbances caused by the hypertonic nature of this solution. It has been recently recommended the use of succilinated gelantine, a very cheap plasma expander, whose only limitation is that it can not be used in patients with hypersensitivity to gelatin. This study asserts that the lift is more lasting and that the number of injections, the total volume injected and the time consumed in the resection are lower. Additionally, the size of the resected fragments is larger and, consequently, lesions of the same size are removed in a smaller number of fragments. Finally, the en bloc resections are almost double that when the lesion is raised just with saline. In our experience, with a saline, methylene blue and epinephrine 1/10,000 mixture most lesions are successfully completely removed. We have recently started to use succilinated gelantine (Gelafundina®), instead of saline, with good results. Apparently, the lift that it provides is more lasting, requiring less number of injections to complete the resection of the lesions. However, in this moment we do not have enough experience to ensure the superiority of a solution over the classic one.

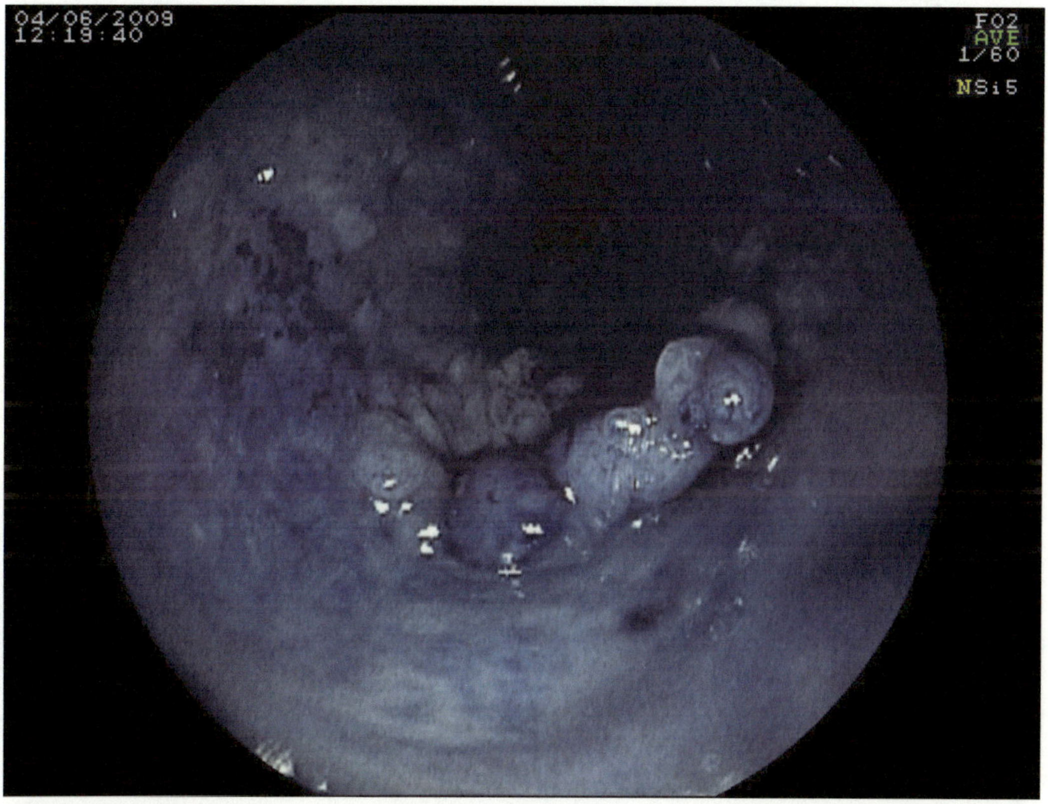

Fig. 7. Computed virtual chromoendoscopy (CVC) is useful for the characterization of colorectal lesions, avoiding the use of coloring agents, catheters and only requiring the use of an endoscope.

Submucosal injection has to be done very carefully, in small aliquots distributed all over the extent of the lesion to achieve a correct elevation (Figure 8). Especially in lesions located on a fold, it is essential to start lifting the distal part to ensure the lesion gets "closer" to the endoscope, instead of being placed in positions that can difficult the visibility. When a lesion that has not been previously biopsied does not lift ("non lifting sign) it fairly predicts the infiltration of the submucosa by a possible focus of adenocarcinoma (Figure 9). However, biopsies, especially in flat or very small lesions, can cause fibrosis in the submucosa and difficult its correct lift. In the absence of previous biopsies, the "non lifting sign" has a sensitivity of 100% and a specificity of 99% in predicting invasive growth. In any case, no elevation of the lesion, just because it is a malignant lesion or because the high risk of perforation, make it reasonable to not perform an endoscopic resection of the lesion.

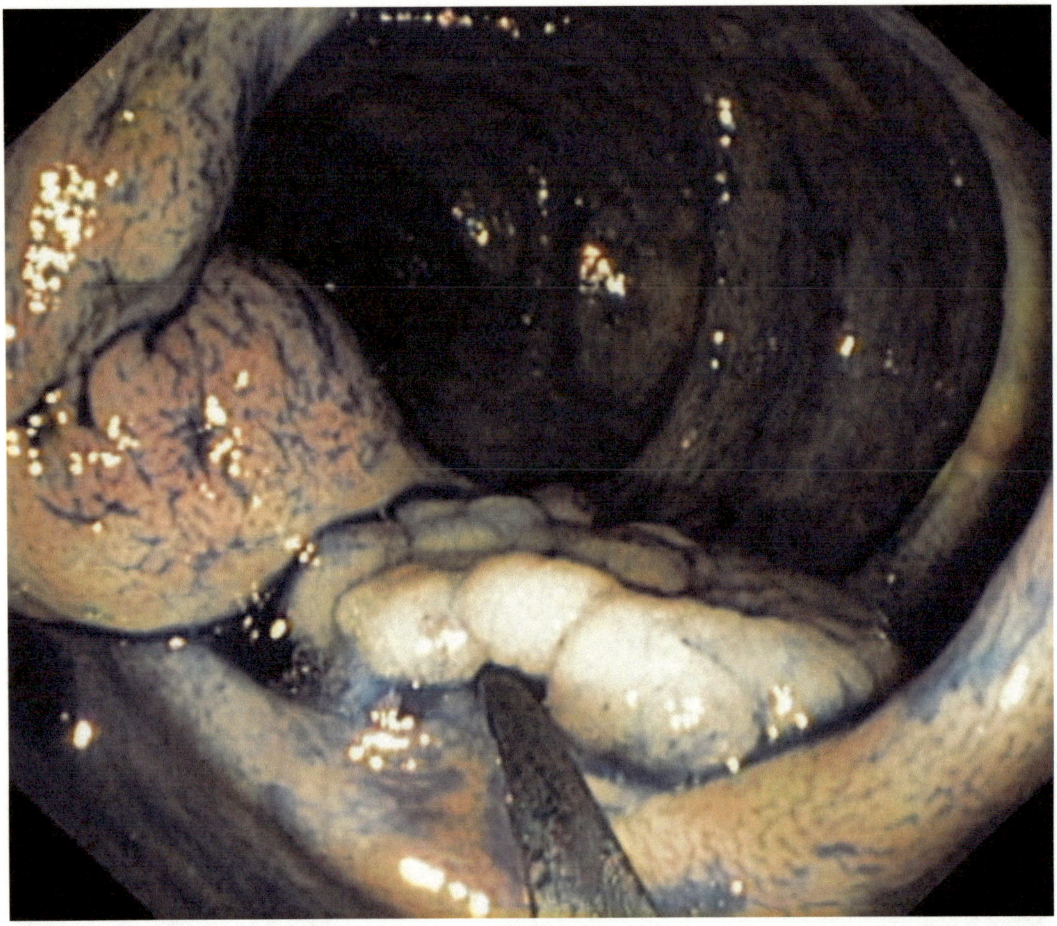

Fig. 8. Submucosal injection, with an adequate lift of the lesion prior to its removal. It is recommended to start injecting at the distal part of the lesion to avoid losing perspective and also to avoid not to see that part of the lesion during the excision. Otherwise, we may be forced to confront the farthest part of it to us in retroversion.

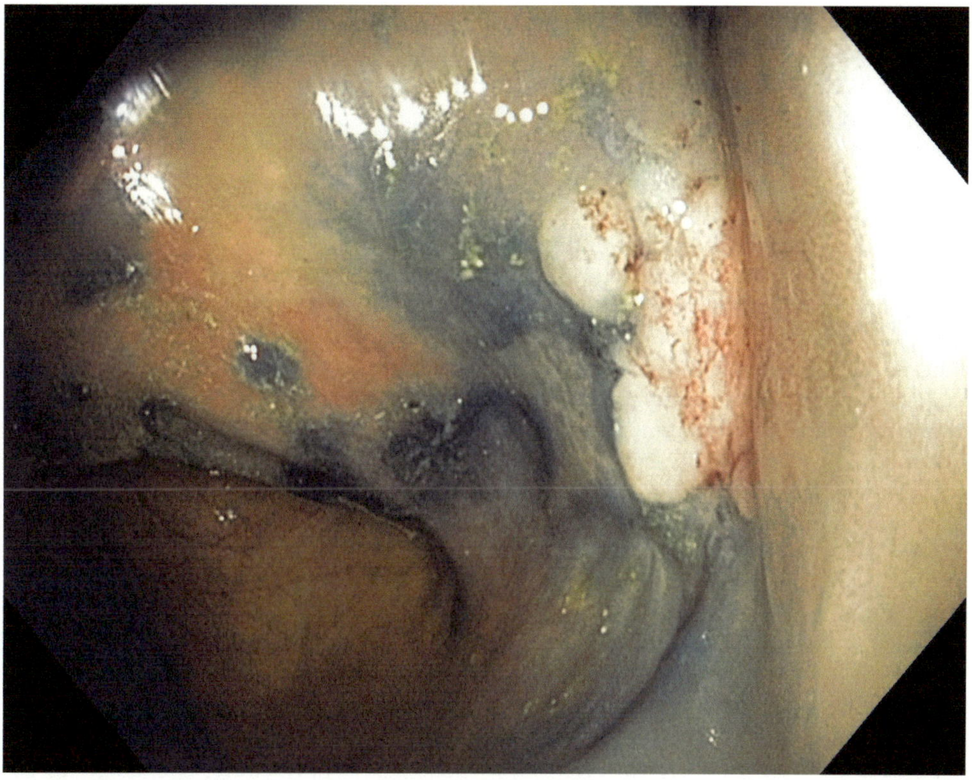

Fig. 9. "Non lifting sign": The lesion is not lifted after submucosal injection. This, if there is no submucosal fibrosis caused by previous attempts of resection, sugests submucosal invasive growth

2.1.4 Endoscopic mucosal resection technique

The most commonly technique used is the conventional one consistent on lifting and cutting. After submucosal injection of different substances, the lesion is totally or partly included on a typical polypectomy snare and it is removed in one or more fragments. As we have stated, performing en bloc resection of lesions larger than 2 cm is neither possible nor desirable, due to the high risk of perforation. If a piecemeal resection is needed, it must be done in the lowest number of fragments as possible in order to restore and "reset" the lesion as close as possible to reality. Thus resection can be achieved for the vast majority of the lesions identified in the colon. Even in a study presented by experienced endoscopists, remarkable results were achieved without making any submucosal injection. It is essential to keep a carefully systematic resection to prevent the persistence of viable tissue areas at the confluence of the different fragments resected. Some authors suggest the possibility of APC ablation of this tissue to prevent recurrence of the lesion, although this practice could increase the possibility of developing postpolypectomy syndrome. Some authors also suggest coagulating the edges of the lesion with APC, thus reducing the risk of recurrence. However, in opinion of leading experts and also ours, this is not necessary if you perform a wide resection including at least 1-2 mm of healthy mucosa in the resected specimen.

In general, with this simple technique of lifting and cutting, most authors report a technical success rate above 90%. That is, with a simple technique we can achieve resection of most lesions. However, some authors have reported small series of cases in which the resection of colorectal lesions is achieved with great success and low risk of complications, using suction and cutting techniques, especially Cap assisted mucusectomy. In our opinion, on a regular basis, it would not be necessary to add complexity to a simple and effective technique in most situations; although this might be a good alternative in case of lesions where the loop can not be placed over them. To facilitate the inclusion of the lesion inside the loop it is often useful to suck as much gas as possible, almost to collapse the lumen. This causes lower intestinal wall tension and this facilitates catching the lesion.

Some authors, in both animal and patients models , have suggested making a circumferential incision at the edges of the lesion before using the snare, allowing it to be snared, thus achieving en bloc resection of large lesions in lesser time. In animal models specimens have been achieved up to 50 mm in diameter, excised by en bloc resection, without a great risk of perforation. This technique, known as IT-EMR (EMR-incision technique) or as CSI-EMR (circunferential submucosal incision-EMR) could be an alternative to ESD as a tool to achieve en bloc resection of some lesions.

For resection of these lesions we usually use mixed stream, cutting and coagulation, with the Endo-cut system. We use a 120W cutting power in rectum and left colon and 80W in the right colon, and a coagulation power of 60W in both right and left colon. When argon plasma is needed, we use power 100W and a flow of 2 liters / min in rectum and power 60W and a flow of 1 to 1.2 liters / min in right colon. Some authors have suggested that the use of pure cutting power causes lesser thermal artifact on the specimen, facilitating the study and a more accurate pathological staging in case of lesions with an infiltrative growth pattern. This would increase the risk of bleeding, which could be controlled using hemoclips as a preventive treatment.

It is essential to complete successful resection of the lesion performing it in a single session. The removal of the lesions, the coagulation of the scar produces fibrosis that would make impossible to lift the lesion in a second time, adding an increasing risk of complications. If in consecutive endoscopic examinations adenomatous tissue is detected, it has to be removed. However, in these cases, the elevation of the lesion with submucosal injection is usually very difficult, and due to the submucosa fibrosis it usually spreads to the lateral areas, lifting more healthy mucosal tissue than residual adenomatous tissue. In one of the largest series published, which belongs to an Australian multicenter group, including 479 patients, it was established an eradication rate of lesions in a single session of 89.2%. Failure factors were involvement of the ileocecal valve by the lesion and the existence of a previous attempt to resection. Submucosal injection is considered an attempted resection, even without resection just because submucosal injection results in submucosal fibrosis. In this case, the probability of failure in the resection is multiplied by 6. In the same series, it is established as predictors of relapse of the lesion an initial size greater than 40 mm and the need of using APC to eradicate adenomatous tissue.

2.1.5 Medium and long term results

Large lesions (> 20 mm) can rarely be en bloc resected, with an estimated recurrence rate of 20% (0-52% in different series published). However, in very large series recurrence rates of lesions have been reported below 10%.

To ensure the success of the procedure, it is essential to perform a systematic resection of the lesions, but also a strict monitoring system of the scars, especially when a piecemeal resection has been carried out. Most authors recommend a first review of the scar 3 months after resection. . In case of detecting residual tumor tissue, resection must be attempted and, if it is not possible, we should apply argon plasma. We perform a review and biopsy of the scar at 3 months after initial resection. We perform quarterly reviews until the scar biopsies are negative, making then a review after 6 and 12 months. If after one year of the last examination in which neoplastic tissue was removed there is no evidence of recurrence we consider that we have achieved the cure of the lesion. Some authors believe that a NBI, chromoendoscopy or magnification endoscopy study could be performed to review the scar, so the presence of residual tumor could be ruled out fairly confidently. We combine the study with NBI and biopsy of the scar, especially in large scars where biopsies may not be representative of the entire surface of it. As recently reported normal appearance of the scar and negative biopsies, performed three months after resection, predict with a negative predictive value of 97.4% freedom from relapse during follow-up. On contrast, it is the size of the lesions (> 4 cm), the most strongly factor associated with a possible recurrence of the lesion. In recent years the term late relapse has been established to define those relapses that can be seen after one or more revisions with negative biopsy scar. In some series, they represent more than half of all recurrences, so patients must be followed for long periods of time. This may be a limiting factor, because if it is impossible to make a correct follow-up this may be the cause of the failure. Therefore, the need for repeating colonoscopy several times is something that should be clearly discussed with the patient before make the decision to choose this form of treatment.

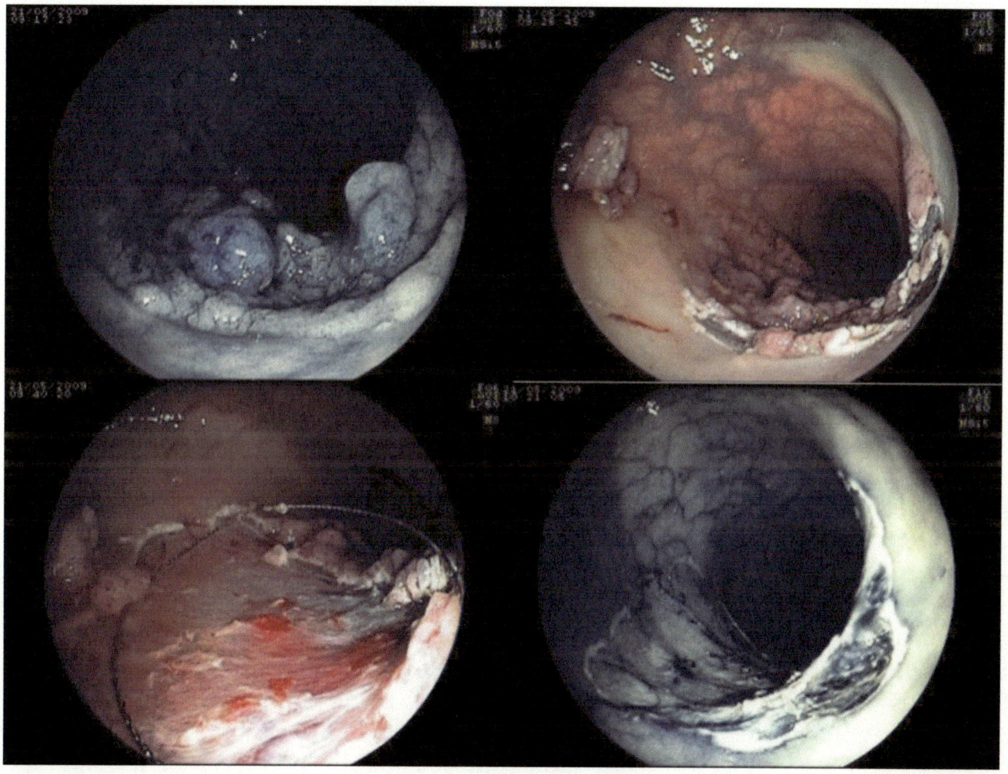

Fig. 10. Piecemeal resection of a large lesion of 6 cm in diameter, located in the upper rectum. After finishing the resection, CVC is used to check the absence of residual adenomatous tissue in the scar.

The results of endoscopic resection of large lesions, make that this could be the best therapeutic approach in properly selected patients. The development of laparoscopic techniques for segmental colon resection has questioned the usefulness of such complex endoscopic procedures. There is no doubt that in patients with extremely complex lesions, where a complete resection is not possible, like in case of lesions involving the appendiceal orifice, those affecting two consecutive folds, or those that fail to raise properly, are serious candidates for surgical treatment. However, we must not forget that the surgical resection, even in case of laparoscopic surgery, it is not free of morbidity and mortality, especially in patients with high surgical risk. Secondly, cost of laparoscopic surgery and hospitalization are significantly higher than the cost of endoscopic procedures, even if it is necessary to perform several colonoscopies during follow-up period. Obviously, if endoscopic treatment represents a serious alternative to surgery, it must be safe and effective, so it is necessary to concentrate the most complex cases in expert hands. This is especially interesting in rectum, where the risks of endoscopic resection are lower and potential consequences of surgery are greater. Thus, an Australian group was able to avoid surgery in 90% of patients that were referred to them from centers where endoscopists had refused endoscopic resection, and they achieved a saving of $ 7,000 per patient that could be endoscopically managed.

2.1.6 Complications

The most common complications of endoscopic resection of colorectal lesions, regardless complications due to sedation when performing endoscopy, are bleeding and perforation of the intestinal wall. Bleeding is the most common complication. It is estimated that it occurs in 1 of every 100 procedures. Proper lift of the lesion allows us to avoid the section of the thick vessels of the submucosa, achieving prevention of bleeding. In case that these vessels get exposed or are partially damaged by resection, its coagulation can be performed with thermal methods (coagulation forceps, APC, heat probe) or mechanical ligation can also been performed with hemoclips; although some authors doubt about the profitability of performing prophylactic coagulation of these vessels. What is important, surely, is to make the cut with sufficient calm to properly coagulate the vessels of submucosa. If bleeding occurs, immediate treatment must be done with the same methods described to prevent this complication. Once bleeding is controlled, resection can be continued. We must avoid, obviously, the contact of the polypectomy snare with metal clips, as they can transmit power through the colonic wall and perforate it in the area where they have been inserted. In most cases bleeding is controlled immediately, having no impact on patient. However, bleeding is not always immediate as it can be deferred (between the 24 hours after the procedure, even up to 14-21 days later). In this case, patient usually presents anemia, so admission and blood transfusion can be required.

Perforation is less frequent, but a much more serious complication. It happens when in a fragment of the lesion that has to be resected it is included the muscular layer or the whole wall, damaging it. It can produce a frank perforation or simply the interruption of the muscular layer. To prevent this complication is essential to make a correct lift of the lesion, allowing us to obtain a cutting plane large enough to avoid the muscular layer. It is also essential to recognize the "non lifting sign" because if the lesion is not correctly raised we should not proceed to resection. Once the lesion is inside the loop it can be useful to make traction of it towards the intestinal lumen, achieving to separate the cutting plane from the muscular layer. We can also liberate the muscular layer, if it has been trapped, making soft forward and backward movements. It is also recommended to to suck as much gas as possible because this causes lower intestinal wall tension. Most authors also recommend, as a preventive measure, to avoid performing multiple resections of large lesions located on the same place. Finally, it is essential to be extremely careful when removing lesions located on a fold, because its section results in transmural resection. Sometimes, it is difficult to fully recognize the situation of the fold as the anatomy of the colon can be altered by the lesion and submucosal injection.

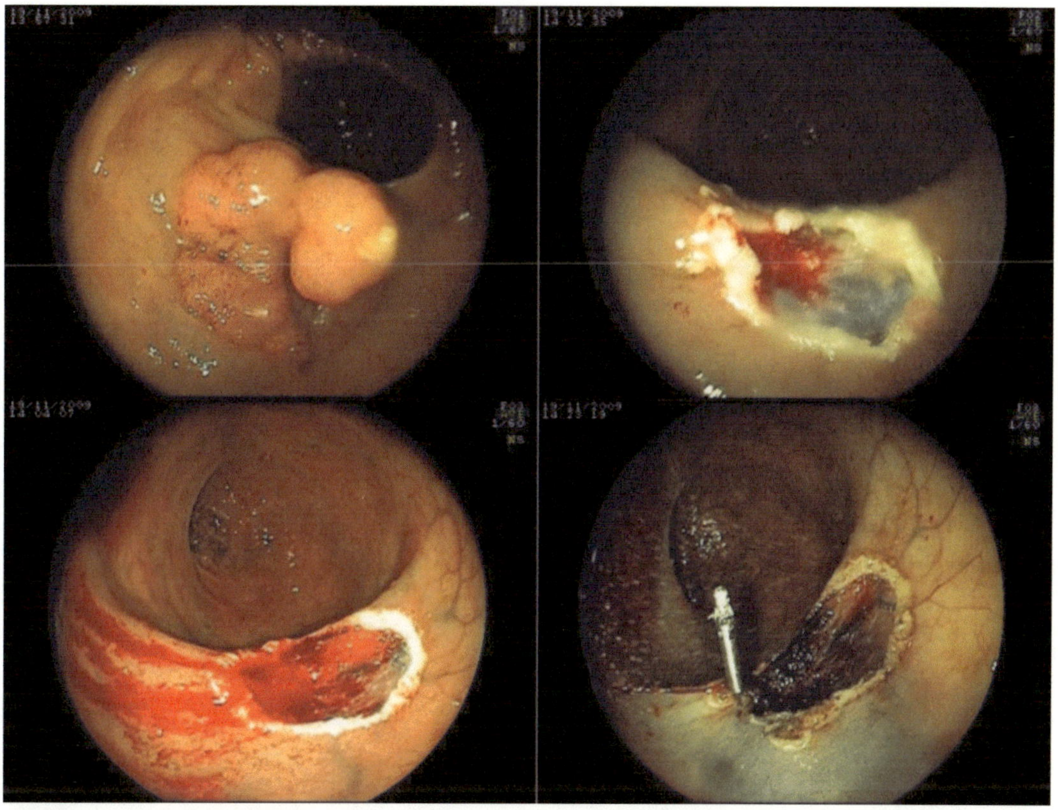

Fig. 11. Resection of a large lesion in the sigmoid colon with hemorrhage during the procedure, controlled by the placement of several hemoclips.

Perforation can occur immediately, being recognized during the procedure so it can be directly solved, not having serious consequences for the patient. On other occasions, perforation can be deferred or delayed, produced by a spontaneous "rupture" of the wall under a large scar. In these cases the colon is not clean, so the patient would present symptoms. It usually requires systematically surgical repair, and it is usually needed to perform a temporal colostomy. In case that perforation is detected during resection of the lesion it can be endoscopically managed, covering the defect by suturing using hemoclips. Modern Ovesco devices ("over the scope hemoclips ") or different tools to perform endoscopic suturing could allow closing large defects. Indeed, the possibility of transmural sutures would allow closing large defects, providing a security level that would allow endoscopists face larger or more complex lesions. If there has been a transection of the muscular layer without frank perforation, this can be sufficient, but if there is a complete perforation of the wall, it is usually necessary to restrict oral intake, to establish broad-spectrum antibiotics and, depending on the magnitude of the pneumoperitoneum, to drain it. In most cases, we can solve problem and so avoid surgery. Consequently, it is essential to immediately detect the complication. Some authors define "target sign" as a whitish lesion on a muscular layer stained in blue (methylene blue) and "mirror target sign" on the surgical specimen that includes a section of the muscular layer. If this sign is observed, we should act accordingly.

Sometimes there is a transmural burn in the colonic wall, without frank perforation. The patient can present abdominal pain and signs of peritoneal irritation, but in the absence of pneumoperitoneum. This is called postpolypectomy syndrome. Conservative management, based on analgesics, broad spectrum antibiotics and fluid therapy is usually enough.

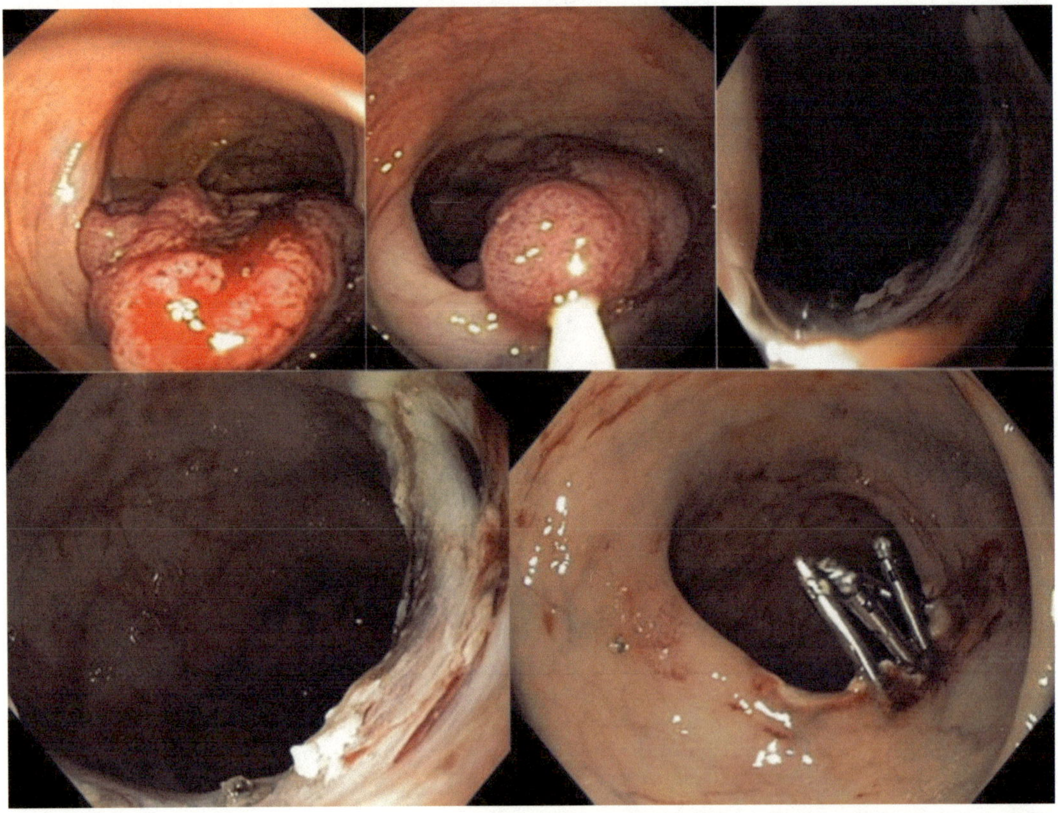

Fig. 12. Resection of large sessile lesion in sigmoid colon. After completing the resection it is clearly seen a lesion of the muscular layer, approximately 10 mm in length, which is completely closed by applying hemoclips. The patient remained in hospital during 48 hours and after restarting oral intake he was discharged without complications.

Resection of large colorectal lesions involves performing submucosal injection through a non-sterile system. In addition, a huge defect in the mucosa will persist over a long time. Both situations could represent the entry point for infections. However, it has not been observed a significant incidence of bacteremia after these procedures, so it is not justified a systematic antibiotic prophylaxis.

In conclusion, complications are rare on endoscopic resection of large colorectal lesions and, in most cases; these can be solved in a conservative way, endoscopically.

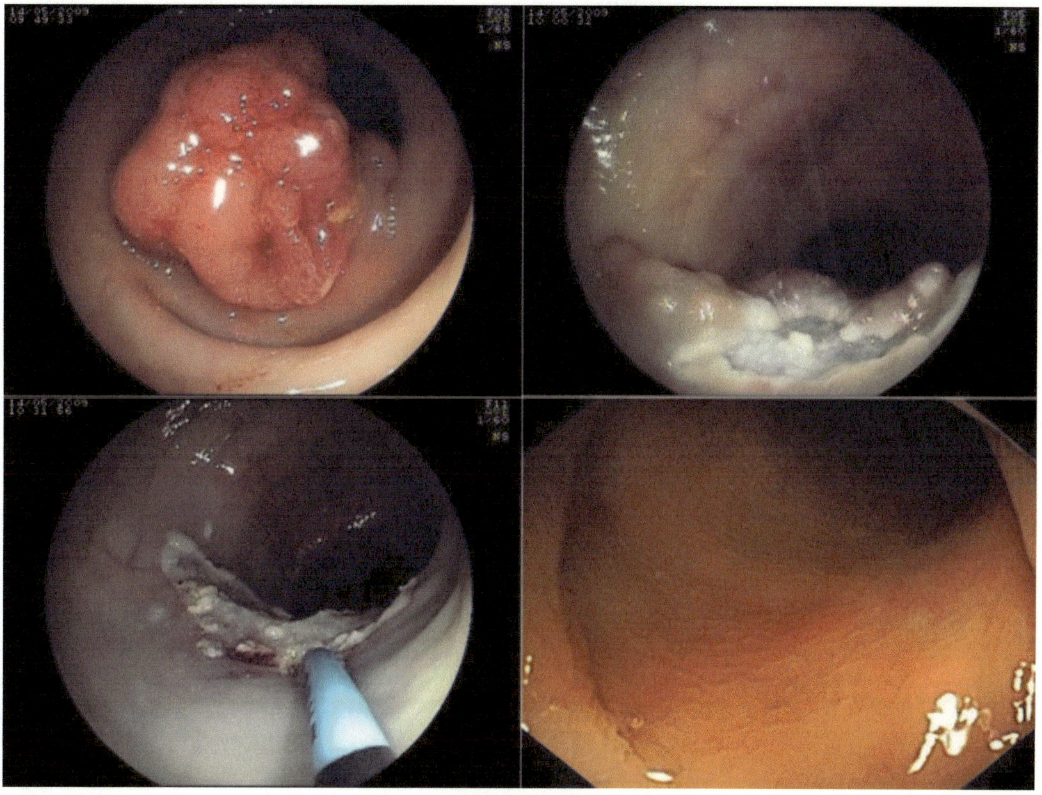

Fig. 13. In the picture we can visualize the piecemeal resection of a large sesile lesion, in the distal sigmoid colon. In this particular case we completed the resection with the coagulation of the lesion edges with argon plasma. In the last image, we can see the scar of the lesion, without recurrence.

2.2 Endoscopic Submucosal Dissection

Resection of large lesions generates uncertainty in the physician and patient, especially in those that are more likely to have invasive growth. En block resection of the lesions results in more certain of achieving a complete resection, a lower recurrence rate, and facilitates a better interpretation of the spcimen by the pathologist, achieving a correct classification of lesions that present an infiltrative growth.

The Endoscopic Submucosal Dissection (ESD) is a technique originally designed for the resection of gastric lesions, but later it was adapted to esophageal lesions and ultimately it was used for en bloc removal of large colorectal lesions. The great attraction of this technique is that, in fact, it allows the resection of large lesions in a single piece. The great inconvenient is its technical complexity, with an increased risk of complications, so its use in the Western countries is quite restricted.

As it has been already explained, it is in lesions that are more likely to have an invasive growth where it is more important to perform an en bloc resection. Then, the pathologist would be able to study the whole specimen, to perform accurate staging and, consequently, to establish the cure of the lesion or the need for surgery. It is considered that endoscopic removal of a lesion presenting adenocarcinoma with infiltration of submucosa can be curative if the following conditions are present:

- Well or moderately differentiated adenocarcinoma
- Absence of lymphatic and vascular permeation
- Presence of intramucosal adenocarcinoma
- Adenocarcinoma that infiltrates submucosa, but only in the most superficial portion (invasive growth of no more than 1000 microns from the muscularis mucosae)
- Edges of resection free of lesion

Endoscopic resection can be considered curative if lesions fulfil these conditions because the risk of lymphatic metastasis is minimal.

Given this, it could be said that indications of ESD in colon could be the following:

- Colonic polyps or lesions presenting intramucosal adenocarcinoma
- Early Neoplasms IIa (Paris classification) with a diameter less than 2 cms
- Neoplasms IIb IIc (Paris classification) with a diameter less than 10 mms
- Laterally spreading tumors

2.2.1 Endoscopic Submucosal Dissection technique

The procedure is very similar, in the majority of the phases, to endoscopic mucosa resection. It begins, as it is logical, with a correct identification, visualization, demarcation and characterization of lesions. Everything explained in EMR is valid now. Using chromoendoscopy, NBI and all the available technology are helpful. The characterization of the lesion according to morphology, Paris classification, and crypts pattern should lead us to the final decision to proceed or not to perform endoscopic resection and also to choose the most appropriate technique. After considering endoscopic treatment, firstly we have to demark the edges of the lesion in the same way as for EMR. In this case, submucosal injection is more important than in EMR, since it is necessary to achieve a good level of separation of the outer layers of the wall respecting to the muscular layer to avoid injury. For this reason, glycerol or hyaluronic acid are preferable because they remain longer in the submucosa. Then, a circumferential incision is performed, which isolates the lesion from the rest of the surrounding mucosa and it allows to open a space to introduce the endoscope and finally to start the dissection. This incision can be made using a conventional needle knife or material especially designed for that purpose. The placement of a transparent cap on the tip of the endoscope is essential to facilitate the visibility at the submucosa level and to permit the management of the material used for dissection. Finally, the lesion is dissected until complete the resection of the lesion in only one fragment.

Various instruments have been designed for the dissection of the submucosa, all of them with common and differentiating elements. They all have advocates and detractors, and each expert recommends the use of the one that best suits to the way of working of the endoscopist. However, experts also recommend mastering more than one of them, because in some lesions an instrument can be adapted better than another. Today there is a wide variety of instruments available: the IT knife (isolated tipped knife), the flex knife, the hook knife (needle point hook-shaped) and the triangle tip knife (triangular-tipped). In addition, recently new instruments have been designed such as the flush knife, which allows submucosal injection and cutting with a single device, allowing saving time by not having to exchange instruments.

In addition, there are specially designed coagulation forceps to coagulate vessels in the submucosa, either as bleeding prevention or as treatment. However, coagulation of vessels can be performed with the same cutting instrument, as long as there is a good domain of the technique.

2.2.2 Medium and long term results

In Japan there are already quite large series of colorectal neoplasms removed by ESD. In all cases, they are great experts in the technique, with many hundreds of procedures performed in the upper gastrointestinal tract. In all cases the results are quite similar. The en bloc resection rate is 85-94%, with a cure rate of 80-90%. As expected the en bloc resection rate is clearly superior to the one achieved with the conventional mucusectomy, and the cure rate is also slightly higher, not being necessary in this case to perform several sessions to complete the treatment of the lesion. In contrast, as expected in a more technically demanding and complex procedure from a technical standpoint, the time spent on each patient is significantly higher than used in EMR.

2.2.3 Complications

Complications, both in the case of perforation or bleeding, are considerably higher in the ESD than in EMR. This fact, together with the time consumed by each procedure, makes that the technique has not spread too much in Europe. If in upper gastrointestinal tract the number of procedures performed in Europe is reduced to a few hundreds of patients, in the colorectal area, theoretically more complex due to the reduced thickness of the wall and with an increased risk of complications, the number is even lower.

Complications related to ESD are the same as for EMR, but considerably more frequent, even in the case of Japanese experts. After reviewing the different series there is a perforation rate of around 5% and bleeding occurs with a frequency of 2-3%. In most cases, as in EMR, these complications can be resolved by endoscopic treatment, being exceptional the need to refer the patient for surgery to solve the complication.

3. Conclusions

The vast majority of benign lesions of the colon and lesions that present malignant degeneration, but without a massive infiltration of the submucosa by cancer, can be endoscopically managed and endoscopic resection may be considered curative. However, endoscopic resection of these lesions is not always simple and sometimes it requires great technical skill and perfect mastery of technique and material used. In addition, it is essential to properly master the different hemostatic techniques as well as the available devices to close perforations in order to be able to solve complications that could happen during the procedure. The security and confidence in resolving complications, makes these less feared, so indications for endoscopic procedures would be extended.

ESD and EMR are complementary techniques in colorectal disease. ESD is much more complex and it is associated with a greater number of complications and requires considerably more time consuming. EMR is easier, and involves the use of material with which the endoscopists are usually familiar; it presents a lower risk of complications but in contrast, it presents a major limitation in en bloc resection of large lesions. However, EMR can keep its place: we believe that it is the ideal technique for resection of all those lesions that can be en bloc resected using this technique and it may not be unreasonable to perform a piecemeal resection of those lesions with very low risk of developing invasive growth (laterally spreading tumors with granular surface). By contrast, those lesions more likely to present invasive component always without breaking the clearly established indications for endoscopic resection and fulfilling the curative criteria of lesions, should be resected using the ESD.

Finally, as we have seen, the adecuate selection of patients for the endoscopic procedure and its results, require a great domain of it. This is only possible if the management of these patients is carried out in the context of specialized units, by expert endoscopists and with special dedication to this type of pathologies.

4. Acknowledgements

We especially thank the whole team of the Endoscopy Unit of the Complejo Hospital Universitario de Vigo.

5. References

Khashab M, Eid E, Rusche M, Rex DK. Incidence and predictors of "late"recurrences after endoscopic piecemeal resection of large sessile adenomas. Gastrointest Endosc. 2009; 70:344-9.

Conio M, Ponchon T, Blanchi S, Filiberti R. Endoscopic mucosal resection. Am J Gastroenterol. 2006; 101: 653-63.

Kaltenbach T, Friedland S, Maheshwari A, Ouyang D, Rouse RV, Wren S, Soetikno R. Short- and long-term outcomes of standardized EMR of nonpolypoid (flat anddepressed) colorectal lesions > or = 1 cm (with video). Gastrointest Endosc. 2007;65:857-65.

Swan MP, Bourke MJ, Moss A, Williams SJ, Hopper A, Metz A. The target sign: an endoscopic marker for the resection of the muscularis propria and potential perforation during colonic endoscopic mucosal resection. Gastrointest Endosc. 2011; 73:79-85.

Niimi K, Fujishiro M, Kodashima S, Goto O, Ono S, Hirano K, Minatsuki C, Yamamichi N, Koike K. Long-term outcomes of endoscopic submucosal dissection for colorectal epithelial neoplasms. Endoscopy. 2010; 42: 723-9.